The Human Oncogenic Viruses

Molecular Analysis and Diagnosis

The Oncogenes

The Human Oncogenic Viruses: *Molecular Analysis and Diagnosis*
edited by *Albert A. Luderer* and *Howard H. Weetall,* 1986

The Human Oncogenic Viruses

Molecular Analysis and Diagnosis

Edited by
ALBERT A. LUDERER
AND
HOWARD H. WEETALL

Humana Press • Clifton, New Jersey

Library of Congress Cataloging in Publication Data
Main entry under title:

© 1986 The Humana Press Inc.
Crescent Manor
PO Box 2148
Clifton, NJ 07015

Printed in the United States of America

Library of Congress Cataloging-in-Publication Data

The Human oncogenic viruses.

(The Oncogenes)
Includes bibliography and index.
1. Encogenic viruses. 2. Oncogenes. I. Luderer,
Albert A. II. Weetall, Howard H. III. Series.
[DNLM: 1. Oncogenic Viruses. QW 166 H918]
QR372.06H86   1986   616.99′4071   86-7518
ISBN 0-89603-088-1

Preface

The early, organ-specific diagnosis of malignancy continues to be a major unmet medical need. Clearly the ability to establish an early diagnosis of cancer is dependent upon an intimate knowledge of the cancer's biology, which if understood at the molecular level should identify key diagnostic and therapeutic manipulation points. Advances in recombinant gene technology have provided significant understanding of the mechanisms of action of oncogenic viruses, as well as of cancer-associated genomic sequences (oncogenes). This text will explore the known molecular genetic, biological, and clinical knowledge of selected human neoplasms that demonstrate association with suspected oncogenic virus and those cytogenetic alterations that either cause or are caused by oncogene activation.

The text first reviews the cytogenetics of human cancers linking classical cytogenetics and molecular genetics. Avery A. Sandberg (Roswell Park Memorial Institute, Buffalo, New York) reviews the leukemias and lymphomas, followed by S. Pathak (M. D. Anderson Hospital and Tumor Institute, Houston, Texas), who reviews solid tumors. Functional consideration of oncogenes is highlighted by Keith C. Robbins and Stuart A. Aaronson (NCI, Bethesda, Maryland) through their description of the v-*sis* locus and its gene product p.28^{sis}; a protein that closely resembles human platelet-derived growth factor (PDGF).

In the following chapters, the molecular biology of those human viruses associated with human cancer are carefully reviewed in relation to disease natural history. Herpes simplex type 2 (HSV-2) genes and gene products in cervical neoplasia are described by Cecilia M. Fenoglio-Preiser (Veteran's Administration Medical Center, Alberquerque, New Mexico) and James K. McDougall (Fred Hutchinson Cancer Research Center, Seattle, Washington), followed by a discourse on anogenital neoplasms and papillomaviruses by Wayne D. Lancaster et al. (Georgetown University Medical School, Washington, DC). Toyoro Osato et al. (Hokkaido University School of Medicine, Sapporo, Japan) review the molecular biology of the Epstein-Barr virus and its associated cancers, including Burkitt's, nasopharyngeal, and opportunistic lymphoma. Hepatitis B and its relationship with hepatocellular carcinoma is reviewed by Hubert E. Blum et al. (UCSF, San Francisco, California). In the last chapter, Kaposi's sarcoma is reviewed by Thomas J. Spira (CDC, Atlanta, Georgia) relative to human T-cell leukemia virus (HTLV) types 1 and 3, as well as cytomegalovirus (CMV).

It is our hope that this work will provide a reference point for the merging of molecular and clinical knowledge of human malignancies. It is only through the thorough understanding of the molecular process of malignancy that more realistic therapeutic regimens will evolve and earlier specific diagnosis be achieved.

Albert A. Luderer
Howard H. Weetall
Ciba Corning Diagnostic Corp.
Cambridge, Massachusetts

Acknowledgment

The authors gratefully acknowledge the patience and support extended to our work by Thomas Lanigan, President, Humana Press; Fran Lipton and Deborah Epstein, Humana Press; the secretarial work of Ruth Dhionis and Pamela Velie, and, finally, the continued support of Ciba Corning Diagnostics Corp., all of which have aided the editors immeasurably in the completion of this work.

Contents

Cytogenetics of Solid Tumors: Renal Cell Carcinoma, Malignant Melanoma, Retinoblastoma, and Wilms' Tumor
S. Pathak

Elucidation of a Normal Function for a Human Proto-Oncogene
Keith C. Robbins and Stuart A. Aaronson

Detection of HSV-2 Genes and Gene Products in Cervical Neoplasia

Cecilia M. Fenoglio-Preiser and James K. McDougall

Papillomaviruses in Anogenital Neoplasms

Wayne D. Lancaster, Robert J. Kurman, and A. Bennett Jenson

Human Epstein-Barr Virus and Cancer

Toyoro Osato, Fumio Mizuno, Shigeyoshi Fujiwara, and Shigeki Koizumi

Hepatitis B Virus and Hepatocellular Carcinoma

Hubert E. Blum, Myron J. Tong, and Girish N. Vyas

Kaposi's Sarcoma: *Acquired Immunodeficiency Syndrome (AIDS) and Associated Viruses*

Thomas J. Spira

Contributors

STUART A. AARONSON • *Laboratory of Cellular and Molecular Biology, National Cancer Institute, National Institutes of Health, Bethesda, Maryland*

HUBERT E. BLUM • *Hepatitis Research Unit, Department of Laboratory Medicine and Liver Center, University of California, San Francisco, California*

CECILIA M. FENOGLIO-PREISER • *Veterans Administration Medical Center, Albuquerque, New Mexico*

SHIGEYOSHI FUJIWARA • *Department of Virology, Cancer Institute, Hokkaido University School of Medicine, Sapporo, Japan*

A. BENNETT JENSON • *Department of Pathology, Georgetown University Medical Center, Washington, DC.*

SHIGEKI KOIZUMI • *Department of Virology, Cancer Institute, Hokkaido University School of Medicine, Sapporo, Japan*

ROBERT J. KURMAN • *Departments of Obstetrics and Gynecology and Pathology, Georgetown University Medical Center, Washington, DC*

WAYNE D. LANCASTER • *Departments of Obstetrics and Gynecology and Pathology, Georgetown University, Washington, DC*

JAMES K. MCDOUGALL • *Fred Hutchinson Cancer Research Center, Seattle, Washington*

FUMIO MIZUNO • *Department of Virology, Cancer Institute, Hokkaido University School of Medicine, Sapporo, Japan*

TOYORO OSATO • *Department of Virology, Cancer Institute, Hoddaido University School of Medicine, Sapporo, Japan*

S. PATHAK • *Section of Cellular Genetics, M. D. Anderson Hospital and Tumor Institute, Houston, Texas*

KEITH C. ROBBINS • *Laboratory of Cellular and Molecular Biology, National Cancer Institute, National Institutes of Health, Bethesda, Maryland*

AVERY A. SANDBERG • *Roswell Park Memorial Institute, Buffalo, New York*

THOMAS J. SPIRA • *Division of Host Factors, Center for Infectious Diseases, Centers for Disease Control, Atlanta, Georgia*

MYRON J. TONG • *Huntington Memorial Hospital and University of Southern California School of Medicine, Pasedena, California*

GIRISH N. VYAS • *Hepatitis Research Unit, Department of Laboratory Medicine and Liver Center, University of California, San Francisco, California*

Cytogenetics of the Leukemias and Lymphomas

Avery A. Sandberg

1. Introduction

This chapter addresses those chromosomal (karyotypic, cytogenetic) changes and aberrations in human leukemia and lymphoma that have found application in the analysis and diagnosis of malignant conditions, and that will undoubtedly serve in the future as a basis for further molecular analysis and diagnostic approaches in human neoplasia. This contention is based on the observation that chromosomal changes, particularly translocations, when they involve those chromosomal segments that are the sites of proto-oncogenes, often lead to the displacement of such genes and their activation at new chromosomal sites, resulting in the expression, often abnormal, of such oncogenes (Bishop, 1983; Varmus, 1984; Weinberg, 1984). Though such oncogenes have not been shown to be directly responsible for human neoplasia, the evidence obtained in lower animals and in vitro studies would seem to indicate that oncogenes probably play a crucial role in malignant transformation (Greenberger et al., 1979; Raschke et al., 1978; Rosenberg et al., 1975; Scher and Siegler, 1975), and, furthermore, that they may interact with genes of another nature, thus leading to abnormal or excessive expression (Canaani et al., 1984; Collins et al., 1984; Leibowitz et al., 1984, 1985) and possibly setting off a cascade of gene, including oncogene, activations that may play a crucial role in the biology of neoplasia (Slamon et al., 1984). In addition, the demonstration of specific (primary) chromosomal changes in leukemia and lymphoma may be indicative of the possible location of oncogenes hitherto not characterized or known to exist (Chaganti, 1983; Rowley, 1983; Yunis, 1983). Thus, this chapter will summarize the known, nonrandom, particularly specific (primary) karyotypic changes observed in the various human lymphomas and leukemias and attempt to correlate these findings with some of the clinical, laboratory, and molecular parameters.

2. Methodologic Background and Considerations

For a decade and a half prior to the introduction of banding techniques, the human chromosomes were identified on the basis of their size, location of centromere (defining metacentric, submetacentric, acrocentric, and subtelocentric chromosomes) and presence of satellites (Sandberg, 1980b). It is of interest that only rare errors were made on the basis of these criteria, though undoubtedly the banding techniques increased not only the accuracy of identification of chromosomes, but also led to the recognition of many karyotypic changes that could not be seen without banding.

The introduction of various banding techniques made possible the recognition and identification not only of individual chromosomes (Standardization in Human Cytogenetics, 1971), but also of subchromosomal structures and changes (Sandberg, 1980b). These banding techniques thus afforded cytogeneticists the opportunity to define rigorously the chromosomes, their bands and subbands involved in various translocations, as well as the location and extent of deletions, insertions, additions, and breaks. Furthermore, refinement in cellular in vitro methodologies (Berger et al., 1983b; Fitzgerald et al., 1982; Knuutila et al., 1981), particularly methotrexate synchronization (Hagemeijer et al., 1979; Yunis, 1976), have led to higher yields of metaphases and, hence, cytogenetic results, an improved quality of chromosome preparations, and an ever-increasing number of conditions in which specific cytogenetic changes are being described. Thus, the utilization of banding approaches has resulted in an almost explosive description of many specific (primary) chromosomal changes in leukemia and lymphoma, with new entities and subentities being added regularly.

The recent introduction into cytogenetics of molecular probes capable of establishing the presence, location, and activation of genes, particularly cancer genes (oncogenes) (Emanuel et al., 1984; Rigby et al., 1977; Shows et al., 1982), has further expanded the scope and breadth of information yielded through chromosome analysis. What appears clear now is that the application of molecular techniques will allow the recognition of karyotypic events (e.g., translocations, oncogene locations) not readily ascertained through presently available cytogenetic methodologies and will undoubtedly result in another leap forward of chromosomal information on leukemia and cancer akin to those brought about by the introduction of other techniques in the past.

A few words must be said about the nature of the cells involved in the chromosomal changes in human leukemia and lymphoma. These changes are confined to the affected cells and, thus, are not seen in such cellular elements as skin fibroblasts, normal blood cells, and other unaffected tissues. In leukemia, particularly of the acute type, the cytogenetic changes must usually be established on bone marrow material, since this is often the source of the abnormal cells. Though under some circumstances leukemic cells may be found in the circulation, peripheral blood generally constitutes a rather poor source of leukemic metaphases for chromosome analysis. In the case of lymphoma, only the affected tissues, such as the lymph nodes, lymphomatous tumors, and, rarely, marrow and blood, yield cells with chromosomal changes. Thus, it can be stated that in leukemia the best source of cells for cytogenetic analysis is generally the marrow and for lymphoma, the affected lymph nodes or tumors.

3. Chromosome Changes in Chronic Myelocytic Leukemia (CML)

3.1. The Philadelphia (Ph) Chromosome

A discussion of the karyotypic changes in human leukemia and lymphoma invariably directs one to begin with chronic myelocytic leukemias (CML) (Table 1), since it was the first human neoplastic disease in which a specific cytogenetic change, consisting of the Ph chromosome, was established (Nowell and Hungerford, 1960) (Figs. 1 and 2). Furthermore, more information is available on the chromosome changes in this disease and its various phases than in any other human condition (Sandberg, 1980b).

Table 1
Common Chromosome Changes in CML

Chromosome changes	Stage of CML
t(9;22) (q34;q11)	CML[a]
i(17q)	BP[b] of CML
+8	BP of CML
+19	BP of CML

[a] CML, Chronic myelocytic leukemia.
[b] BP, Blastic phase.

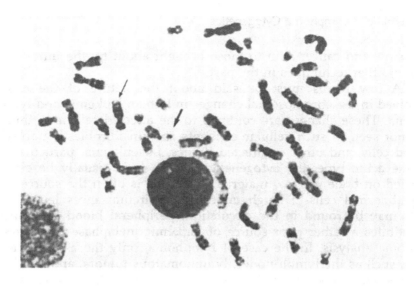

Fig. 1. G-banded metaphase of a cell from a patient with CML showing the Ph translocation, i.e., the thick arrow pointing to the Ph chromosome and the thin arrow pointing to the chromosome #9 to which the material from chromosome #22 (now the Ph) had been translocated. (See text for further details regarding the Ph translocation.)

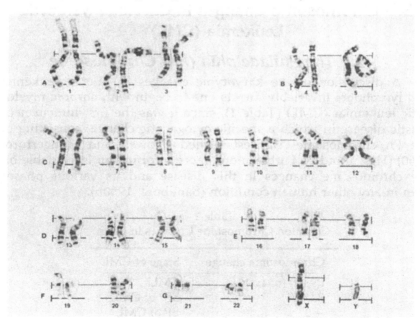

Fig. 2. G-banded high-resolution karyotype of a normal male blood cell showing the chromosomal bands. Each chromosome can be identified by its unique banding pattern. The methotrexate synchronization technique was used to obtain this karyotype.

The exact identity and origin of this abnormal chromosome were not realized until 1973 when banding techniques revealed it to be an abbreviated chromosome #22 (Rowley, 1973b) involved in what appeared to be a reciprocal and balanced translocation with chromosome #9, i.e., t(9;22)(q34;q11) in about 95% of the cases with CML. Ph-negative CML, if such an entity truly exists, may contain within it a number of subentities, including chronic mono-cytoid or myelomonocytic leukemia.

The Ph chromosome is invariably an abbreviated chromosome #22, with the break occurring at band q11. This has not only been defined cytogenetically, but also on a molecular basis (de Klein et al., 1982; Geurts van Kessel et al., 1981). In about 5% of the cases, it appears that chromosomes other than #9 are involved in the Ph translocation, some involving only another chromosome (variant simple Ph translocations), and others involving more than one (complex Ph translocations) (Sandberg, 1980a) (Figs. 3 and 4). To date, every chromosome in the human set except the Y has been shown to be involved in variant Ph translocations of one type or another (Sandberg, 1980a). Some chromosomes appear to be involved more often than others, e.g., chromosome #1 is often involved in complex Ph translocations, whereas chromosome #18 is only rarely involved in either simple or complex Ph transloca-tions. An evaluation of survival and other laboratory and clinical parameters of cases with variant Ph translocations vs those with the standard Ph translocation have generally not revealed major differences (Potter et al., 1981; Sandberg, 1980a) (Fig. 5), again pointing to the crucial role played by the initial change on chromo-some #22 in establishing the nature and course of the disease.

The introduction of various DNA probes has led to the excit-ing finding of the translocation of an oncogene (c-abl) from chro-mosome #9 to the Ph chromosome (Bartram et al., 1983; Groffen et al., 1983a, 1984; Heisterkamp et al., 1983) (Fig. 6). In fact, a rela-tively small region on chromosome #22, bcr, consisting of a small number of kilobases (kb), has been shown to be the site of the break on chromosome #22 in the genesis of the Ph (Groffen et al., 1983a). Furthermore, abnormal messenger RNAs (mRNA) have been shown to be produced by the combination of c-abl and the bcr on the Ph chromosome, i.e., 8- and 9-kb mRNA produced by the Ph versus 6- and 7-kb mRNA generated in normal marrow cells (Canaani et al., 1984; Collins et al., 1984; Leibowitz et al., 1984, 1985). In addition to establishing whether the molecular events related to c-abl apply to CML with complex and unusual Ph translocations, it also remains to be ascertained whether other

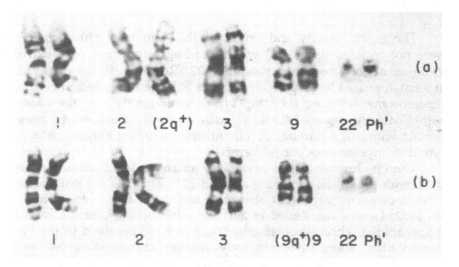

Fig. 3. Partial karyotypes based on G banding in which the genesis of Ph chromosome is shown to be caused by the standard (common) type of translocation in (b), i. e., t(9;22)(q34;q11), and that caused by a variant (simple) translocation in (a), i. e., t(2;22)(q37;q11). Chromosome #9 in (a) appears to be normal with G banding performed in 1975; however, recent publications indicate that the utilization of high-resolution R banding affords a means of visualizing involvement of chromosome #9 in variant translocations, such involvement not being readily seen with other banding methods. Since *in situ* hybridization has shown translocation of the oncogene *abl* to the Ph, it is possible that chromosome #9 is involved in all Ph translocations in CML. (*See* text for more details.)

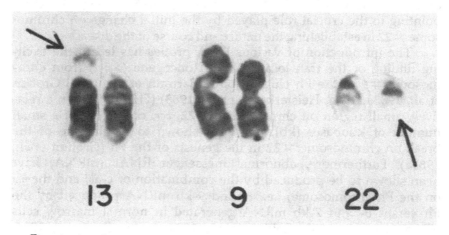

Fig. 4. Another variant (simple) Ph translocation between chromosomes #22 and #13 (arrows), i. e., t(13;22)(p13;q11). Chromosomes #9 appear normal with G banding. (*See* Fig. 3 for comments.)

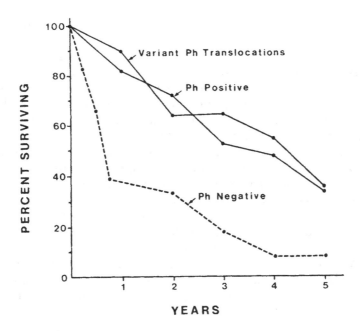

Fig. 5. Median survival of patients with Ph-positive or Ph-negative CML. In addition, the survival of patients with variant Ph translocations is also shown; no significant difference was seen from that of CML patients with a standard Ph.

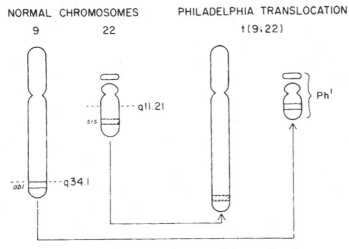

Fig. 6. Schematic presentation of some of the molecular events associated with the standard Ph translocation in CML. The oncogene *abl* is translocated to the Ph and *sis* to chromosome #9. Since the break in chromosome #9 is in the locus of *abl*, this oncogene is activated, whereas *sis*, not being involved in a break, apparently remains inactive. (See text for further discussion.)

oncogenes are activated and expressed, temporarily or permanently, and the relation of such events to the karyotypic changes, both in the chronic and blastic phases. The effects of therapy on oncogene expressions are yet to be established. Even more exciting is the fact that in variant translocations, in which microscopically the chromosomes #9 appear to be normal and apparently not involved in Ph translocations, molecular probing has revealed the presence of the c-*abl* oncogene on the Ph, indicative of a molecular translocation occurring that is not discernible cytologically (unless special techniques are used) (Bartram et al., 1983). This field is now being actively investigated and the significance and exact incidence of this and other molecular events will undoubtedly be established in the future. For example, some variation from the events in CML have been reported in Ph-positive ALL (acute lymphoblastic leukemia) and other translocations affecting chromosome #22, e.g., t(11;22) in Ewing's sarcoma and t(8;22) in Burkitt's lymphoma (Cannizzaro et al., 1985).

3.2. Cytogenetics of the Blastic Phase

Though a small proportion of cases with CML shows karyotypic changes in the chronic phase similar to those observed in the blastic phase (i.e., +8, +Ph, +19), generally the disease is characterized by the presence of the Ph as the sole karyotypic anomaly over a number of years before the blastic phase appears. The blastic phase, which has many of the biologic and clinical characteristics of acute leukemia, may be heralded by the appearance of additional chromosomal changes weeks, months, and occasionally a year prior to the appearance of laboratory and clinical aspects of the blastic phase. The most common changes observed in the blastic phase are those already mentioned, +Ph, +8, +19, including an isochromosome for the long arm of chromosome #17, i(17q), the latter being rather characteristic for that phase. Seldom does the i(17q) appear without other additional karyotypic changes.

The blastic phase of CML may assume either myeloblastic or lymphoid cytologic characteristics, and though cytogenetically these two entities have not been defined to date (Sandberg, 1980b), it is possible that the lymphoid phase is not associated with as many karyotypic aberrations, in addition to the Ph, as is the myeloblastic phase, though this remains to be established on a firmer basis. In some patients, the origin of the abnormal cells in the blastic phase of CML is not in the marrow but in other organs or tissues, such as the spleen, lymph nodes, and testes. Under these circumstances, the cells generated by these organs or tissues find themselves in the circulation prior to being established in the marrow; in these cases, examining the circulating leukemic cells may, in fact, offer more information than examining the bone marrow. This is one of the few exceptions in a hematologic disease in which examination of extramedullary cells affords the cytogeneticist and clinician the possibility of yielding more information than examining the marrow cells.

4. Oncogenes, the Ph, and CML

Events connected with the generation of the Philadelphia (Ph) chromosome can serve as an example of oncogene involvement in a human malignancy (Tables 2A and B). In the preponderant number of cases with CML, the Ph is the result of a reciprocal translocation between chromosomes #9 and #22, with the breaks occurring at bands q34 and q11, respectively (Sandberg et al., 1985). The break on chromosome #9 involves a proto-oncogene that is ultimately expressed as the oncogene c-abl when translocated to chromosome #22. The break in chromosome #22 occurs within a relatively confined area of 5 kb known as bcr, whereas that on chromosome #9 appears to involve a more extensive area, but apparently always affecting the proto-oncogene abl (Groffen et al., 1984). Of interest is the fact that the mRNA produced by c-abl under normal circumstances appears to consist of 6 and 7 kb elements, whereas an abnormal size mRNA of 8 and 9 kb appears to be produced as a result of the Ph translocation (Canaani et al., 1984; Collins et al., 1984; Leibowitz et al., 1984, 1985). Apparently, the interaction of c-abl with the bcr moiety left on chromosome #22 after the Ph translocation leads to the production of abnormal mRNA. Whether the latter plays a key role in the genesis of CML has not been ascertained to date.

Another interesting facet of the Ph translocation is related to so-called variant translocations in which on a cytologic basis it appeared that chromosome #9 was not involved in a translocation with #22—so-called simple variant Ph translocations—and those in which in addition to chromosomes #9 and #22, other chromosomes may be involved—so-called complex Ph translocations (Sandberg, 1980a). As recently demonstrated with molecular studies related to variant Ph translocations, in all of these translocations c-abl appears to be translocated from chromosome #9 to chromosomes #22, whether cytologic evidence exists for it or not (Hagemeijer et al., 1984). That in some cases anomalies of chromo-

Table 2A
Chromosomal Oncogene Locations in the Human Genome

Chromosome	Location	Oncogene
1	1p32	c-B*lym*-1
1	1p13–p22	c-N-*ras*
1	1q12–qter	c-*sk*
2	2q22–q34	c-*fos*
3	3p25	c-*raf*-1
4		c-*raf*-2
5	5q34	c-*fms*
6	6q23–q12	c-K-*ras*-1
6	6q22–24	c-*myb*
7	7p11–13	c-*erb* B
8	8q22	c-*mos*
8	8q24	c-*myc*
9	9q34.1	c-*abl*
11	11p15	c-H-*ras* 1
11	11q13	c-*bcl*-1
11	11q23–24	c-*ets*
12	12p12	c-K-*ras* 2
12	12pter–q14	c-*int*
15	15q26.1	c-*fes*
17	17p12–q21	c-*erb* A
18	18q21	c-*bcl*-2
18		c-*erv* 1
20	20q12–q15	c-*src*
22	22q13.1	c-*sis*
X		c-H-*ras* 2

some #9 may have been present but missed microscopically may be a result of failure to utilize the most optimal staining techniques, as has been recently demonstrated in several studies (Hagemeijer et al., 1984; Ishihara et al., 1985). Still to be determined is which event is crucial in the genesis of CML, that at 9q34 or that at 22q11, for there are those who believe that activation of the oncogene c-*abl* as a result of the break at 9q34 may constitute the primary molecular event in CML (Sandberg et al., 1985). However, this remains to be demonstrated and until such time it would appear that events at both locations, 9q34 and 22q11, one affecting the oncogene c-*abl* and the other the locus *bcr*, may constitute key events in the genesis of CML.

Activation of the oncogene *sis* does not occur with these translocations since the chromosomal breaks do not affect the locus of this gene.

Table 2B
Chromosomal Location of Oncogenes and List of Diseases
(and Associated Karyotypic Changes) of Possible Relevance to the Oncogenes

Putative oncogene	Chromosomal location of oncogene	Associated disease	Chromosomal change
c-B*lym*-1	1p32	Neuroblastoma, malignant melanoma	del(1)(p32)
			del(1)(p22)
c-*sk*	1q11–qter	Carcinomas	trisomy 1q
c-*raf*-1	3p25	Partoid tumors,	
		lung cancer,	3p–
		renal cancer,	3p–
		prolymphocytic	3p–(p15)
		leukemia (B cell),	
		ANLL	3p–
c-*fms*	5q34	ANLL,	5q–
		refractory anemia,	5q–
		ANLL	–5
c-*myb*	6q22–24	ALL,	6q–
		lymphoma,	+6
		ovarian cancer	t(6;14)
c-*erb*-B	7p11–13	ANLL,	7q–
		ANLL	–7
c-*mos*	8q22	AML	t(8;21)
c-*myc*	8q24	Burkitt's lymphoma,	t(8;14)
		ANLL	t(8;14)
			t(8;22)
			t(2;8)
			+8
c-*abl*	9q34	CML,	t(9;22)
		ANLL	t(6;9)
c-Ha-*ras*-1	11p15	Ewing's sarcoma,	t(11;22)
		Wilm's tumor,	11p–
c-*bcl*-1	11q13	Lymphoma	t(11;14)
c-Ki-*ras*-2	12p12	Testicular tumors,	i(12p)
		leukemia,	12p–
		colon cancer,	12q– and/or +12
		CLL	+12
c-*fes*	15q26	APL	t(15;17)
c-*erb* A	17q21–p12	APL, CML (BP)	t(15;17)
c-*cbl*-2	18q21	Lymphoma	t(14;18)
c-*src*	20q12–15	Myeloproliferative diseases	20q–
c-*sis*	22q13	CML,	t(9;22)
		Burkitt's lymphoma,	t(8;22)
		meningioma	–22

5. Karyotypic Aspects of the Acute Leukemias

The acute leukemias have been divided on the basis of their cellular morphology into two categories: acute nonlymphocytic leukemia (ANLL) and acute lymphoblastic leukemia (ALL). Each category has been further subdivided according to the FAB classification (Bennett et al., 1976), into subentities, primarily according to the morphologic criteria of the cells. Immunologic and enzymatic characteristics of the leukemic cells have in recent years added another dimension in defining the nature of the leukemic cells, though they have not led to a definition of specific subentities within the major FAB groups; however, some correlations between the immunologic and enzymatic characteristics of the leukemic cells and the clinical, particularly prognostic, aspects of some acute leukemias have been reported.

A major contribution of cytogenetics has been to further define unique types of leukemias within ANLL and ALL (First, Second, Third, and Fourth International Workshops on Chromosomes in Leukemia, 1978, 1980, 1981, 1984) (Fig. 7). These are shown in Tables 3 and 4. Of importance is not only the fact that each of these subentities of leukemia is associated with a specific cytogenetic event, but also the observation that prognostic and clinical features, and in some, cellular and laboratory aspects, characterize each of the subentities. For example, ALL with t(4;11) is possibly a pluripotent stem cell disorder with lymphoid as well as monocytoid differentiation (Arthur et al., 1982; Kocova et al., 1985; Nagasaka et al., 1983; Weh and Hossfeld, 1982), and pre-B-cell ALL with t(1;19)(q23;q13) may have a much poorer prognosis than cases of ALL without this translocation in the leukemic cells (Carroll et al., 1984); ANLL cases with either an inversion of chromosome #16 or 16q− have an associated bone marrow eosinophilia (Arthur and Bloomfield, 1983; LeBeau et al., 1983) (Fig. 8). In addition to defining diagnostic and clinical parameters of these leukemias, the involved chromosomes may point to the possible location of genes responsible for eosinophil or basophil (Pearson et al., 1983) production and physiology. There is also evidence that chromosome #3, particularly its short arm, may be related to megakaryocytic physiology and platelet production (Bernstein et al., 1982; Sweet, 1979). Cases of leukemia with involvement of chromosome #3 may show megakaryocyte immaturity and abnormal platelet morphology, number, and function.

The cytogenetic delineation of subentities within the acute leukemias indicates that those cases thought to belong to one of the FAB groups are, in fact, heterogeneous and possibly represent different entities etiologically and clinically (Tables 3 and 4). This is particularly true, for example, of the M2 group of ANLL. A similar situation may apply to preleukemia and myelodysplastic disorders (Table 5).

Table 3
Common Chromosome Changes in ANLL

Chromosome changes	Type of leukemia
t(3;5)(q21;q31)	ANLL (M2)[a]
t(6;9)(p23;q34)	AML (M2)[b]
t(8;21)(q22;q22)	AML (M2)with Auer rods
t(9;11)(p21;q23)	AMoL (M5)[c]
t(9;22)(q34;q11)	ANLL Ph+ (M1,M2,M4,M6)[d]
t(11;21)(q22;q21)	ANLL (M4)
t(11;19)(q23;q12 or p12)	ANLL (M5)
t(15;17)(q22;q12)	APL (M3)
3p−, 3q−	Secondary leukemia
5q−, −5	Secondary leukemia
7q−(q33q36), −7	Secondary leukemia
+8	ANLL
11q−(q23)	AMMol (M4)[e], AMoL (M5)
12p−	Secondary leukemia
12q−	ANLL
inv(16)(p13q22) or 16q−(q22)	ANLL with eosinophilia (M4)
21q−	ANLL
+22	ANLL

[a] ANLL, Acute nonlymphocytic leukemia.
[b] AML, Acute myeloblastic leukemia.
[c] AMoL, Acute monoblastic leukemia.
[d] M1– M6, FAB classification of ANLL.
[e] AMMoL, Acute myelomonocytic leukemia.

5.1. Acute Nonlymphocytic Leukemia (ANLL)

The FAB classification of the group of leukemias known as ANLL and the cytogenetic findings in these are shown in Table 6. It is clear that cytogenetically each FAB group contains within it two or more subentities, thus demonstrating that the cytogenetic approach is capable of differentiating leukemias not readily discerned by cytologic, immunologic, enzymatic, and clinical evaluations (Rowley, 1973a; Yunis et al., 1981) (Figs. 8 and 9). Undoubt-

Table 4
Common Chromosome Changes in ALL

Chromosome changes	Type of leukemia
t(1;19)(q21;q23)	ALL (L1)[a,b]
t(1;19)(q23;p13.3)	Pre-B-cell ALL
t(2;8)(p11–13;q24)	ALL (L3)
t(4;11)(q21;q23)	ALL (also myelomonocytic acute leukemia)
t(8;14)(q24;q32)	ALL (L3)
t(8;22)(q24;q11)	ALL (L3)
t(9;22)(q34;q11)	ALL–Ph+ (L1 and L2)
t(11;14)(q13;q32)	ALL
6q–	ALL
9p–	T-cell ALL
12p–(p12)	ALL
14q+(q32)	Adult T-cell acute leukemia
14q–(q11)	Adult T-cell acute leukemia
+21	ALL

[a] ALL, Acute lymphoblastic leukemia.
[b] L1–L3, FAB classification of ALL.

Table 5
Chromosome Changes in Myelodysplastic
and Myeloproliferative Syndromes and Preleukemic States

Chromosome changes	Hematologic Disorder
t(1;3)(p36;q21)	Myelodysplastic syndrome
t(1;7)(p11;p11)	Dysmyelopoeitic disorder (induced)
t(2;11)(p21;q23)	Dysmyelopoeitic preleukemia
t(3;17)(q26;q22)	Acute disease in myeloproliferative disorders?
t(6;9)(p23;q34)	Myeloproliferative diseases
t(11;21)(q22;q21)	Myeloproliferative diseases
5q– (interstitial)	Refractory anemia
–7	Preleukemia with infection
+8	Preleukemia
20q–	Polycythemia vera
21q–	Preleukemia

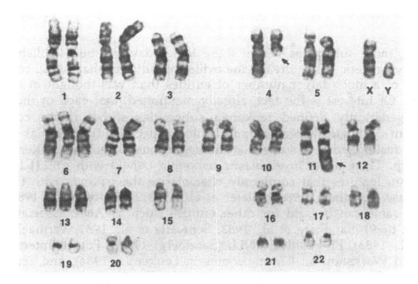

Fig. 7. G-banded karyotype of a cell from a patient with ALL showing t(4;11)(q21;q23). This type of translocation is now thought to be often associated with a myelomonocytoid leukemia, at least in a subgroup of patients with acute leukemia. The prognosis in patients with t(4;11) is poor. A +13 is also present in this karyotype.

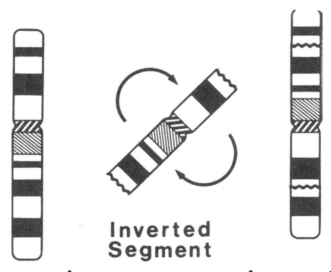

Inverted Segment

Normal   **Inversion**

Inversion of Chromosome No. 16

Fig. 8. Schematic presentation of an inversion of chromosome #16 with the breaks at bands p13 and q22. This karyotypic anomaly is seen in a subgroup of patients with ANLL (often M4 in the FAB classification) with bone marrow eosinophilia and a rather poor prognosis.

edly, more subgroups within these leukemias will be established on cytogenetic basis; already the evidence indicates that ANLL consists of a much larger number of entities than was thought in the past. Of interest is the fact, already mentioned, that each of these cytogenetically defined leukemia subentities shows rather consistent cytologic, laboratory, and clinical aspects, indicating that we are dealing with a somewhat homogeneously defined leukemic group. Thus, acute myeloblastic leukemia (AML) with t(8;21) has certain features that commonly characterize the patients with this disease (Sandberg, 1980b; Slater et al., 1983; Swirsky et al., 1984). The same can be said for other entities, such as AML associated with t(6;9) (Sandberg et al., 1983; Schwartz et al., 1983; Vermaelen et al., 1983), Ph-positive ANLL (Sandberg, 1980b; Fourth International Workshop on Chromosomes in Leukemia, 1984), and acute promyelocytic leukemias associated with t(15;17) (Fitzgerald et al., 1983; Fraser et al., 1981; Fourth International Workshop on Chromosomes in Leukemia, 1984).

Table 6
FAB Classification of ANLL and Common Chromosome Changes

Classification	Cytologic characteristics	Common chromosomal changes
M1	Myeloblastic leukemia without maturation	Includes t(9;22), Ph-positive AML
M2	Myeloblastic leukemia with maturation	t(8;21) with Auer rods; t(6;9) with possible marrow basophilia; involvement of chromosomes 3, 5, 7, and 12 in secondary leukemia t(3;5) (q26;q22)
M3	Hypergranular promyelocytic leukemia	t(15;17)
M4	Myelomonocytic leukemia	Chromosome #11 often involved; inv(16)(p13q22) or 16—(q2̇2)
M5	Monocytic leukemia	t(9;11) and 11q—; t(11;19) (q23;q12 or p12)
M6	EL	Ph[1]-positive EL, often AA and MAKA[a]; high chromosome counts

[a] AA, Cytogenetically abnormal cells; EL, erythroleukemia; MAKA, major karyotypic changes.

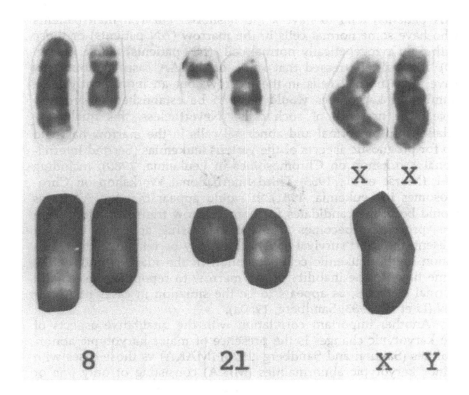

Fig. 9. Q- and G-banded partial karyotypes showing t(8;21)(q22;q22), a karyotypic anomaly usually associated with M2 types of AML, Auer bodies in the cells, good response to therapy, and relatively long survival. Missing sex chromosomes are not uncommon.

As in the case of Ph-positive CML, it is possible that the primary (specific) karyotypic events in these leukemias are capable of activating genes that may have a direct relevance to the disease, including its genesis. In some instances, proto-oncogenes are known to be located in the area of the chromosomal change, whereas in others the karyotypic events may, in fact, point to the location of hitherto possibly unrecognized oncogenes.

A quantitative evaluation of the chromosome changes in ANLL has revealed a definite correlation with the prognostic aspects of the disease (Berger et al., 1983a; Bernard et al., 1980; First International Workshop on Chromosomes in Leukemia, 1978; Sakurai and Sandberg, 1973; Second International Workshop on Chromosomes in Leukemia, 1980). Thus, it has been shown that those cases in which the bone marrow contains no cytogenetically normal cells (AA patients) tend to have a much shorter survival than patients who have some normal cells in the marrow (AN patients) or those with only cytogenetically normal cells (NN patients) (Table 7) (Fig. 10). It must be stressed that some of the AA cases undoubtedly have some normal cells in the marrow, but an inordinantly large number of karyotypes would have to be established in order to reveal the presence of such cells. Nevertheless, this qualitative relationship of normal and abnormal cells in the marrow has held up for prognostic aspects of the various leukemias (Second International Workshop on Chromosomes in Leukemia, 1980), including ALL (Morse et al., 1983; Third International Workshop on Chromosomes in Leukemia, 1981). It would appear that the AA cases would be prime candidates for bone marrow transplantation when this procedure becomes a more successful approach than at present; the short survival of AA cases may be related to the eradication of the leukemic cell population in the marrow and, at the same time, to the inability of the marrow to repopulate itself with normal elements, as appears to be the situation in cases of AN or NN (Li et al., 1983; Sandberg, 1980a).

Another important correlation with the qualitative aspects of the karyotypic changes is the presence of major karyotypic abnormalities (Sakurai and Sandberg, 1976) (MAKA) vs those cases with minor karyotypic abnormalities (MIKA) consisting of only one or two cytogenetic events. Generally, MAKA cases tend to have a much shorter survival because of failure of the patients to respond to therapy or achieve long, complete remissions, vs MIKA cases who respond to therapy more readily and achieve long-lasting, complete remission. This situation appears to apply in particular to cases of erythroleukemia, which are often of the MAKA variety (Sandberg, 1980a).

The presence of double minute chromosomes (DMS) appears to be associated with a poor prognosis in leukemia when they are

Table 7
Median Survival of ANLL Patients According to Karyotypic Status

Number of patients	Karyotypic classification	Median survival, mo
136	NN	7.9
79	AN	5.9
51	AA	2.4

SURVIVAL AFTER FIRST SYMPTOMS OF AML

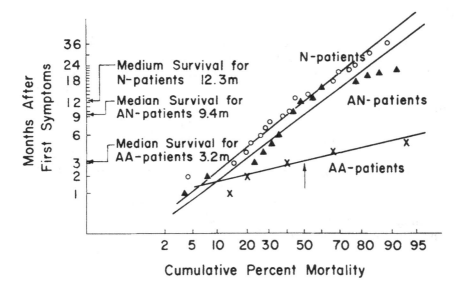

Fig. 10. Survival of NN, AN, and AA patients with AML. The AA patients, who essentially have no cytogenetically normal cells in the marrow, have a much shorter survival than the two other groups, who do have such cells in the marrow. (See text for discussion of these parameters.)

seen in the leukemic cells of the marrow (Cooperman and Klinger, 1981; Marinello et al., 1980), though such experience has not been universal (Hartley and Toolis, 1980).

5.2. Acute Lymphoblastic Leukemia (ALL)

The cytogenetic findings in acute lymphoblastic leukemia (ALL) (Tables 4 and 8) have also led to a definition of subgroups within presently established entities according to the FAB classification (Third International Workshop on Chromosomes in Leukemia, 1981). Thus, as mentioned previously, it may be that ALL with t(4;11) is a common progenitor stem cell disorder capable of differentiating also as a myelomonocytoid leukemia, at least in a subgroup of patients (Fig. 7). Other subentities within ALL have recently been pointed to, such as a subgroup of L1 with t(1;19)(q21;q13) (Michael et al., 1984), a subentity of T-cell ALL with t(11;14)(p13;q13) (Williams et al., 1984), pre-B cell ALL with t(1;19)(q23;p13) (Williams et al., 1984), and 9p— in T-cell ALL (Kowalczyk and Sandberg, 1983).

In T-cell diseases (leukemias and lymphomas), besides the 9p— anomaly in T-cell ALL, it appears that a break at 14q11 may be a nonrandom event, particularly in adult T-cell acute leukemia. In those leukemias with a high association with a virus, the possibility exists that the integration of a viral part into a specific chromosomal locus may constitute the primary karyotypic event, thus explaining the variability in the chromosomal changes seen in these states. Undoubtedly other subentities will be described that will have definite correlations with clinical and laboratory parameters. Thus, the cytogenetic findings have added to our diagnostic armamentarium in ALL, as well as in ANLL.

Other cytogenetic parameters in ALL, related to prognostic and diagnostic parameters in ALL, include the number of chromosomes in the leukemic cells (Fig. 11), i.e., the higher the chromosome number the better the prognosis, and the more prevalent the

Table 8
FAB Classification of ALL and Common Chromosome Changes

Classification	Cytologic characteristics	Common chromosomal changes
L1	Small blasts, nucleoli not present, scanty cytoplasm, regularly shaped nucleus	6q—; t(1;19) (q23;13) t(11;14) (q13;q32), high chromosome counts, Ph[1]-positive ALL
L2	Large blasts; heterogenous in size, 1–2 large nucleoli, Moderately abundant cytoplasm, irregularly shaped nucleoli	Includes Ph[1]-positive ALL; near-haploid ALL; t(4;11); 12p-
L3	Large and homogeneous blasts, 1–2 prominent nucleoli, cytoplasmic vacuolation, Moderately abundant cytoplasm, regularly shaped (oval or round) nucleus	t(8;14), t(2;8) t(8;22)

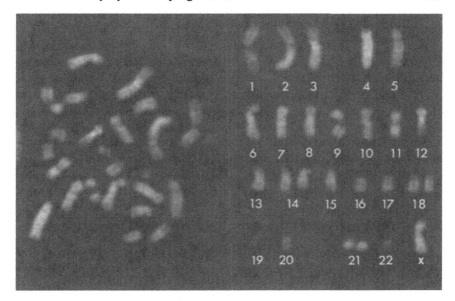

Fig. 11. Near-haploid (26 chromosomes) ALL with a marrow meta-phase (Q banded) shown on the left and the karyotype on the right. This type of ALL is associated with a rather poor prognosis. Except for a few chromosomes, all others were represented by only one member.

normal cells in the marrow (Secker-Walker et al., 1982; Williams et al., 1982). The latter situation is apparently associated with a better prognosis that when such cells are not encountered during the usual cytogenetic analysis. As in the case of ANLL, in about one third of the patients with ALL, the chromosome picture appears to be normal, at least with presently utilized cytogenetic methodologies. There is a possibility that the cytogenetic events in these so-called diploid ALL cases may occur at the molecular level, involving an oncogene or other genetic material whose nature can only be established with specialized probes. Thus, it will be of interest to ascertain in the future whether diploid leukemias exist at all.

Ph-positive ALL, though it may affect other varieties of ALL, appears to be most commonly associated with the pre-B cell type of ALL. As more and more cases of Ph-positive ALL are accumulated, this correlation will hopefully be established on a firmer basis than now exists.

6. Preleukemia and Myelodysplastic Disorders

In addition to the chromosomal changes already established in most of the acute and chronic leukemias, a group of diseases consisting of preleukemic states and myelodysplastic disorders (Bennett et al., 1982) has recently received much cytogenetic attention. Of interest is the fact that some of these states have been shown to be characterized by specific chromosomal changes (Table 5), such as t(1;7)(p11;p11) in some myelodysplastic disorders (Geraedts et al., 1980; Mecucci et al., 1985; Scheres et al., 1984; Smadja et al., 1985), and since these states often procede to ANLL, it would appear that such karyotypic changes may hold a significance similar to that ascribed to the established changes in various forms of leukemia.

7. Cytogenetic Changes in Chronic Lymphocytic Leukemia (CLL)

7.1. B- and T-Cell Mitogenic Stimulants

Chromosome changes in chronic lymphocytic leukemia (CLL) were not established on a firm basis until mitogens (Table 9) capable of stimulating the leukemic (as well as normal B) cells into mitosis became available (Gahrton and Robert, 1982; Moller, 1972; Morita et al., 1981). Thus, before such mitogens were introduced the usual results in B-cell CLL consisted of a diploid picture probably comprised of normal T cells present among the leukemic cells and stimulated by PHA (Sandberg, 1980a).

Phytohemagglutinin (PHA), though capable of stimulating normal T cells into mitosis, has not been proven to be a successful stimulant of malignant T cells. The availability of a T-cell growth factor (Poisez et al., 1980) may afford the opportunity to induce into mitosis the leukemic cells of T-type CLL.

In both chronic and acute T-cell leukemias, with the exception of 14q– and inv(14q), to be mentioned below, specific karyotypic changes have not been established. This may be a result of the failure to stimulate the cells with the primary change into mitosis or the existence of a chromosomal change beyond the resolution of presently used cytogenetic techniques and possibly requiring molecular DNA probing for its establishment.

7.2. B- and T-Cell CLL

With the availability of various mitogenic agents capable of stimulating B cells, including the leukemic type, the karyotypic picture in B-cell CLL has become much clearer (Table 10). Thus, the most common change appears to be trisomy 12 (+12) (Fig. 12),

Table 9
Mitogenic Stimulators of Blood Lymphocytes

Mitogen	Cell type stimulated	Concentrations used
Phytohemagglutinin (PHA)	T lymphocytes	$25-100 \ \mu g/mL$
Pokeweed mitogen (PWM)	B and T lymphocytes	Up to $150 \ \mu g/mL$
Concanavalin (Con A)	T lymphocytes (mouse)	$1-5 \ \mu g/mL$
Calcium ionophore-A23187	B and T lymphocytes	$5 \times 10^{-7}-10^{-6}M$ $(0.5-2.0 \ \mu g/mL)$
Sodium metaperiodate	T lymphocytes	$2-4 \times 10^{-3}M$
EB virus (EBV)	B lymphocytes	10–20% supernatant; 1:9 v/v of culture
Lipopolysaccharide W (E. coli 055:B5)	B lymphocytes	$100 \ \mu g/mL$
Staphylococcus Bacteria strain, Cowan I protein	B lymphocytes	$100 \ \mu g/mL$
Conditioned medium from PHA-stimulated T cells (PHA-induced soluble factors)	B lymphocytes	1:2 dilution
Protein A	B lymphocytes	$20-100 \ \mu g/mL$
T-cell growth factor (Interleukin-2)	T lymphocytes	10%

with 14q being the second most common aberration (Gahrton and Robert, 1982; Morita et al., 1981). The possibility will have to be explored (e.g., more cases studied and more precise and informative definitions of the cell type involved and the nature of the genes activated) that each specific karyotypic change in CLL defines a subentity within CLL related to differences in etiology or cell type. Establishment of a relation of cytogenetic changes to prognostic aspects of CLL has been attempted (Robert et al., 1982), and it appears that additional chromosomal changes, besides trisomy 12, carry a poorer prognosis and a more aggressive picture of the disease than in patients without the additional karyotypic changes (Han et al., 1984). Much remains to be accomplished cytogenetically in B-cell CLL, and undoubtedly the refinement and use of various mitogenic agents will greatly enhance the success of establishing the karyotypic changes and their relationship to various clinical parameters.

The chromosomal picture in T-cell chronic lymphocytic leukemia (as well as the acute variety of the disease) has not been

Table 10
Common Chromosome Changes in CLL[a]

Chromosome changes	Type of leukemia
t(6;12) (q15;p13)	Prolymphocytic (B-cell) leukemia
t(11;14) (q13;q32)	CLL
3p−(p13)	Prolymphocytic (B-cell) leukemia
+12	CLL
14q+(q32)	CLL
inv(14) (q11q32)	T-cell CLL

[a] CLL, Chronic lymphocytic leukemia.

established with certainty, with reports indicating considerable variability in the karyotypes, though some changes appear to occur more frequently than others (Ueshima et al., 1984). Nevertheless, a specific chromosome change, at least in some cases of T-cell CLL, has been established recently (Zech et al., 984), i.e., inversion of the long arm of chromosome #14, inv(14)(q11q32).

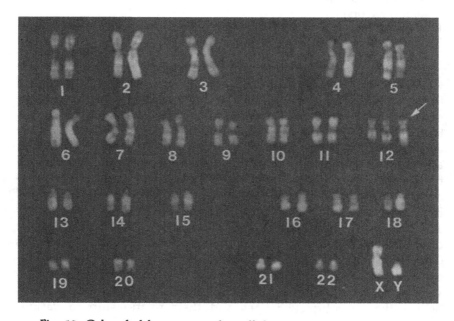

Fig. 12. Q-banded karyotype of a cell from a patient with CLL showing a common and specific karyotypic change in this disease, i. e., +12 (arrow).

Chromosome studies in adult acute T-cell leukemia (ATL), a disease associated with viral parameters and background, have not yielded a specific karyotypic change. One group in Japan has reported frequent involvement of chromosome #7 (+7) and to a lesser extent that of #14 (14q+) (Ueshima et al., 1981). Another Japanese group (Miyamoto et al., 1983), on the other hand, stressed the lack of consistent chromosome abnormalities in ATL, though some common changes affecting chromosomes #1 (duplication of the segment q21q32), #3 (translocations, trisomy), #6 (deletions of the long arm), #10, #14 (14q+), and #18, in order of their frequency, were seen. The donor chromosomes for the 14q+ were Yq, 5p, 5q, 9q, 10q, and 12q. Some evidence is emerging that at least a subgroup of patients with ATL may have a deletion at 14q11 in the affected cells and, hopefully, future studies will reveal the nature and characteristics of these cases (Fifth International Workshop on Chromosomes in Leukemia/Lymphoma, 1985). Whether the use of specific mitogenic stimulators for the involved T cells will lead to the establishment of the specific changes in ATL, or whether the specific karyotypic event is incorporation of a virus into a specific locus of the genome with the cytogenetic changes described to date being of a secondary nature, will have to await more definitive studies in the future.

7.3. Prolymphocytic Leukemia

Prolymphocytic leukemia of the B-cell type appears to be characterized, at least in a subgroup of cases, by t(6;12) (Sadamori et al., 1983). The T-cell variety of prolymphocytic leukemia is accompanied by a variety of chromosome changes (Ueshima et al., 1984), and it will be of interest to ascertain whether the specific change described in T-cell CLL will also be observed in the pro-lymphocytic leukemia.

8. Cytogenetic Aspects of Lymphoma

8.1. Burkitt's Lymphoma

The first consistent karyotypic anomaly in lymphoma was the description of a 14q+ change in Burkitt's lymphoma, established shortly following the introduction of banding techniques (Manolov and Manlova, 1972) and subsequently shown to be caused by a translocation between chromosomes #8 and #14 (Zech et al.,

1976) (Fig. 13). This translocation has now been more clearly defined, with the bands and subbands involved in t(8;14) now established, i.e., 8q24.13 and 14q32.33 (Yunis, 1984). The translocation is then reciprocal and balanced. Variant translocations, though always involving chromosome #8 at band q24, were also described, and these involved either chromosome #2 or #22 (Fig. 14), i.e., t(2;22) or t(8;22) (Sandberg, 1984a). It should be pointed out that secondary chromosome changes, in addition to these primary events, have almost invariably been found in these tumors, and that these secondary chromosome changes possibly play a role in affecting the anatomic and biologic nature of the disease, e.g., frequent involvement of the area of the neck and head in endemic areas of the disease and less frequently in the nonendemic areas. The karyotypic changes in Burkitt's lymphoma have served as an important basis for establishing some of the molecular events in the disease. These include the translocation of an oncogene, c-*myc* (ar-Rushdi et al., 1983; Leder et al., 1983), from chromosome #8 and the expression of only certain light chains of surface immunoglobulins (Bernheim et al., 1981; Sandberg, 1984a) (Fig. 15). Thus, in the disease characterized by a translocation between chromo-

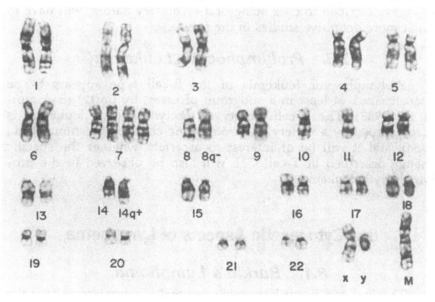

Fig. 13. G-banded karyotype of a cell from a Burkitt's lymphoma with the often seen t(8;14)(q24.1;q32.5). Other changes are also present: +7, +7, −10, −11, and a marker chromosome (M).

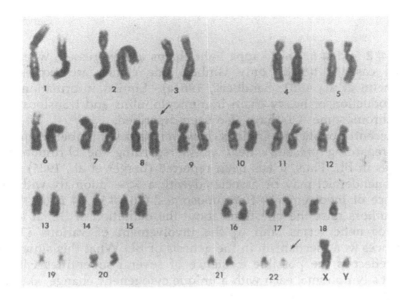

Fig. 14. G-banded karyotype of a cell from a Burkitt's type acute leukemia (L3) with a variant translocation, i. e., (8;22)(q24;q12) (arrows). This type of translocation is usually accompanied by the production of lambda light chain surface immunoglobulins, pointing to the possible location of the gene for the production of these immunoglobulins on the long arm of chromosome #22.

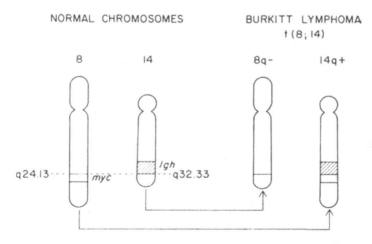

Fig. 15. Schematic presentation of some of the molecular events associated with Burkitt's lymphoma cells. The oncogene *myc* is translocated to a new site on the 14q, this also leading to stimulation of the IgH locus responsible for heavy chain immunoglobulin production, as well as activation of the *myc* oncogene.

some #2 and #8, only kappa light chains are expressed, whereas in the case of t(8;22), only lambda side chains are expressed (Bernheim et al., 1981; Sandberg, 1984a). Similar information on the production of heavy chain immunoglobulins and translocation onto chromosome #14 have also been described.

Recently published findings, however, raise a number of questions regarding presently held views regarding the chromosome changes in BL. Thus, it has been reported (Berger et al., 1985) that BL (nonendemic) may be associated with a 6q— anomaly without evidence of involvement of chromosomes #8, #14, #2, or #22. The authors raise the questions about the definition of BL, at least in cytogenetic terms, and of the involvement of various DNA sequences as a mechanism in the genesis of BL. What this situation may reflect is the possible existence of several subentities within Burkitt's lymphoma, each with a unique cytogenetic change, akin to the situation in the acute leukemias. In another report (Chaganti et al., 1983), cell lines derived from a homosexual patient with probable acquired immunodeficiency syndrome and BL and with a consistent t(8;22) produced kappa light chains rather than the expected lambda chains. The findings indicated to the authors that the translocation in BL may occur as a separate event from immunoglobulin gene rearrangement or that the proposed hierarchial sequence of immunoglobulin gene rearrangement is not always adhered to. Furthermore, the authors (Chaganti et al., 1983) indicated that in cells containing a translocation between the long arm of chromosome #8 and a chromosome bearing an immunoglobulin gene, activation and expression of the cellular *myc* oncogene may occur regardless of the immunoglobulin gene that is expressed.

The frequent involvement of chromosome #1 in the karyotypic changes of Burkitt's lymphoma, as it is in other lymphomas, leukemias, and cancers, was related to EBV status. All nine BL cell lines not associated with EBV were shown to contain an abnormality of the long arm (bands 1q23–q24) of chromosome #1. The authors hypothesized (Bernheim et al., 1983) that genetic information resembling that contained within the viral genome was present on the long arm of chromosome #1 and may bear upon the relationship between BL cell proliferation and EBV.

It has been shown that the part of chromosome #14 that breaks during the genesis of the t(8;14) in Burkitt's lymphoma is situated precisely within the area of chromosome #14 that encodes the immunoglobulin heavy chain (Croce et al., 1979). Using hybrids between mouse and human cells, it was demonstrated that cells containing a normal #14 possessed genes for antibody production, whereas those with a normal #8 did not (Croce et al., 1983). In contrast, hybrid cells with a chromosome #14 that had been involved in the above translocation, a 14q+, contained the genes for the constant regions of heavy chains but not for the variable regions. Chromosome #8 that had taken part in the translocation contained the genes for the variable regions. The results indicate that chromosome #14 breaks between the genes coding for the variable region and constant regions of the heavy chain and that the genes coding for the variable region move to chromosome #8. The heavy-chain locus on chromosome #14 is thus directly involved in one of the translocations that is characteristic of Burkitt's lymphoma.

Though the oncogene *myc* became translocated from chromosome #8 to #14 in t(8;14) of Burkitt's lymphoma, the c-*myc* protein product is the same as in normal and Burkitt's lymphoma cells (Croce et al., 1984). This contrasts with the abnormal mRNA (and hence one can assume protein products) associated with the c-*abl* translocation in CML with a Ph chromosome (Canaani et al., 1984; Collins et al., 1984; Leibowitz et al., 1984, 1985). The question naturally arises as to what is the oncogenetic consequence of the chromosome translocation or Burkitt's lymphoma. It is possible that the translocation somehow causes the c-*myc* gene product, small quantities of which are required for the cells normal function, to be expressed at abnormally high levels.

8.2. Malignant Lymphomas (Other Than Burkitt's)

A meaningful correlation of the cytogenetic findings in malignant lymphomas has been hampered to a large extent by the lack of a uniform system of nomenclature. The introduction of the new formulation for the classification of human lymphomas (Non-Hodgkin's Lymphoma Pathologic Classification Project, 1982) should help considerably in correlating the chromosome changes with histology and other aspects of the lymphomas. In fact, at the Fifth International Workshop on Chromosomes in Leukemia/ Lymphoma held at Saitama in October 1984, an attempt was made at such a correlation, and though much remains to be accomplished in that regard, the recommendations of this workshop should go a long way in stimulating correlations between the karyotypic changes and the types of lymphoma.

In lymphomas other than those of the Burkitt's variety, certain karyotypic changes appear to be commonly associated with a particular type of lymphoma (Tables 11 and 12) (Bloomfield et al., 1983; Yunis et al., 1982). Thus, t(8;14), of apparently the same genesis as in Burkitt's lymphoma, appears often in the diffuse type of disease, including small noncleaved non-Burkitt's lymphoma, as well as immunoblastic lymphoma. On the other hand, t(14;18)(q32.3;q21.3) appears to be commonly associated with follicular types of lymphoma (Fig. 16), such as small-cleaved and mixed small- and large-cleaved cell lymphomas. This translocation has also been seen in rare cases of diffuse large-cell lymphoma. In addition, 6q− (q21q25) has been commonly associated with diffuse large- (noncleaved) cell lymphoma, as well as in some cases of follicular lymphoma of the mixed small- and large-cell variety. 6q− has also been seen in rare cases of T-cell lymphoma, as well as in transformed small-cell lymphocytic lymphoma and immunoblastic lymphoma. The anomalies t(11;14)(q13.1;q32.3) and +12 have been seen most commonly in small-cell lymphocytic lymphoma or, as mentioned previously, in chronic lymphocytic leukemia. These chromosome changes are retained when a small-cell lymphocytic

Table 11
Type of Lymphoma and Chromosome Changes

Chromosome changes	Type of leukemia
t(8;14)(q24;q32)	Diffuse large cell
t(14;18)(q32;q21)	Follicular
t(11;14)(q13;q32)	Diffuse small cell
del(6)(q21)	Large cell, diffuse
+7	Diffuse, large cell, or follicular
11q−	Diffuse small cell
+12	Diffuse small cell

Table 12
Common Numerical and Morphologic Karyotypic Changes in
Malignant Lymphomas (in Order of Their Frequency)

Morphologic	Numerical
14q	+12
18q	+18
6q	+7
1p	+21
8q	

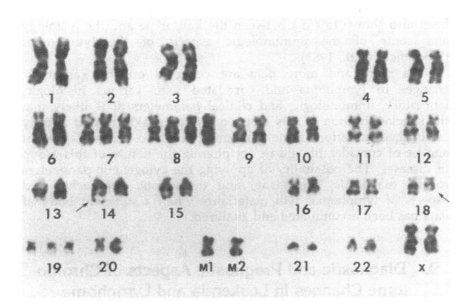

Fig. 16. G-banded karyotype from a lymphoma (follicular) showing a t(14;18)(q32;q21), a translocation commonly seen in follicular types of lymphoma. Several numerical changes (+7, +8, +8, +19) and two marker chromosomes (M1 and M2) of unknown origin are also present.

lymphoma is transformed to a diffuse large-cell variety. To date, the nonrandom or specific chromosome changes have not been established in diffuse cleaved-cell lymphoma, lymphoblastic lymphoma, and diffused T- or B-cell mixed-cell lymphoma. Of interest is the involvement of 9p13 either in translocation or inversions in some cases of T-cell mixed-cell lymphomas (Yunis et al., 1982).

In more recent reports (Bloomfield et al., 1983) on a large series of lymphomas, it was shown that among the numerical chromosome changes, the most frequent are of #12, #18, #7, and #21 (in order of frequency), the +12 being seen most frequently in small-cell lymphocytic lymphoma, an entity that has much in common with CLL. In the latter leukemia, the +12 is the most frequent karyotypic change observed (Gahrton and Robert, 1982; Morita et al., 1981). Structural abnormalities most frequently involved 14q, 18q, 6q, 1p, and 8q (in order of frequency). The long arm of chromosome #14, which is often involved in translocations, was involved in more than 70% of the lymphomas. The most frequent translocation was t(14;18)(q32;q21), followed by t(8;14)(q24;q32) and t(1;14)(q42;q32). Deletions most frequently involved chromosome #6 at band q21 or q23. Correlations have been also shown to exist between the karyotype and the histology and some of the immunologic aspects of the lymphomas (Bloomfield et al., 1983).

As more and more data are collected on the karyotypic changes in lymphoma and correlated with various histologic, laboratory, immunologic, and clinical parameters, it is likely that the subclassification of this group of diseases, akin to that already established in various acute leukemias, will also become apparent and be of considerable aid in deciphering the nature of this group of diseases. The possibility of applying the cytogenetic parameters to the diagnostic, prognostic, and therapeutic approaches and aspects of lymphomas will materialize when a sufficient body of data has been accumulated and analyzed.

9. Diagnostic and Prognostic Aspects of Chromosome Changes in Leukemia and Lymphoma

9.1.   Specific (Primary) Changes

It is possible that in most, if not all, human cancers, lymphomas, and leukemias, a specific (primary) karyotypic change in human neoplasia is responsible and/or necessary for the development of malignant transformation (Sandberg, 1983, 1984b). Such a karyotypic event, microscopic or submicroscopic (molecular), may or may not involve known oncogenes, but appears nevertheless to be of crucial importance in initiating the malignant process within a cell. However, very frequently the primary karyotypic change is followed by the development of secondary chromosome changes that may play an important role in the biology of the leukemia or lymphoma (Sandberg, 1982).

9.2.   Primary vs Secondary Chromosome Changes

Most of the leukemias and lymphomas have been shown to be characterized by primary (specific chromosome changes that have been tabulated in this chapter. These primary changes, as mentioned above, are possibly related to, if not necessary for, the process of malignant transformation, which occurs in the affected cells, as a result of which the ultimate manifestations of these diseases become clinically evident when the bulk of the abnormal cells affect normal physiology. Generally, a leukemia or lymphoma is at its lowest level of malignancy when only the primary chromosome change exists, since when other secondary karyotypic changes appear (Sandberg, 1982, 1985), the disease becomes more progressive and often resistant to therapy. In some instances, these secondary changes are of a nonrandom variety (e. g., +Ph, +8, and i(17q) in CML). On the other hand, in the lymphomas the secondary chromosome changes are often of a complex nature, with the secondary changes differing from one patient to another. Thus, in the future it will be important to ascertain which of these secondary karyotypic changes are related to the phenotypic manifestations of the leukemia or lymphoma, so that a better understanding of these diseases may be achieved. It is also possible that the secondary karyotypic changes may decide some of the clinical and phenotypic manifestations, e. g., the anatomic distribution of Burkitt's lymphoma in the neck and head in Africa vs that in the Western world. The possibility exists that some of the phenotypic variations of the lymphomas with the same primary karyotypic change, i. e., t(14;18), may also be related to the secondary changes that may be reflected in such parameters as whether the cells are cleaved or noncleaved and large or small in the organs affected by lymphoma.

The secondary chromosome changes may also be responsible for activation and expression of oncogenes (and other genes) not involved in the primary karyotypic event and may, in fact, result in a "cascade" of oncogene activations of an either permanent or transient nature. Crucial to our understanding of these events will be to be ascertain which of these activations are related to karyotypic changes and which are not. Since such "cascades" of oncogene activations may play an important role in the biology of leukemia and lymphoma, with some of these activations being possibly transient or reversible, correlations between the karyotypic changes in these diseases and gene functions and expressions should yield key information of value diagnostically and basically.

Mention should be made of the relationship between chromosomal fragile sites (Glover et al., 1984) and the development of cytogenetic changes in leukemic or lymphoma cells, since often chromosome breaks involved in translocations or deletions appear to be located in such fragile site areas (LeBeau and Rowley, 1984; Yunis and Soreng, 1984). To date, fragile sites have not been demonstrated in all chromosome areas involved by specific karyo-typic events, e.g., 9q34 and 22q11 in the Ph translocation (Table 13). Furthermore, it remains to be shown that sites affected by chromosomal changes in neoplastic cells are invariably associated with constitutional fragile sites in the same patients.

Table 13
Classification of Fragile Sites on Human Chromosomes That
May Be Related to Translocation or Other
Morphologic Karyotypic Changes[a]

Group	Methods of induction	Chromosomal locations	Population incidence
Folate-sensitive	Thymidylate stress: Folate and thymidine deficient medium Inhibition of dihydrofolate reductase (methotrexate, aminopterin, etc.) Inhibition of thymidylate synthetase (FUdR)	2q11, 2q13, 6p23, 7p11, 8q22, 9p21, 9q32, 10q23, 11q13, 11q23, 1q213, 16p12, 2p11, Xq27	Rare
Distamycin A inducible	Distamycin A Novobiocin Bromodeoxyuridine (BrdU)	16q22, 17p12	Rare
BrdU inducible	BrdU	10q25	2–3%
Common or aphidicolin inducible	DNA polymerase alpha inhibition: Aphidicolin Thymidylate stress	2q31, 3p14, 6q26, 7q32 16q23, Xp22 Possible: 1p22, 1p32, 1p36, 1q25, 2p13, 2q33, 3p24, 3q27, 5q31, 7p31, 7q22, 8q22, 9q32, 11p13, 14q24, 22q12, Xq22	Very common

[a] This table is based primarily on published data of Glover et al. (1984), as well as on private communications from Dr. T. W. Glover.

References

ar-Rushdi, A., Nishikura, K., Erikson, J., Watt, R., Rovera, G., and Croce, C. M. (1983), Differential expression of the translocated and the untranslocated c-myc oncogene in Burkitt lymphoma. *Science* **222**, 390–393.

Arthur, D. C., and Bloomfield, C. D. (1983), Partial deletion of the long arm of chromosome 16 and bone marrow eosinophilia in acute nonlymphocytic leukemia: A new association. *Blood* **61**, 994–998.

Arthur, D. C., Bloomfield, C. D., Lindquist, L. L., and Nesbit, Jr., M. E. (1982), Translocation 4;11 in acute lymphoblastic leukemia: Clinical characteristics and prognostic significance. *Blood* **59**, 96–99.

Bartram, C. R., de Klein, A., Hagemeijer, A., van Agthoven, T., Geurts van Kessel, A., Bootsma, D., Grosveld, G., Ferguson-Smith, M. A., Davies, T., Stone, M., Heisterkamp, N., Stephenson, J. R., and Groffen, J. (1983), Translocation of the human c-abl oncogene occurs in variant Ph-positive but not Ph-negative chronic myelocytic leukaemia. *Nature* **306**, 277–280.

Bennett, J. M., Catovsky, D., Daniel, M. T., Flandrin, G., Galton, D. A. G., Gralnick, H. R., and Sultan, C. (1976), Proposals for the classification of the acute leukaemias. *Br. J. Haematol.* **33**, 451–458.

Bennett, J. M., Catovsky, D., Daniel, M. T., Flandrin, G., Galton, D. A. G., Gralnick, H. R., and Sultan, C. (1982), Proposals for the classification of the myelodysplastic syndromes. *Br. J. Haematol.* **51**, 189–199.

Berger, R., Bernheim, A., Flandrin, G., Daniel, M. T., Valensi, F., Ochoa, M. H., Marty, M., Schaison, G., and Boiron, M. (1983a), Valeur pronostique des anomalie chromosomiques dans les leucemies aigues non lymphoblastiques. *Nouv. Rev. Fr. Hematol.* **25**, 87–90.

Berger, R., Bernheim, A., Le Coniat, M., Vecchione, D., Pacot, A., and Flandrin, G. (1983b), Cytogenetique et leucemies aigues non lymphoblastiques interet des cultures a court terme. *Nouv. Rev. Fr. Hematol.* **25**, 81–86.

Berger, R., Bernheim, A., Sigaux, F., Valensi, F., Daniet, M. -T., and Flandrin, G. (1985), Two Burkitt's lymphomas with chromosome 6 long arm deletions. *Cancer Genet. Cytogenet.* **15**, 159–167.

Bernard, P. H., Reiffers, J., Boisseau, M. R., and Broustet, A. (1980), Leucemies aigues granuleuses de l'adulte: Valeur pronostique du caryotype medullaire. *Nouv. Presse Medicale* **9**, 499–503.

Bernheim, A., Berger, R., and Lenoir, G. (1981), Cytogenetic studies on African Burkitt's lymphoma cell lines: t(8;14),t(2;8) and t(8;22) translocations. *Cancer Genet. Cytogenet.* **3**, 307–315.

Bernheim, A., Berger, R., and Lenoir, G. (1983), Cytogenetic studies on Burkitt's lymphoma cell lines. *Cancer Genet. Cytogenet.* **8**, 223–229.

Bernstein, R., Pinto, M. R., Behr, A., and Mendelow, B. (1982), Chromosome 3 abnormalities in acute nonlymphocytic leukemia (ANLL) with abnormal thrombopoiesis: Report of three patients with a "new" inversion anomaly and a further case of homologous translocation. *Blood* **60**, 613–617.

Bishop, M. J. (1983), Cellular oncogenes and retroviruses. *Ann. Rev. Biochem.* **52**, 301–354.

Bloomfield, C. D., Arthur, D. C., Frizzera, G., Levine, E. G., Peterson, B. A., and Gajl-Peczalska, K. J. (1983), Nonrandom chromosome abnormalities in lymphoma. *Cancer Res.* **43**, 2957–2984.

Canaani, E., Gale, R. P., Steiner-Saltz, D., Berrebi, A., Aghai, E., and Januszewicz, E. (1984), Altered transcription of an oncogene in chromic myeloid leukaemia. *Lancet* i, 593–595.

Cannizzaro, L. A., Nowell, P. C., Croce, C. M., and Emanuel, B. S. (1985), The breakpoint in 22q11 for a t(9;22) acute lymphoblastic leukemia differs from the breakpoint of t(8;22) Burkitt's lymphoma. *Cancer Genet. Cytogenet.*, in press.

Carroll, A. J., Crist, W. M., Parmley, R. T., Roper, M., Cooper, M. D., and Finley, W. H. (1984), Pre-B cell leukemia associated with chromosome translocation 1;19, *Blood* 63, 721–724.

Chaganti, R. S. K. (1983), Significance of chromosome changes to hematopoietic neoplasms. *Blood* 62, 515–524.

Chaganti, R. S. K., Jhanwar, S. C., Koziner, B., Arlin, Z., Mertelsmann, R., and Clarkson, B. D. (1983), Specific translocations characterize Burkitt's-like lymphoma of homosexual men with the acquired immunodeficiency syndrome. *Blood* 61, 1269–1272.

Collins, S. J., Kubonishi, I., Miyoshi, I., and Groudine, M. T. (1984), Altered transcription of the c-*abl* oncogene in K-562 and other chronic myelogenous leukemia cells. *Science* 225, 72–74.

Cooperman, B. S., and Klinger, H. P. (1981), Double minute chromosomes in a case of acute myelogenous leukemia resistant to chemotherapy. *Cytogenet. Cell Genet.* 30, 25–30.

Croce, C. M., Shander, M., Martinis, J., Cicurel, L., D'Ancona, G. G., Dolby, T. W., and Koprowski, H. (1979), Chromosomal location of the genes for human immunoglobulin heavy chains. *Proc. Natl. Acad. Sci. USA* 76, 3416–3419.

Croce, C. M., Thierfelder, W., Erikson, J., Nishikura, K., Finan, J., Lenoir, G. M., and Nowell, P. C. (1983), Transcriptional activation of an unrearranged and untranslocated c-myc oncogene by translocation of a C locus in Burkitt lymphoma cells. *Proc. Natl. Acad. Sci. USA* 80, 6922–6926.

Croce, C. M., Tsujimoto, Y., Erikson, J., and Nowell, P. (1984), Biology of Disease: Chromosome translocations and B Cell Neoplasia. *Lab. Invest.* 51, 258–267.

de Klein, A., Geurts van Kessel, A., Grosveld, G., Bartram, C. R., Hagemeijer, A., Bootsma, D., Spurr, N. K., Heisterkamp, N., Groffen, J., and Stephenson, J. R. (1982), A cellular oncogene is translocated to the Philadelphia chromosome in chronic myelocytic leukaemia. *Nature* 300, 765–767.

Emanuel, B. S., Selden, J. R., Wang, E., Nowell, P. C., and Croce, C. M. (1984), In situ hybridization and translocation breakpoint mapping. *Cytogenet. Cell Genet.* 38, 127–131.

Fifth International Workshop on Chromosomes in Leukemia/Lymphoma (1985), in press.

First International Workshop on Chromosomes in Leukemia (1978), Helsinki, Finland, Aug. 25–28, 1977. *Cancer Res.* 38, 867–868.

Fitzgerald, P. H., Morris, C. M., Fraser, G. J., Giles, L. M., Hamer, J. W., Heaton, D. C., and Beard, M. E. J. (1983), Nonrandom cytogenetic changes in New Zealand patients with acute myeloid leukemia. *Cancer Genet. Cytogenet.* 8, 51–66.

Fitzgerald, P. H., Morris, C. M., and Giles, L. M. (1982), Direct versus cultured preparation of bone marrow cells from 22 patients with acute myeloid leukemia. *Hum. Genet.* 60, 281–283.

Fourth International Workshop on Chromosomes in Leukemia: A Prospective Study of Acute Nonlymphocytic Leukemia (1984), Chicago, Illinois, USA, Sept. 2–7, 1982. *Cancer Genet. Cytogenet.* 11, 249–360.

Fraser, J., Hollings, P. E., Fitzgerald, P. H., Day, W. A., Clark, V., Heaton, D. C., Hamer, J. W., and Beard, M. E. J. (1981), Acute promyelocytic leukemia: Cytogenetics and bone-marrow culture. *Int. J. Cancer* **27,**

Gahrton, G., and Robert, K. -H. (1982), Chromosomal aberrations in chronic B-cell lymphocytic leukemia. *Cancer Genet. Cytogenet.* **6,** 171–181.

Geraedts, J. P. M., den Ottolander, G. J., Ploem, J. E., and Muntinghe, O. G. (1980), An identical translocation between chromosome 1 and 7 in three patients with myelofibrosis and myeloid metaplasia. *Br. J. Haematol.* **44,** 569–575.

Geurts van Kessel, A. H. M., ten Brinke, H., Boere, W. A. M., den Boer, W. C., de Groot, P. G., Hagemeijer, A., Meera Khan, P., and Pearson, P. L. (1981), Characterization of the Philadelphia chromosome by gene mapping. *Cytogenet. Cell Genet.* **30,** 83–91.

Glover, T. W., Berger, C., Coyle, J., and Echo, B. (1984), DNA polymerase inhibition by aphidicolin induces gaps and breaks at common fragile sites in human chromosomes. *Hum. Genet.* **67,** 136–142.

Greenberger, J. S., Davisson, P. B., Gans, P. Y., and Moloney, W. C. (1979), In vitro induction of continuous acute promyelocytic leukemia cell lines by Friend or Abelson murine leukemia virus. *Blood* **53,** 987–1001.

Groffen, J., Heisterkamp, N., Reynolds, F. H., Jr., and Stephenson, J. R. (1983a), Homology between phosphotyrosine acceptor site of human c-*abl* and viral oncogene products. *Nature* **304,** 167–169.

Groffen, J., Heisterkamp, N., Stephenson, J. R., Geurts van Kessel, A., de Klein, A., Grosveld, G., and Bootsma, D. (1983b), C-sis is translocated from chromosome 22 to chromosome 9 in chronic myelocytic leukemia. *J. Exp. Med.* **158,** 9–15.

Groffen, J., Stephenson, J. R., Heisterkamp, N., de Klein, A., Bartram, C. R., and Grosveld, G. (1984), Philadelphia chromosomal breakpoints are clustered within a limited region, bcr, on chromosome 22. *Cell* **36,** 93–99.

Hagemeijer, A., Bartram, C. R., Smit, E. M. E., van Agthoven, A. J., and Bootsma, D. (1984), Is the chromosomal region 9q34 always involved in variants of the Ph1 translocation? *Cancer Genet. Cytogenet.* **13,** 1–16.

Hagemeijer, A., Smit. E. M. E., and Bootsma, D. (1979), Improved identification of chromosomes of leukemic cells in methotrexate-treated cultures. *Cytogenet. Cell Genet.* **23,** 208–212.

Han, T., Ozer, H., Sadamori, N., Emrich, L. Gomez, G. A., Henderson, E. S., Bloom, M. L., and Sandberg, A. A. (1984), Prognostic importance of cytogenetic abnormalities in patients with chronic lymphocytic leukemia. *N. Eng. J. Med.* **310,** 288–292.

Hartley, S. E., and Toolis, F. (1980), Double minute chromosomes in a case of acute myeloblastic leukemia. *Cancer Genet. Cytogenet.*

Heisterkamp, N., Stephenson, J. R., Groffen, J., Hansen, P. F., de Klein, A., Bartram, C. R., and Grosveld, G. (1983), Localization of the c-abl oncogene adjacent to a translocation breakpoint in chronic myelocytic leukaemia. *Nature* **306,** 239–242.

Ishihara, T., Minamihisamatsu, M., and Tosuji, M. (1985), Chromosome 9 in variant Ph translocations. *Cancer Genet. Cytogenet.* **14,** 183–184.

Knuutila, S., Vuopio, P., Elonen, E., Siimes, M., Kovanen, R., Borgstrom, G. H., and de la Chapelle, A. (1981), Culture of bone marrow reveals more cells with chromosomal abnormalities than the direct method in patients with hematologic disorders. *Blood* **58,** 369–375.

Kocova, M., Kowalczyk, J. R., and Sandberg, A. A. (1985), Translocation t(4;11) acute leukemia: Three case reports and review of the literature. *Cancer Genet. Cytogenet.* **16**, 21–32.

Kowalczyk, J., and Sandberg, A. A. (1983), A possible subgroup of ALL with 9p–. *Cancer Genet. Cytogenet.* **9**, 383–385.

LeBeau, M. M., Larson, R. A., Bitter, M. A., Vardiman, J. W., Golomb, H. M., and Rowley, J. D. (1983), Association of an inversion of chromosome 16 with abnormal marrow eosinophils in acute myelomonocytic leukemia. *N. Eng. J. Med.* **309**, 630–636.

Le Beau, M. M., and Rowley, J. D. (1984), Heritable fragile sites in cancer. *Nature* **308**, 607–608.

Leder, P., Battey, J., Lenoir, G., Moulding, C., Murphy, W., Potter, H., Stewart, T., and Taub, R. (1983), Translocations among antibody genes in human cancer. *Science* **222**, 765–771.

Leibowitz, D., Cubbon, R., and Bank, A. (1985), Increased expression of a novel c-*abl*-related RNA in K562 cells. *Blood* **65**, 526–529.

Leibowitz, D., Schaefer-Rego, K., Popenoe, D., and Mears, J. G. (1984), Variable position of the breakpoint of the Ph1 translocation in chronic myelogenous leukemia (CML). *Blood* **64**, 203a (abstract).

Li, Y. S., Khalid, G., Hayhoe, F. G. J. (1983), Correlation between chromosomal pattern, cytological subtypes, response to therapy, and survival in acute myeloid leukemia. *Scand. J. Haematol.* **30**, 265–277.

Manolov, G., and Manlova, Y. (1972), Marker band in one chromosome 14 from Burkitt lymphomas. *Nature* **237**, 33–34.

Marinello, M. J., Bloom, M. L., Doeblin, T. D., and Sandberg, A. A. (1980), Double minute chromosomes in human leukemia. *N. Eng. J. Med.* **303**, 704.

Mecucci, C., Ghione, F., Tricot, G., and Van den Berghe, H. (1985), Combined trisomy 1q and monosomy 7q due to translocation t(1;7) in myelodysplastic syndromes. *Cancer Genet. Cytogenet.*, in press.

Michael, P. M., Levin, M. D., and Garson, O. M. (1984), Translocation 1;19-A new cytogenetic abnormality in acute lymphocytic leukemia. *Cancer Genet. Cytogenet.* **12**, 333–341.

Miyamoto, K., Sato, J., Kitajima, K., Togawa, A., Suemaru, S., Sanada, H., and Tanaka, T. (1983), Adult T-cell leukemia: Chromosome analysis of 15 cases. *Cancer* **52**, 471–478.

Moller, G. (1972), Lymphocyte activation by mitogens. *Transplant. Rev.* **11**, 1–267.

Morita, M., Minowada, J., and Sandberg, A. A. (1981), Chromosomes and causation of human cancer and leukemia. XLV. Chromosome patterns in stimulated lymphocytes of chronic lymphocytic leukemia. *Cancer Genet. Cytogenet.* **3**, 293–306.

Morse, H. G., Odom, L. F., Tubergen, D., Hays, T., Blake, M., and Robinson, A. (1983), Prognosis in acute lymphoblastic leukemia of childhood as determined by cytogenetic studies at diagnosis. *Med. Pediat. Oncol.* **11**, 310–318.

Nagasaka, M., Maeda, S., Maeda, H., Chen, H. L., Kita, K., Mabuchi, O., Misu, H., Matsuo, T., and Sugiyama, T. (1983), Four cases of t(4;11) acute leukemia and its myelomonocytic nature in infants. *Blood* **61**, 1174–1181.

Non-Hodgkin's Lymphoma Pathologic Classification Project (1982), National Cancer Institute sponsored study of classification of non-Hodgkin's lymphomas: Summary and description of a working formulation for clinical usage. *Cancer* **49**, 2122–2135.

Nowell, P. C., and Hungerford, D. A. (1960), A minute chromosome in human granulocytic leukemia. *Science* **132**, 1497.

Pearson, M. G., Vardiman, J. W., Le Beau, M. M., and Rowley, J. D. (1983), T(6;9): A new cytogenetic subset in acute non-lymphocytic leukemia (ANLL) associated with bone marrow basophilia. *Blood* **62**, 180 (abstract).

Poisez, B. J., Ruscetti, R. W., Mier, J. W., Woods, A. M., and Gallo, R. C. (1980), T-cell lines established from human T-lymphocytic neoplasias by direct response to T-cell growth factor. *Proc. Natl. Acad. Sci. USA* **77**, 6815–6819.

Potter, A. M., Watmore, A. E., Cooke, P., Lilleman, J. S., and Sokol, R. J. (1981), Significance of non-standard Philadelphia chromosomes in chronic granulocytic leukaemia. *Br. J. Cancer* **44**, 51–54.

Raschke, W. C., Baird, S., Ralph, P., and Nakoinz, I. (1978), Functional macrophage cell lines transformed by the Abelson leukemia virus. *Cell* **15**, 261–267.

Rigby, P. W. J., Dickman, M., Rhodes, G., and Berg, P. (1977), Labeling deoxyribonucleic acid to high specific activity in vitro by nick translation with DNA polymerase I. *J. Mol. Biol.* **113**, 237–251.

Robert, K. -H., Gahrton, G., Friberg, K., Zech, L., Nilsson, B. (1982), Extra chromosome 12 and prognosis in chronic lymphocytic leukaemia. *Sand. J. Haematol.* **28**, 163–168.

Rosenberg, N., Baltimore, D., and Scher, C. D. (1975), In vitro transformation of lymphoid cells by Abelson murine leukemia virus. *Proc. Natl. Acad. Sci. USA* **72**, 1932–1936.

Rowley, J. D. (1973a), Identification of a translocation with quinacrine fluorescence in a patient with acute leukemia. *Ann. Genet.* **16**, 109–112.

Rowley, J. D. (1973b), A new consistent chromosomal abnormality in chronic myelogenous leukaemia identified by quinacrine fluorescence and Giemsa staining. *Nature* **243**, 290–293.

Rowley, J. D. (1983), Human oncogene locations and chromosome aberrations. *Nature* **301**, 290–291.

Sadamori, N., Han, T., Minowada, J., Bloom, M. L., Henderson, E. S., and Sandberg, A. A. (1983), Possible specific chromosome change in prolymphocytic leukemia. *Blood,* **62**, 729–736.

Sakurai, M., and Sandberg, A. A. (1973), Prognosis in acute myeloblastic leukemia: Chromosomal correlation. *Blood* **41**, 93–104.

Sakurai, M., and Sandberg, A. A. (1976), Chromosomes and causation of human cancer and leukemia. XI. Correlation of karyotypes with clinical features of acute myeloblastic leukemia. *Cancer* **37**, 285–299.

Sandberg, A. A. (1980a), Chromosomes and causation of human cancer and leukemia. XL. The Ph[1] and other translocations in CML. *Cancer* **46**, 2221–2226.

Sandberg, A. A., ed. (1980b). *The Chromosomes in Human Cancer and Leukemia,* Elsevier North-Holland, New York, New York.

Sandberg, A. A. (1982), Chromosomal Changes in Human Cancer: Specificity and Heterogeneity in *Tumor Cell Heterogeneity: Origins and Implications,* Vol. 4, (Owens, A. H., Jr., Coffey, P. S., and Baylin, S. B., eds.) Academic, New York.

Sandberg, A. A. (1983), A chromosomal hypothesis of oncogenesis. *Cancer Genet. Cytogenet.* **8**, 277–285.

Sandberg, A. A. (1984a), Cytogenetic Abnormalities in Lymphoid Neoplasia in *Pathogenesis of Leukemias and Lymphomas: Environmental Influences* (Magrath, I. T., O'Connor, G. T., and Ramot, B., eds.) Raven, New York.

Sandberg, A. A. (1984b), Chromosomal Changes and Cancer Causation: Chromatin's Reawakening in *Accomplishments in Cancer Research* (Fortner, J. G., Rhoads, J. E., eds.) Lippincott, Philadelphia, Pennsylvania.

Sandberg, A. A. (1985), Secondary chromosome changes in cancer: Their nature and significance. *Cancer Genet. Cytogenet.*, submitted.

Sandberg, A. A., Gemmill, R. M., Hecht, B. K., and Hecht, F. (1985), The Philadelphia chromosome: A model of cancer and molecular cytogenetics. *Cancer Genet. Cytogenet.*, in press.

Sandberg, A. A., Morgan, R., McCallister, J. A., Kaiser-McCaw, B., and Hecht, F. (1983), Acute myeloblastic leukemia (AML) with t(6;9)(p23;q34): A specific subgroup of AML? *Cancer Genet. Cytogenet.* 10, 139–142.

Scher, C. D., and Siegler, R. (1975), Direct transformation of 3T3 cells by Abelson murine leukaemia virus. *Nature* 253, 729–731.

Scheres, J. M. J. C., Hustinx, T. W. J., Holdrinet, R. S. G., Geraedts, J. P. M., Hagemeijer, A., and van der Blij-Philipsen, M. (1984), Translocation 1;7 in dyshematopoiesis: Possibly induced with a nonrandom geographic distribution. *Cancer Genet. Cytogenet.* 12, 283–294.

Schwartz, S., Jiji, R., Kerman, S., Meekins, J., and Cohen, M. M. (1983), Translocation (6;9)(p23;q34) in actue nonlymphocytic leukemia. *Cancer Genet. Cytogenet.* 10, 133–138.

Secker-Walker, L. M., Swansbury, G. J., Hardisty, R. M., Sallan, S. E., Garson, O. M., Sakurai, M., and Lawler, S. D. (1982), Cytogenetics of acute lymphoblastic leukaemia in children as a factor in the prediction of long-term survival. *Br. J. Haematol.* 52, 398–399.

Second International Workshop on Chromosomes in Leukemia (1980), Leuven, Belgium, Oct. 2–6, 1979. *Cancer Genet. Cytogenet.* 2, 89–113.

Shows, T. B., Sakaguchi, A. Y., and Naylor, S. L. (1982), Mapping the human genome, cloned genes, DNA polymorphisms, and inherited disease. *Adv. Hum. Genet.* 12, 341–452.

Slamon, D. J., deKernion, J. B., Verma, I. M., and Cline, M. J. (1984), Expression of cellular oncogenes in human malignancies. *Science* 224, 256–262.

Slater, R. M., Behrendt, H., and De Waal, F. C. (1983), Chromosome studies on acute nonlymphocytic leukaemia in children. *Pediatr. Res.* 17, 398–405.

Smadja, N., Krulik, M., de Gramont, A., Audebert, A. A., and Debray, J. (1985), Translocation 1;7 in de novo preleukemic states. *Cancer Genet. Cytogenet.*, in press.

Standardization in Human Cytogenetics, Paris Conference (1971), 1975 Birth Defects: *Orig. Art. Ser.* XI, 9, The National Foundation, New York.

Sweet, D. L., Golomb, H. M., Rowley, J. D., and Vardiman, J. M. (1979), Acute myelogenous leukemia and thrombocythemia associated with an abnormality of chromosome No. 3. *Cancer Genet. Cytogenet.* 1, 33–37.

Swirsky, D. M., Li, Y. S., Matthews, J. G., Flemans, R. J., Rees, J. K. H., and Hayhoe, F. G. J. (1984), 8;21 translocation in acute granulocytic leukaemia: Cytological, cytochemical and clinical features. *Br. J. Haematol.* 56, 199–213.

Third International Workship on Chromosomes in Leukemia (1981), Lund, Sweden, July 21–25, 1980. *Cancer Genet. Cytogenet.* 45, 95–142.

Ueshima, Y., Fukuhara, S., Hattori, T., Uchiyama, T., Takatsuki, K., and Uchino, H. (1981), Chromosome studies in adult T-cell leukemia in Japan: Significance of trisomy 7. *Blood* 58, 420–425.

Ueshima, Y., Rowley, J., Variakojis, D., Winter, J., and Gordon, L. (1984), Cytogenetic studies on patients with chronic T-cell leukemia/lymphoma. *Blood* 63, 1028–1038.

Varmus, H. E. (1984), The molecular genetics of cellular oncogenes. *Am. Rev. Genet.* 18, 533–612.

Vermaelen, K., Michaux, J. -L., Louwagie, A., and Van den Berghe, H. (1983). Reciprocal translocation t(6;9)(p21;q33): New characteristic chromosome anomaly in myeloid leukemias. *Cancer Genet. Cytogenet.* **10**, 125–131.

Weh, H. J., and Hossfeld, D. K. (1982), Translocation t(4;11) in acute lymphocytic leukemia (ALL). *Blut* **44**, 271–274.

Weinberg, R. A. (1984), *Ras* oncogenes and the molecular mechanisms of carcinogenesis. *Blood* **64**, 1143–1145.

Williams, D. L., Look, A. T., Melvin, S. L., Roberson, P. K., Dahl, G., Flake, T., and Stass, S. (1984), New chromosomal translocations correlate with specific immunophenotypes of childhood acute lymphoblastic leukemia. *Cell* **36**, 101–109.

Williams, D. L., Tsiatis, A., Brodeur, G. M., Look, A. T., Melvin, S. L., Bowman, W. P., Kalwinsky, D. K., Rivera, G., and Dahl, G. V. (1982), Prognostic importance of chromosome number in 136 untreated children with acute lymphoblastic leukemia. *Blood* **60**, 864–871.

Yunis, J. J. (1976), High resolution of human chromosomes. *Science* **191**, 1268–1270.

Yunis, J. J. (1983), The chromosomal basis of human neoplasia. *Science* **221**, 227–236.

Yunis, J. J. (1984), Clinical Significance of High Resolution Chromosomes in the Study of Acute Leukemias and Non-Hodgkin's Lymphomas in *Current Hematology*, Vol. 3, (Fairbanks, V. F., ed.) John Wiley, New York.

Yunis, J. J., Bloomfield, C. D., and Ensrud, B. S. (1981), All patients with acute nonlymphocytic leukemia may have a chromosomal defect. *N. Eng. J. Med.* **305**, 135–139.

Yunis, J. J., Oken, M. M., Kaplan, M. E., Ensrud, K. M., Howe, R. R., and Theologides, A. (1982), Distinctive chromosomal abnormalities in histologic subtypes of non-Hodgkin's lymphoma. *N. Eng. J. Med.* **307**, 1231–1236.

Yunis, J. J., and Soreng, A. L. (1984), Constitutive fragile sites and cancer. *Science* **226**, 1199–1204.

Zech, L., Gahrton, G., Hammarstrom, L., Juliusson, G., Mellstedt, H., Robert, K. -H., and Smith, C. I. E. (1984), Inversion of chromosome 14 marks human T-cell chronic lymphocytic leukaemia. *Nature* **308**, 858–860.

Zech, L., Haglund, U., Nilsson, K., and Klein, G. (1976), Characteristic chromosomal abnormalities in biopsies and lymphoid-cell lines from patients with Burkitt and non-Burkitt lymphomas. *Int. J. Cancer* **17**, 47–56.

Cytogenetics of Solid Tumors

Renal Cell Carcinoma, Malignant Melanoma, Retinoblastoma, and Wilms' Tumor

S. Pathak

1. Introduction

The concept that irregular mitosis and an abnormal genetic constitution in cells play an important role in neoplastic transformation is not a new one. As early as 1890 von Hansemann first observed abnormal mitosis in human carcinomas. Later, a German embryologist named Boveri (1912) proposed his famous hypothesis of malignancy. According to this hypothesis the abnormal distribution of chromatin in a cell is responsible for that cell becoming neoplastic. At that time, even the exact chromosome constitution of normal human cells was not yet known. Boveri's hypothesis of malignancy, as it is called now, has been described by Wolf (1974) as follows: (1) malignant cells can be derived from normal tissue cells; (2) the cause of the abnormal behavior lies within the tumor cell itself and not in its environment; (3) the tumor cell is a defective cell in the sense that it has lost the properties of a normal cell; (4) typically, each tumor cell originates from one cell (monoclonal origin); and (5) the cells of the malignant tumor contain certain abnormal chromatin. Each process that brings about this variable chromatin constitution would result in the origin of a malignant tumor. Boveri's hypothesis could not be tested effectively before 1970 because adequate cytogenetic techniques were not available. Since that time, the development of various cytogenetic techniques has made it possible to accumulate a large amount of data concerning the role(s) of chromosomes in human and animal neoplasms. Cytogenetic data accumulated from various leukemias, lymphomas, and some solid tumors have thrown light on the structural and numerical alternations of chromosomes. The discovery of the Phil-

43

adelphia (Ph1) chromosome in bone marrow cells of patients with chronic granulocytic leukemia (CGL) actually laid the foundation for the specific chromosome anomaly associated with a particular neoplasm (Nowell and Hungerford, 1960).

With the invention of various chromosome banding techniques (Hsu, 1974), rapid progress has been made in the field of cytogenetic oncology. The exact nature of the Ph1 chromosome, a reciprocal translocation between chromosomes 22 and 9, and not a deletion of a chromosome 21, was quickly determined (Rowley, 1973), and other specific chromosome anomalies in leukemias and lymphomas were discovered (Yunis, 1982). The nonrandom chromosome alterations in hematopoietic neoplasms are described in detail in this book by Sandberg. The rapidly growing understanding of the role(s) of viral and cellular oncogenes in the genesis of cell transformation and tumor induction has provided further credence to the study of chromosome alterations in tumorigenesis because such oncogenes are being mapped on specific chromosome segments that are involved in specific alterations (Klein, 1983).

Although a large body of cytogenetic data has been collected for the leukemias and lymphomas with the exception of multiple myelomas, progress in the field of solid tumor cytogenetics has been unsatisfactory and frustrating. The lack of suitable techniques to obtain sufficient high-quality metaphase spreads of solid tumors is the major problem. Even when metaphase plates are present, their chromosomes are highly condensed, have a fuzzy morphology, and are poorly spread. Adding a mitotic arrestant such as Colcemid to increase the number of metaphase spreads only further condenses the chromosomes and induces precocious sister chromatid separation, a condition that is most often seen in tumor chromosomes and is highly unsatisfactory for banding analysis. Another problem in chromosome analysis of solid tumors is that many tumors tend to exhibit highly altered chromosome morphology and chromosome numbers. Many tumors have hyperdiploid ranges of chromosome numbers (close to 100), with a number of highly altered chromosomes whose origin could not be traced even with excellent banded preparations. However, some solid tumors have been reported to have stem line numbers within hypodiploid range. The lowest stem line number of 24 chromosomes has been reported in a malignant melanoma (Atkin and Baker, 1981). In human breast tumors, the lowest chromosome number reported is 35 (Pathak et al., 1979). Since most solid tumor biopsies are obtained from metastatic lesions or effusions, and rarely from the primary tumor, it is not unreasonable to find a wide array of chromosome anomalies.

Recently, some progress has been made in the area of solid tumor cytogenetics, with the bulk of information derived from established long-term cell lines. A number of such cell lines have been established from human tumor biopsies. However, most cell lines from human tumors were established from pleural effusions or other body fluids because biopsies of solid tumors invariably provided cultures of normal fibroblasts.

The cytogenetic information derived from established tumor cell lines may be flawed because chromosome alterations take place frequently in vitro and therefore the chromosome data collected may or may not have the characteristics of the original tumor cells in vivo (Cruciger et al., 1976). For this reason the primary genetic change of a given neoplasm may not be present in permanent cell lines. An alternative procedure is to analyze tumor metaphases suspended in body fluids (pleural and peritoneal effusions) (Ishihara et al., 1963). The body fluid has one advantage; cells are suspended in the fluid and therefore no dissociation of tissues is needed. The only disappointment is that not every body fluid yields ample mitotic spreads for banding analysis. Our experience with breast carcinoma, renal cell carcinoma, and malignant melanoma patients' body fluids has been rewarding to some extent. The chromosome data obtained from renal cell carcinoma patients has been rather useful (Pathak et al., 1982a), and will be described in detail later. However, it should be borne in mind that tumor cells in body fluids are found only in advanced stages of neoplastic development, and, therefore, extensive chromosome changes may have taken place. In spite of this shortcoming, the chromosome characteristics at least represent the in vivo constitution. The primary tumor is the ideal material for studying cancer chromosomes, but adequate techniques for processing such materials remain to be developed.

The purpose of this chapter is to review the inherited constitutional and acquired tumor-specific chromosome alterations in selected human neoplasms, i. e., renal cell carcinoma, malignant melanoma, retinoblastoma, and Wilms' tumor, with a discussion on the role(s) of chromosomes in human cancers.

2. Materials and Procedures

Because cytogenetic analysis requires cells in metaphase, tissue with a high mitotic index is desirable. Bone marrow, body fluids (pleural effusion, ascitic fluid, and so on), some tumors, and lymph nodes may be processed directly (without culture) for metaphase chromosome preparations. On the other hand, peripheral blood samples, skin, and most tumor biopsies must be cultured in vitro to obtain sufficient metaphase spreads. As stated earlier, the direct processing is certainly more representative of in vivo chromosome constitution for neoplastic cells because it provides an instant chromosomal characteristic that contains primary genetic changes. In contrast, the cell culture method can introduce cell selection and chromosome alterations, providing a potentially false chromosomal picture of the in vivo condition.

2.1. Tissue Culture Techniques

Some individuals have a constitutionally abnormal karyotype, i. e., deletion, reciprocal translocations, and mosaicism, that has no obvious phenotypic effects. Such constitutional anomalies exist in tumor cells as well. Some congenital anomalies may be closely related to the neoplastic transformation, e. g., the 13q interstitial deletion in retinoblastoma, 11p interstitial deletion in Wilms' tumor, and so on. However, such deletions apparently have no deleterious effects on tissues other than the retina and kidney, respectively. The chromosome anomalies of neoplasms, therefore, may be either inherited and/or acquired, but in the majority of instances, the genetic alterations occur in the target cells as acquired anomalies. Peripheral lymphocyte culture is an excellent source for the study of congenital chromosome anomalies.

2.1.1. Peripheral Lymphocyte Culture

A 5–10 mL sample of peripheral blood is aseptically drawn in a sodium heparinized syringe or collected directly into a green-top heparin tube. Approximately 5–6 drops of the whole blood is seeded in each culture tube containing 5 mL of RPMI-1640 culture medium supplemented with 15% fetal calf serum, 50 U/mL penicillin, 50 μg/mL streptomycin, and 0.5 mL phytohemagglutinin (from Burroughs Wellcome Co.). Normal lymphocyte cultures are incubated for 72 h at 37°C. Parker-199 and 1a blood culture media are used as well.

2.1.2. Solid Tumor Culture

Most solid tumors do not yield ample metaphases in direct chromosome preparation. Investigators have therefore turned to established cell lines, human tumors grown in nude mice, and, finally, tumors grown following the soft-agar cloning procedure to obtain adequate chromosome preparations.

2.1.2.1. Establishing Cell Lines. A number of permanent cell lines have been established successfully from human tumor biopsies. At the time of initiation in culture, tumor cells start proliferating first. Such cells should be separated from the rest of the cell types to prevent normal fibroblasts quickly taking over the entire culture flask. Some tumor cells have been grown on suitable fibroblast feeder layers.

In our laboratory we sometimes carry out short-term culture of tumor specimens before they are harvested for chromosome preparations. Most tumor biopsies are collected into sterile medium (RPMI-1640 or L-15) containing 15% fetal calf serum, 50 U/mL penicillin, and 50 μg/mL streptomycin. In the tissue culture laboratory the tumor is minced or cut into smaller pieces to obtain a single-cell suspension. For certain tumor types the collagenase technique is used to obtain a single-cell suspension (Kusyk et al., 1979). Some tumors, such as retinoblastoma, break easily into a single-cell suspension without collagenase treatment. The single-cell suspension, as well as the remaining smaller tumor pieces, are washed in sterile medium and then placed into plastic tissue culture flasks containing complete L-15 medium and incubated at 37°C for 24–48 h. Some bottles can then be harvested for chromosome preparations and others used for establishing cell lines.

2.1.2.2. Soft-Agar Cloning Procedure. The soft-agar procedure, originally developed for the bioassay of human tumor stem cells, has been used successfully to directly clone certain human tumor cells (Hamburger et al., 1978). Tumor clones developed by this procedure have yielded some usable metaphases for banding analysis. The tumor biopsy is cleaned, minced with a scalpel, then filtered through sterile gauze to remove larger pieces. The filtered tumor cells are washed in the culture medium. The cell suspension, which may contain normal cells as well as tumor cells, is cultured in a layer of soft-agar and liquid culture medium (Hamburger and Salmon, 1977; Courtenay et al., 1978). Tumor stem cells divide and form colonies in the soft-agar matrix, whereas fibroblasts do not grow under such culture conditions.

2.1.2.3. Growth of Tumors in Nude Mice and Rats. Athymic nude mice and rats have provided an excellent in vivo incubator system for growing human tumors. Retinoblastoma tumor cells have been successfully injected intraocularly or subcutaneously into nude mice and the resultant human tumors have been used for cytogenetic analysis (Gallie et al., 1977, 1982; Gardner et al., 1982). Tumor development depends upon the malignancy of the cells injected, the in vivo incubation period, and the site of inoculation. Once the tumor develops, it can be processed directly or put into tissue culture and then processed for chromosome preparations. In the direct chromosome preparation technique, the metaphases obtained are often of poor quality. Tumors from nude animals may contain host cells transformed by the human tumor (Bowen et al., 1983). Sometimes, metaphases from both host and injected tumor cells coexist in the excised tumor material (Pathak, 1984). In spite of these shortcomings, a number of Burkitt's lymphomas and other human tumors have been grown in nude mice for cytological analyses.

2.2. Harvesting and Chromosome Preparation

Harvesting of cell cultures for chromosome preparation is essentially the same for peripheral blood, body fluids, and cell lines with slight variations of hypotonic treatments.

2.2.1. Peripheral Blood Culture

For routine chromosome analysis, harvest blood cultures after 72 h of incubation at 37°C. Approximately 0.06 μg/mL of Colcemid is added 1 h prior to termination of culture. KCl (0.075M) is used as the hypotonic solution for 20 min at 37°C. The cells are fixed in methanol and acetic acid (3:1 v/v) for 15 min, washed three times in the fixative, and finally air dried on glass slides.

For prophase chromosome morphology, we have adapted the procedure of Rybak et al. (1982).

2.2.2. Body Fluids

Pleural effusions or ascitic fluids obtained from cancer patients are harvested directly for chromosome preparation. Such fluids are not treated with a mitotic arrestant (colchicine or Colcemid) because chromosome morphology becomes too condensed. In some cases excellent results have been obtained (Pathak et al., 1979, 1982a). Sodium citrate (1.0%) is used as a hypotonic solution before fixation.

2.2.3. Solid Tumors

The technique of Rønne (1984) has been adapted for making chromosome preparations from solid tumors. The tumor biopsies are collected in cold medium containing 15% fetal calf serum, heparin, gentamycin (30 μg/mL), and colchicine (0.1 μg/mL). Tumor biopsies are cut into smaller pieces and a fine cell suspension is obtained by aspirating the supernatant, then mincing the larger pieces. After centrifugation, the cell pellet is resuspended in fresh culture medium (L-15), incubated at 37°C for 30 min, followed by 2–3 h at 10–12°C. At the lower temperature, cells are able to enter mitosis, but chromosome contraction is retarded or partly delayed. Cells are centrifuged and suspended in a hypotonic solution (in our experience, 0.95% sodium citrate does a better job than regular $0.075M$ KCl) at 37°C for 25–30 min, and then fixed in freshly prepared fixative (methanol and acetic acid, 3:1 v/v). Fixed cells are washed with fixative and finally air dried on glass slides. Leftover fixed cells can be stored at −20°C for future slide preparations. This harvesting procedure has resulted in fairly elongated chromosome morphology quite suitable for banding analyses.

2.3. Chromosome Banding Techniques

For collecting data on spontaneous chromosome aberrations, stain two slides directly with Giemsa (5.0% in $0.01M$ phosphate buffer, pH 7.0). The Q-, G-, C-, and Ag-NOR techniques are used on all samples (Pathak, 1979). One most likely obtains more information by applying a battery of banding techniques than by using just one. Details of these techniques have been published (Pathak, 1976).

3. Renal Cell Carcinoma (RCC)

3.1. General Description

Renal cell carcinoma, which accounts for 2–3% of all malignant tumors, is the cause of approximately 6000 deaths each year in the United States (Cutler and Young, 1975). Close to 30 family aggregates of RCC have been described in the literature, but cytogenetic data in several instances are fragmentary. Renal cell carcinoma may be present in unilateral or bilateral conditions in both familial or hereditary forms. Familial renal cell carcinoma may be caused by genetic factors or exposure to carcinogens among relatives. Environmental studies have demonstrated an association between exposure to Thorotrast, phenacetin, and certain other organic compounds, and the occurrence of renal pelvis carcinomas (Poole-Wilson, 1959; Rathert et al., 1975; Griffiths et al., 1977). Renal cell cancers in general show a median age of 60 yr at diagnosis, but familial RCC has been diagnosed at fairly young ages in some patients (Li et al., 1982). Although the familial Von Hippel-Lindau disease has been associated with the development of RCC, many families with RCC do not carry such genetic defects (Horton et al., 1976). In many families, the susceptibility to develop renal cell carcinoma is dominantly transmitted.

3.2. Chromosome Anomalies in RCC

The first constitutional chromosome translocation involving chromosomes 3 and 8 in the peripheral blood cultures of hereditary RCC patients was reported by Cohen and associates (1979). In this family there were 10 members with a balanced reciprocal translocation between chromosomes 3 and 8. The other 12 non-symptomatic members had normal karyotypes. Not a single family member showed an unbalanced translocation. The reciprocal translocation was present in the five survivors of RCC—one with renal cysts and four other nonsymptomatic members of the family. The balanced translocation was also present in the skin fibroblasts of four patients who had a similar translocation in their peripheral blood cultures. These authors assigned the break points to bands 8q24 and 3p21, respectively, by analyzing metaphase chromosomes. By using high-resolution prophase Giemsa-banding (G-banding), it was demonstrated that the break points occurred at the subbands 3p14.2 (instead of 3p21) and 8q24.1 (Fig. 1) in one male and two female translocation carriers from the same family (Wang and Perkins, 1984). In order to better understand the etiologic importance of either chromosome 3 or 8 in this neoplasm, additional chromosome analysis of both renal tumor cells and peripheral blood cultures should be performed.

Recently, Pathak et al. (1982a) reported a case of familial renal cell carcinoma and identified a translocation involving chromosomes 3 and 11 in tumor cells processed directly from a patient. The lymphocyte cultures of the patient and other relatives of his family were considered normal by G-banding. The break point in the 3p segment observed in the tumor cells was in the p13–14 region. The familial nature of RCC for over three generations in

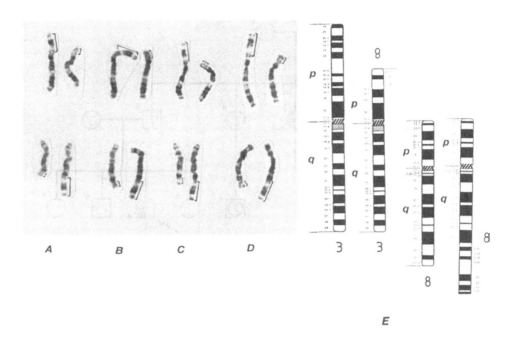

Fig. 1. G-banded partial karyotype (A–D) and ideogram (E) of chromosomes 3 and 8 from the peripheral blood cultures of an RCC patient. The left side of each pair shows a normal no. 3 and 8 chromosome; the right side shows the translocation (from Wang and Perkins, 1984, courtesy of Elsevier Science Publishing).

this family was confirmed through medical records and death certificates (Fig. 2). The majority of metaphases (30) showed a stem-line number of 54 chromosomes. However, a minor peak (eight cells only) had a stem-line number of 52 chromosomes. Thirty G-banded metaphases analyzed showed a number of marker chromosomes. A typical G-banded karyotype of this tumor is shown in Fig. 3. Twenty-two (73.3%) of the metaphases contained a translocation involving 3p and the entire chromosome 11; the remaining metaphases had normal chromosomes 3 and 11. Four marker chromosomes (M1–M4) were identified in the majority of metaphases: M1, the long arm of the altered chromosome 3; M2, the entire chromosome 11 with a translocation in its short arm of 3p; M3, the largest acrocentric involving the entire chromosome 14 and the distal segment of 2q; and M4, a small metacentric, probably an isochromosome of 5p. A diagrammatic explanation of the formation of M1 and M2 chromosomes is shown in Fig. 4. Pathak et al. (1982a) emphasized that the alteration in chromosome 3 could

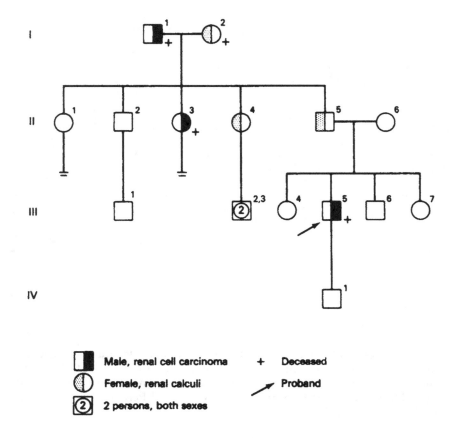

Fig. 2. Pedigree of the RCC family members by their clinical phenotypes (from Pathak et al., 1982a, Country of *Science*).

be specifically associated with renal cell tumor development. This hypothesis could be further supported by observations made on established RCC lines (Table 1). In a human renal carcinoma cell line, Sytkowski et al. (1983) reported a modal chromosome number of 45, XX constitution, and abnormalities in chromosomes 3, 9, and 17. A marker chromosome involving the short arm of no. 3 and 17 was present in this line. Normal chromosomes 3 and 17 were each present in single copy. Further chromosome analyses of eight cell lines and seven fresh RCC tumor samples have also indicated alterations in the short arm of chromosome 3 (Wang et al., 1983). The first detailed analysis of banded chromosomes of an established RCC line from a primary tumor and its lymph node metas-

Table 1
Renal Cell Carcinoma Lines Studied by Banding Techniques

Number of tumors	Presence (+) or absence (−) of chromosome 3 anomaly	Reference
3	+	Hagemeijer et al., 1979
1[a]	−	Matsuda et al., 1979
1	+	Pathak et al., 1982a
1	+	Sytkowski et al., 1983
8	+	Wang et al., 1983

[a] No demonstrable marker chromosome.

tasis showed abnormalities in chromosomes 1, 3, 4, 5, 8, 9, and 17 (Hagemeijer et al., 1979). Their marker M9 was identified as the isochromosome for 3p, and M8 as the isochromosome for 8q. Here again chromosome 3 was involved in alteration, but the breakpoint was not in the short arm.

Cytogenetic analysis of most renal cell carcinoma patients has shown normal chromosome constitutions in their peripheral blood cultures. Since 1979 a total of 138 patients with renal cell tumor have been studied cytogenetically for constitutional anomalies. Only seven individuals (5.0%) have shown some anomaly. None of them possessed an abnormality involving chromosome 3 (Li et al., 1982; Kantor et al., 1982; Asal et al., 1983). In a recent chromosome survey of two unrelated RCC families, however, mosaicism was found in the peripheral blood cultures of two unrelated patients. Two brothers in one family were diagnosed as having RCC. The peripheral blood culture of one of the patients showed metaphases (2.0%) with multiple translocations involving chromosomes 1, 3, 9, 11, and 16. A specific translocation involving chromosomes 3 and 16 showed breaks in the 3p13 and 16p13 regions (Fig. 5). The long arm of the translocated no. 3 with a distinct short arm was retained in the cell. Whether this proband shows genetic instability is presently being addressed. In another family with a similar incidence of renal cell cancer, the proband (whose tumor was not available for analysis) showed a translocation involving chromosomes 3p and 6q in 2.0% metaphase of peripheral blood cultures. Thus, the evidence to support that a break in chromosome 3p might be responsible for renal carcinogenesis is accumulating. Fibroblast cultures and peripheral blood cultures from these patients and their nonsymptomatic family members are under investigation.

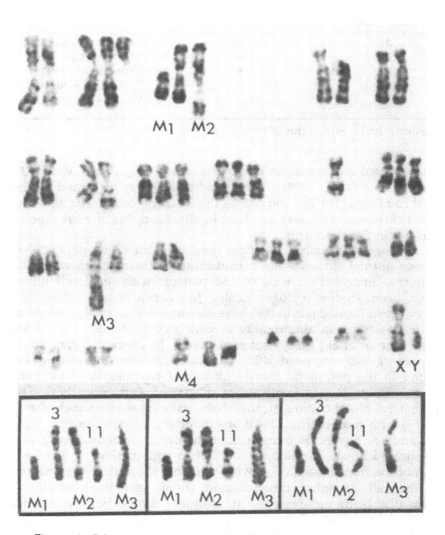

Fig. 3. A G-banded karyotype of a metaphase cell processed directly from an ascitic fluid of RCC patient (BF-22). Four identified marker chromosomes (M1–M4) and two unidentifiable altered chromosomes are shown. Markers M1, M2, M3, and normal chromosomes 3 and 11 from three additional tumor cells are also shown (inset) (from Pathak et al., 1982a, Courtesy of *Science*).

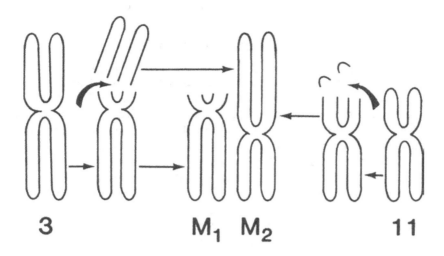

Fig. 4. A diagrammatic representation of chromosomes 3 and 11 and the formation of M1 and M2 markers. A break in the proximal region of 3p and in the extreme distal end of 11p is marked by thick, curved arrows. M1 represents the long arm of chromosome 3, plus the centromere of chromosome 3 with a small piece of 3p. M2 comprises almost the entire chromosome 11 with a translocation of the 3p to its short arm (from Pathak et al., 1982a, Courtesy of *Science*).

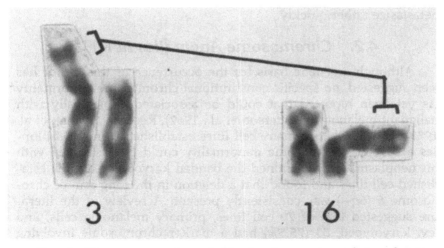

Fig. 5. Chromosomes 3 and 16 showing reciprocal translocation involving their short arms in the peripheral blood culture of a proband with RCC.

4. Malignant Melanoma (MM)

4.1. General Description

According to a report published in 1983 by the American Cancer Society, the most serious skin cancer, malignant melanoma, strikes about 17,000 US men and women annually. The state of Alabama has the highest per capita death rate from melanoma in the US; New South Wales and Queensland in Australia have the highest reported incidence of melanoma in the world (Little et al., 1980, McCarthy et al., 1980). According to a recent report by Balch et al. (1983) on the changing trends in cutaneous melanoma over a quarter century in Alabama, USA and New South Wales, Australia, there was a significant increase in melanomas located on the trunk in men and a corresponding decrease in male head and neck melanomas. On the other hand, they did not find any significant change in the site of melanoma distribution in female patients. Many etiologic factors, such as excessive exposure to the sun and occupational exposure to pitch, creosote, coal tar, radium, and arsenic compounds have been implicated in the development of malignant melanoma in the white population. The incidence of skin cancer in the black population is negligible probably because of heavy skin pigmentation. Melanomas are usually identified by a brown to dark or black pigmentation on a localized area. Initially, they are small, mole-like growths that increase in size, change color rapidly, become ulcerated, and bleed easily. Malignant melanomas metastasize rather quickly.

4.2. Chromosome Anomalies in MM

Although a genetic basis for the occurrence of this tumor has been suggested, no specific constitutional chromosome abnormality has yet been reported that could be associated etiologically with malignant melanoma (Anderson et al., 1967). Recently, Pathak et al. (1983) reported that in many cell lines established from MM biopsies a specific chromosome abnormality could be associated with this neoplasm. They examined the banded karyotypes of nine established cell lines and found that a deletion in the long arm of chromosome 6 (6q−) was consistently present. A review of the literature suggested that of 70 cell lines, primary melanoma cells, and nevi karyotyped, 53 (75.5%) had a marker chromosome involving chromosome 6 (Table 2). The break point observed in the long arm of chromosome 6 was variable in different samples. A typical G-banded karyotype of an MM cell line (TCH #3120) is shown in

Fig. 6, in which the altered chromosomes of this metaphase plate and similar markers from another metaphase of the same tumor line are shown in the two bottom rows, respectively. Marker 3 (m3) showed a deletion in the long arm. Because of the polyploidization of the cell line, two normal-looking chromosome 6's are present in this cell. As mentioned earlier, the break points in the long arms of one chromsome 6 were not the same in all cell lines analyzed (Fig. 7). In some cases the break point was in the centromeric region retaining only the short arm of chromosome 6. A diagrammatic sketch shown in Fig. 8 explains the variable modes of alterations in chromosome 6 observed in these MM cell lines.

Based on these observations, the following hypothesis was proposed by Pathak et al. (1983): The melanoma gene, the gene or genes responsible for the normal development and function of melanocytes, is located in the distal segment of 6q. An interstitial deletion of 6q including this gene would reduce the over all length of this chromosome (Fig. 8A). This interstitial deletion, like the 13q interstitial deletion of retinoblastoma and 11p interstitial deletion of Wilms' tumor, would create a partial monosomy for this segment. If a terminal segment of one 6q is deleted (Fig. 8B) a similar haploid condition occurs. The chromosome may be a true 6q— or another chromosome segment may be translocated onto it to form a marker such as t(6q—;?). If the break point is in the centromeric region, the entire q arm may be lost (Fig. 8C), and an i(6p) or a translocation between 6p and another chromosome segment such as t(1q;6p) may result. Therefore, marker chromosomes with an obvious 6p represent the deletion of the distal segment of 6q that could be etiologically associated with MM.

Recent analyses of freshly processed MM biopsies without a long-term culture have also demonstrated a deletion in the long arm of a chromosome 6 (Fig. 9). A similar case involving a metastatic lesion of MM processed directly for chromosome analysis showed a marker chromosome (m5) involving a translocation of 6p (Atkin and Baker, 1981). These preliminary results indicate that 6q deletion is not caused by in vitro conditions, but is also present in the MM patient.

Recent observations by Balaban et al. (1984) have indicated that in MM other chromosomes, such as no. 1 and 7, in addition to no. 6, may be consistently altered not only in cultured tumors but also in direct preparations. Abnormalities of chromosome 1 and 7 have already been reported in MM cell lines (Kakati et al., 1977; Semple et al., 1982). Determining whether the chromosome 6q deletion or alterations in chromosomes 1 and 7 are etiologically

Table 2
Human Melanomas Showing Involvement of Chromosome 6[a]

Samples	Marker chromosomes[b]	Authors	Pathak (this review)	Reference
			Interpretation of origin	
None	−1			Chen and Shaw (1973)
C9	M5	20q+	t(20q;6p)	Chen and Shaw (1974)
MEL-41	A2	6pi	6q−	Fraccaro et al. (1976)
M-1	12p+	12p+	t(12p;6p)	McCulloh et al. (1976)
M-2	−1			
M-3	6	6	6q−	
M-4	−1			
M-5	6	6	6q−	
M-6	−1			
M-7	1p+	1p+	t(1p;6p)	
73-61	−1			
Case 1	M9	i(17q)	t(5p;6p)	Kakati et al. (1977)
Case 2	Left 6	Normal 6	t(6q−;+?)	
Case 3	M6	17q+del 7	6q−	
Case 4	Second 6	Normal 6	6q−	
RPMI 8252	M3	6q−	6q−	Quinn et al. (1977)
RPMI 7932	M2	6q−	6q−	
COLO 38	M2	t(9q;3p)	t(9q;6p)	
COLO 53	m1	1p−	t(1q;6p)	
COLO 103	−1			
MM 96-1	m3	i(6p)	t(18q;6p)	Muir and Gunz (1979)
MM 96-2	m3	i(6p)	t(18q;6p)	
MM 138	m4	6q−	6q−	
MM 170	−1			
MM 200	−2			
MM 214	m1	t(1q;6p)	t(1q;6p)	
MM 229	−1			
MM253	m2	t(5p;6p)	t(5p;6p)	
None	M5	t(7q;6p)	t(7q;6p)	Atkin and Baker (1981)
COLO 297	M4	t(4q;6p)	t(4q;6p)	Semple et al. (1982)
COLO 298	First m	None	t(1q;6p)	
COLO 324	M2	6q−	6q−	
COLO 349	M6	17p−	6q−	
COLO 381	Third m	None	i(6p)	
COLO 415	M1	i(6p)	i(6p)	
COLO 437	Second 6	Normal 6	t(6q-;+?)	
Case 1	6q−	6q−	6q−	Becher et al. (1983)
Case 2	i(6p)	i(6p)	i(6p)	
Case 3	t(6p;7q)	t(6p;7q)	t(6p;7q)	

(continued)

Table 2 (*continued*)
Human Melanomas Showing Involvement of Chromosome 6[a]

Samples	Marker chromosomes[b]	Interpretation of origin		Reference
		Authors	Pathak (this review)	
RL	t(3p;6q)	t(3p;6q)	t(3p;6q)	Trent et al. (1983)
RW	t(6q;?)	t(6q;?)	t(6q;?)	
MH	t(1q;6q)	t(1q;6q)	t(1q;6q)	
TCH 3116	a	—	t(6q-;?)	Pathak et al. (1983)
TCH 3120	b	—	6q—	
TCH 3118	c	—	6q—	
TCH 3119	d	—	t(1q;6p)	
TCH 3115	e	—	t(6q-;?)	
TCH 3114	f	—	t(6q-;?)	
TCH 3636	g	—	t(6q-;?)	
TCH 3635	h	—	t(6q-;?)	
TCH 3121	i	—	6q—	
WM 245		t(6p;22q)	t(6p;22q)	Balaban et al. (1984)
WM 115		6p—	6p—	
WM 9		6q—	6q—	
WM 28	—1			
WM 46		—6	—6	
WM 47		6q—	6q—	
WM 230	—1			
WM 262		i(6p)	i(6p)	
CCM2B		i(6p)	i(6p)	
SK-MEL-23		6q+	t(6q-;?)	
SK-MEL-37	—1			
SW 691		t(6q;?)	t(6q-;?)	
ML 817	—1			
WM 229	—1			
WM 170	—1			
WM 293	—1			
WM 305	—1			
BF-26		—	6q—	This report

[a] Updated from Pathak et al., 1983.
[b] —1 = A marker chromosome containing 6p or 6q— was not identified because either an incomplete karyotype was presented or the sample lacked such a marker. —2 = Markers m2, m6, and m10 of this cell line are similar to HeLa markers 1, 2, and 4, respectively. —6 = An entire chromosome 6 was missing.

associated with the neoplastic transformation or merely associated with growth and invasiveness of MM will depend on future research on much larger samples of MM.

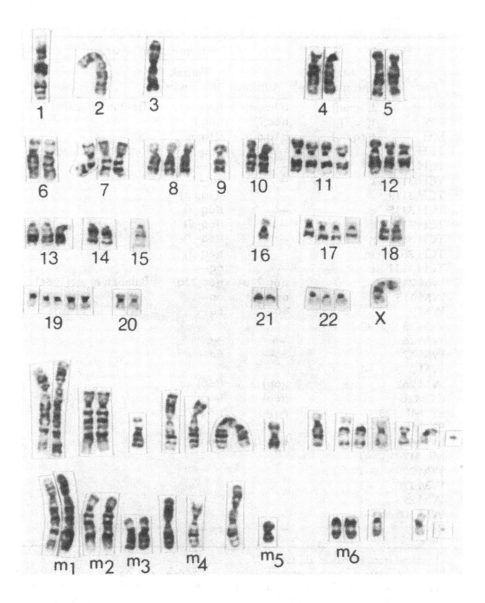

Fig. 6. Karyotype of a G-banded metaphase of a malanoma cell line 3120. The altered chromosomes of this cell and similar altered chromosomes of another cell of the same line are shown on the bottom two rows, respectively. Note the deleted chromosome no. 6 (m3).

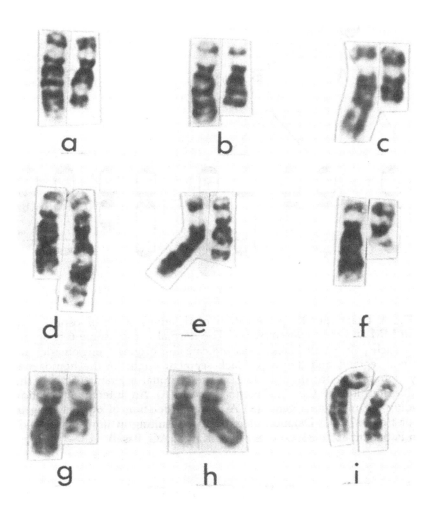

Fig. 7. A G-banded normal chromosome 6 (left) and the marker chromosomes involving the 6 (right) from 9 MM cell lines: (a) 3116, (b) 3120, (c) 3118, (d) 3119, (e) 3115, (f) 3114, (g) 3636, (h) 3635, (i) 3121. All marker chromosomes contain the piece of a chromosome 6 (6p or 6q−) with or without a translocation of a segment of another chromosome (from Pathak et al., 1983, courtesy of S. Karger AG, Basel).

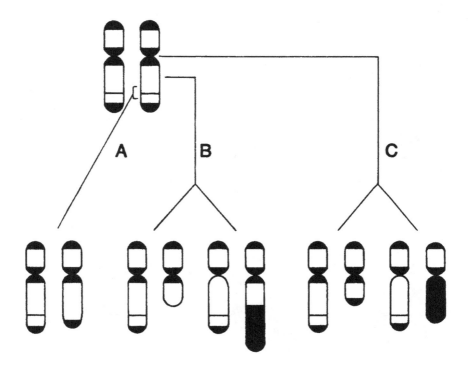

Fig. 8. Diagrammatic presentation of deletions of chromosome 6 in human MM and their consequences. The normal chromosome 6 is on the left in each pair; small black areas indicate the original centromeric and telomeric regions, and the large black segment might be the homogeneously staining region; the thin line in the terminal segment of 6q is the putative location of the "melanoma gene." (A) An interstitial deletion including the melanoma gene; (B) A terminal deletion of 6q, resulting in 6q− or t(q−;+?); (C) Deletion of entire 6q, resulting in i(6p) or t(6p;+?) (from Pathak et al., 1983, courtesy of S. Karger AG, Basel).

5. Retinoblastoma (RB)

5.1. General Description

Retinoblastoma, a childhood tumor of neuroectodermal origin, is the most common intraocular malignancy of infancy. It generally presents in children between 2 and 3 yr of age. Its frequency is approximately 1/20,000 live births, with 95% sporadic and 5% familial cases. The hereditary form of retinoblastoma, present in some

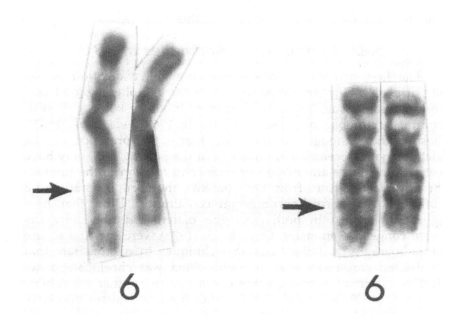

Fig. 9. Two pairs of G-banded chromosome 6 from BF-26 (human MM) processed directly for chromosome preparation. Note the normal morphology of chromosome 6 arranged on left. Chromosome 6 on the right is much smaller and shows an interstitial deletion in the distal segment of the long arm region 6q 22–26 (arrows).

40% of cases, appears to be caused by an autosomal dominant mutation with very high penetrance. The majority of the hereditary forms (68%) are bilateral, whereas 32% are unilateral. Most recently, "trilateral (pineal tumor) retinoblastoma" has also been reported in at least 13 cases (Bader et al., 1980, 1982) in which all patients had bilateral RB. Most nonhereditary forms of RB are unilateral and tend to have higher median ages at diagnosis than do the familial and bilateral cases. Both unilateral and bilateral cases (approximately 1–3% of the total cases) may be associated with a constitutional deletion of chromosome 13.

According to the hypothesis proposed by Knudson (1971), both inherited and noninherited RB are caused by two mutational steps. Individuals with inherited first mutation (germ cell) will require a second mutation (somatic) in the target organ to develop retinoblastoma. If no germ cell mutation was inherited, then two somatic mutational events in a single cell are required for the development of retinoblastoma. So far, the data collected for unilateral and bilateral cases have supported this hypothesis.

5.2. Chromosome Anomalies in RB

The first structural chromosome anomaly, a deletion in the long arm of a D-group chromosome in the peripheral blood culture, dermal tissue, and the tumor cells of a baby girl with confirmed retinoblastoma, was reported in 1963 (Lele et al., 1963). These authors thought at the time that, "the presence of the deleted large acrocentric chromosome in the patient, E.P., may have been a coincidence and of no significance in relation to the tumor." The fibroblast cultures from both parents, the normal sister, and a brother showed normal chromosome constitution. Other than having retinoblastoma in both eyes, the patient did not show any severe congenital anomaly. Orye et al. (1971) were the first to use autoradiography and the banding techniques to demonstrate that the deleted chromosome in retinoblastoma was chromosome no. 13. This observation was quickly confirmed in another retinoblastoma patient (Wilson et al., 1973). Since then several reviews have been published demonstrating retinoblastoma patients with constitutional 13q deletions (Vogel, 1979; Johnson et al., 1982; Francke, 1983; Matsunaga, 1983). A total of approximately 72 patients with interstitial deletion of 13q have been reported, of which 26 (40%) have unilateral and 39 (60%) have bilateral retinoblastoma. Six of the cases were reported in an abstract where detailed information was not available (Turleau et al., 1983). Most of these patients presented with a clinical history of short stature, minor dysmorphic features, and different degrees of mental retardation. The deleted segment differs in length in different patients, but they all involve a part of 13q14. According to Yunis and Ramsay (1978), patients with larger interstitial deletion showed more severe mental retardation and phenotypic anomalies than those with a subband deletion of 13q14. Since most patients with a deletion of 13q14 had this neoplasm, development of retinoblastoma may be closely related with the deletion of this segment.

The deletion of 13q14 may be achieved by different mechanisms that can lead to the neoplastic initiation of RB: (1) in the nonhereditary form, the deletion could originate *de novo* in the prezygotic stage (Francke, 1976; Francke and Kung, 1976; Turleau et al., 1983) or could occur as a postzygotic event leading to mosaicism (Motegi, 1981, 1982). A G-banded karyotype of a *de novo* 13q14 deletion RB patient is shown in Fig. 10; (2) in hereditary forms, one of the unaffected parents with balanced translocation,

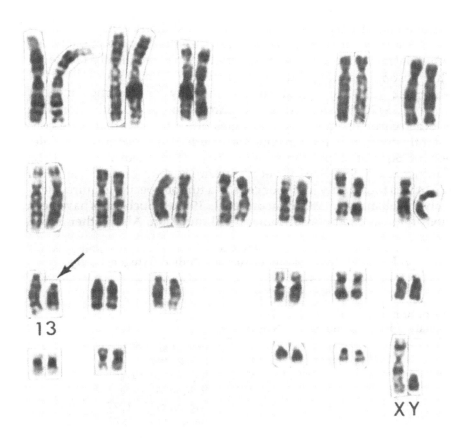

Fig. 10. A G-banded peripheral blood karyotype of a retinoblastoma patient showing deletion in one of the no. 13 chromosomes (arrow). All other chromosomes, including the sex elements, are normal.

involving chromosome 13q14 and any other chromosome, might transmit the deleted 13 to offspring by way of malsegregation in meiosis (Nöel et al., 1976; Hoegerman, 1979; Sparkes et al., 1979; Riccardi et al., 1979; Rivera et al., 1981; Strong et al., 1981; Michalova et al., 1982; Junien et al., 1982; Turleau et al., 1983). Figure 11 represents the partial karyotype of a parent showing insertional-type balanced translocation between chromosomes 13q and 12p. An unbalanced child of this carrier had deletion of 13q 12.3 to 22.1 and bilateral retinoblastoma (Riccardi et al., 1979); (3) *de novo* translocations leading to the inactivation of 13q14 segment (Cross et al., 1977; Davidson et al., 1979; Nichols et al., 1980; Hida et al., 1980; Hata et al., 1982; Motegi et al., 1982; Turleau et al., 1983). Spreading of inactivation in the translocated 13q segment and the inactivation of the esterase-D locus, mapped to the chromosome 13q14 band, have been reported (Mohandas et al., 1982).

A survey of the literature reveals that approximately 91 retinoblastoma tumors have been studied cytogenetically (Table 3). Chromosome banding data were available from 75 cell lines, of which 22 (29.33%) contained an anomaly of chromosome 13, whereas 53 (70.9%) showed normal chromosomes 13, with anomalies of other chromosomes. Chromosomes other than 13 that were consistently involved in rearrangements include 1p+, trisomy of 1q, deletion of 6q− or i(6p), 13q+, and 17q+ (Kusnetsova et al., 1982; Gardner et al., 1982; Benedict et al., 1983a). In some cases a deletion of 13q14 was found only in tumor cells as a tumor-specific acquired anomaly (Balaban et al., 1982; Benedict et al., 1983a). Such cases have been interpreted as examples of somatic cell mutation. Also, either a total

Table 3
A List of 91 Retinoblastoma Tumors Studied Cytogenetically

| No. of tumors analyzed | No. of tumors | | Reference |
	With 13 anomaly	Without 13 anomaly	
1	1	—	Lele et al., 1963
1[a]	?	?	Mark, 1970
1	—	1	Inoue et l., 1974
1[a]	?	?	Reid et al., 1974
1	1	—	McFall et al., 1977
2	—	2	Seeger et al., 1977
1	1	—	Hossfeld, 1978
1	1	—	Balaban-Malenbaum et al., 1981
1	1	—	Gilbert et al., 1981
4	—	4	Phillips et al., 1981
6	5	1	Balaban et al., 1982
10	2	8	Gardner et al., 1982
9	—	9	Kusnetsova et al., 1982
15	6	9	Benedict et al., 1983a
1	1	—	Benedict et al., 1983b
14[a]	?	?	Bogenmann and Mark, 1983
1	1	—	Cavenee et al., 1983
5	—	5	Godbout et al.,, 1983a
1	—	1	Godbout et al., 1983b
13	2	11	Chaum et al, 1983

[a] Banding data was not available.

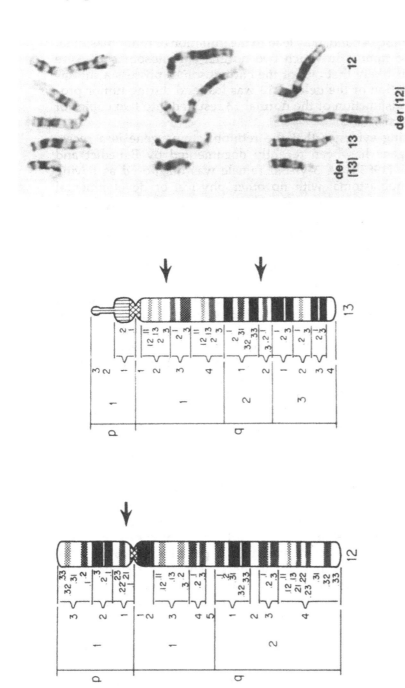

Fig. 11. Partial karyotypes and the ideogram of a parent showing an insertional type translocation involving chromosomes 12p and 13q. In the karyotypes the derivative 13 (der 13) and the normal 13 have been arranged upside down to facilitate comparison with the inserted segment in the derivative 12 (der 12). The breakpoints have been renumbered according to ISCN (1981) (from Francke, 1983, courtesy of Academic Press).

loss of one chromosome 13 or a deletion in one chromosome 13, including the 13q14 band, may lead to the initiation of retinoblastoma. Even in those tumors in which two normal chromosomes 13 were observed, it is likely that one of the chromosomes possess a submicroscopic deletion or the deleted 13 was lost and during tumor progression nondisjunction of the normal 13 resulted into two copies of this chromosome.

Convincing evidence that the retinoblastoma gene is a recessive cancer gene has been recently documented by Benedict and his associates (1983b). A 3-yr-old female was diagnosed as having bilateral retinoblastoma, with no other physical or developmental anomalies previously described with the 13q14 deletion syndrome (Yunis and Ramsay, 1978). The patient had a 50% esterase-D activity in her fibroblasts and peripheral lymphocytes. Both parents had normal activity of esterase-D. The lymphocyte cultures of the parents and proband showed no deletion of 13q14. Because all previously studied patients with RB and a 50% esterase-D activity in their normal tissues had a deletion of 13q14, it was interpreted that in this girl the loss of esterase-D activity was caused by a submicroscopic deletion that included the retinoblastoma and esterase-D gene. Two distinct tumor lines (LA-RB69A and LA-RB69B), established from one eye of this patient, had both lost a chromosome 13. The esterase-D activity in the tumor cells was totally absent. Based on these observations it was concluded that the normal nondeleted chromosome 13 had been lost in each tumor cell line, and the only 13 present in the tumor cells had deletion of both the RB and esterase-D genes. This observation further supports the idea that the retinoblastoma gene is a recessive cancer gene (Benedict et al., 1983b; Cavenee et al., 1983).

Evidence thus far accumulated has also shown that individuals with genetic predisposition to retinoblastoma have a much greater risk for the development of other tumors in the later part of their lives. Occurrence of osteosarcomas, soft tissue sarcomas, and skin carcinomas has been documented in RB patients 10–15 yr after their treatments (Jensen and Miller, 1971). The cancer could occur in the previously irradiated area or often in unirradiated parts of the body. Another tumor, pineoblastoma (tumor of the pineal gland), has been reported in 13 cases of retinoblastoma (Bader et al., 1980, 1982). The incidence of nonradiogenic primary neoplasms in RB survivors is also high (Strong and Knudson, 1973; Kitchin and Ellsworth, 1974), suggesting that the retinoblastoma mutation may act as an "initiator" or has pleiotropic effects (Kitchin and Ellsworth, 1974).

6. Wilms' Tumor (WT)

6.1. General Description

Wilms' tumor (nephroblastoma) is the most common abdominal solid tumor of childhood. The association of WT with other congenital defects, including aniridia, hemihypertrophy, pigmented nevi, genitourinary anomalies, and mental retardation, was first reported by Miller et al. (1964). Epidemiologic studies have indicated that at least one of every 10,000 live births may be expected to develop a malignant kidney tumor by age 15, the most common of which is nephroblastoma. Wilms' tumor occurs in both familial and sporadic forms, and can be unilateral or bilateral. Wilms' tumor occurs at a 1:3 frequency in children with no iris or incomplete development of the ocular iris—a condition called aniridia. It has been suggested that nodular renal blastema, which is found in approximately one-third of patients with WT (Machin, 1980), serves as a precursor lesion in individuals who carry the "Wilms' tumor gene" (Bove and McAdams, 1976).

Knudson and Strong (1972) suggested a hypothetical model for WT development. According to this model, two mutations are required in all cases. They postulated that a hereditary form, present in approximately 38% of cases, has one mutation in the germinal cell of one of the parents. Children born with this germinal mutation develop a second mutation in the somatic cells of the target organ, which ultimately gives rise to WT. The bulk of these children with such a mutation have unilateral tumors (79%), whereas the remaining 21% have bilateral multifocal Wilms' tumor. Only 5% of the sporadic cases of WT are bilateral, and these may be caused by new mutations of the autosomal dominant form. The median age of diagnosis is between 2 and 3.8 yr in most familial cases. Wilms' tumor, if detected very early, can be cured with surgery or chemotherapy.

6.2. Chromosome Anomalies in WT

Although the first report of a boy with mental retardation, aniridia-Wilms' tumor, and a complex translocation between chromosomes 8 and 11 was made by Ladda et al. (1974), they failed to identify the association of aniridia-Wilms' tumor with a specific chromosome anomaly in chromosome 11. Riccardi et al. (1978) were the first to demonstrate a constitutional interstitial deletion in the short arm of a chromosome 11 (11p13) and its association with aniridia-Wilms' tumor syndrome (AWTS) in three unrelated children. Three patients (two white boys and a Mexican-American girl, all with a 46, XY chromosome constitution) who presented with mental retardation, genitourinary anomalies, and aniridia were studied, but only one of them had Wilms' tumor. The peripheral blood cultures of all of them showed interstitial deletion in the 11p arm that had different break points but loss of a partially overlapping region (11p13). Cotlier et al. (1978) reported a pair of twins, but only one had aniridia-Wilms' tumor and the other did not. A gene coding for catalase (CAT) has been mapped on the 11p13 locus (Junien et al., 1980). One of the patients studied by Francke et al. (1977), whose deletion extended into 11p12 region, showed lactate dehydrogenase A (LDHA) deficiency. It therefore appears that CAT and LDHA are linked together in the same region of 11p that shows deletion in AWTS. Since then more than 27 cases have been reported with aniridia and a deletion involving variable regions of 11p; all cases demonstrated a deletion of the distal half of band 11p13. A recent review on aniridia-Wilms' tumor patients has been presented by Francke (1983). Figure 12 demonstrates constitutional deletions in the 11p arms from three patients with aniridia, but only patient B has WT.

Many patients with aniridia-Wilms' tumor syndrome (AWTS) have demonstrated *de novo* deletion in 11p13. There are, however, some cases reported in which a deleted chromosome 11 was inherited from a balanced translocation carrier parent, such as a t(8;11) translocation (Gödde-Salz and Behnke, 1981), a balanced rearrangement within chromosome 11 (Hittner et al., 1979), an insertion of a small region of 11p into a chromosome 2 (Yunis and Ramsay, 1980), and a complex rearrangement between chromosomes 8 and 11 in a patient showing a deletion of 11p (Francke et al., 1979).

Most of the cytogenetic data reported from WT patients are from the peripheral blood cultures, as summarized recently (Gilgendrantz et al., 1982). Only a limited number of Wilms' tumors *per se* have been analyzed cytogenetically. The first report of a deleted 11p in the Wilms' tumor cells of a patient who did not show aniridia and a constitutional 11p deletion in her peripheral blood and the fibroblast cultures was made by Kaneko et al. (1981). As shown in Table 4, 15 (65.1%) out of 23 Wilms' tumors analyzed showed deletion in the short arm of a chromosome 11. A single case studied was rather unusual. This female patient had a normal chromosome constitution, 46, XX, in her repeat peripheral blood cultures. Her Wilms' tumor showed a 46, XX chromosome constitution in the majority of metaphases. Chromosome 11 was present in single copy. A small ring chromosome (11q?), partial trisomy of

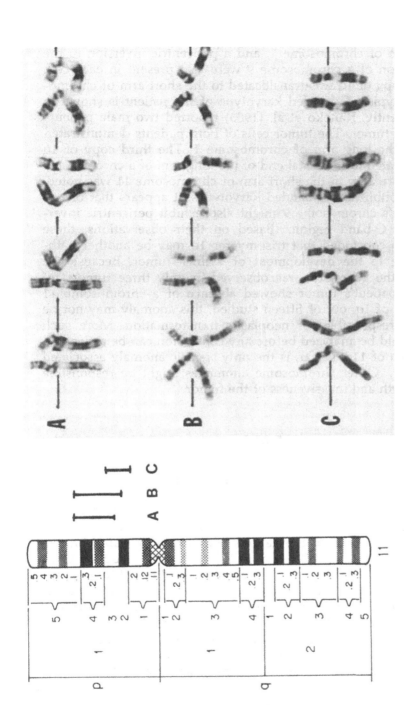

Fig. 12. Four pairs of G-banded chromosome 11 and the ideogram from 3 male patients A, B, and C who had aniridia, genitourinary anomalies, and mental retardation. Only patient B had Wilms' tumor. The right homologues of each pair of chromosomes 11 have the deletion in the short arm. Note the extents of the three different deletions sharing a common band 11p13 (from Francke, 1983, courtesy of Academic Press).

the long arm of chromosome 1, and a pericentric inversion in the C-band region of a chromosome 9 were also present in each cell. The third copy of 1q was translocated to the short arm of chromosome 1. A typical G-banded karyotype of the patient is shown in Fig. 13. Recently, Kaneko et al. (1983) reported two male patients with Wilms' tumor. The tumor cells of both patients demonstrated trisomy of the long arm of chromosome 1. The third copy of 1q was translocated to the distal end of the long arm of a chromosome 16. No abnormality in the short arm of chromosome 11 was noted. From their published Q-banded karyotypes, it appears that one of their patient's chromosome 9 might also exhibit pericentric inversion in the C-band region. Based on their observations, these investigators concluded that trisomy for 1q may be another pathway leading to the development of Wilms' tumor. Because the trisomy of the 1q region was observed in only three tumors, of which our patient's tumor showed absence of a chromosome 11 and trisomy of 1q, out of fifteen studied, this anomaly may not be considered responsible for neoplastic transformation. More such tumors should be analyzed before any conclusion can be arrived at. The deletion of 11p, so far, is the only specific anomaly associated with AWTS. Other chromosome anomalies might be responsible for the growth and invasiveness of the tumor.

7. Discussion

7.1. General Discussion

The study of chromosome anomalies in cancer has become a very exciting field of medicine. This is largely because of the discovery of remarkable correlations between: (1) specific chromosomal rearrangements observed in many human neoplasms; (2) demonstration of "fragile site(s)" on most of these chromosomes; and (3) locations of cellular oncogenes (c-*onc*) on such chromosomes. Examples of specific chromosome alterations are plentiful in leukemias and lymphomas, providing credibility to Boveri's hypothesis of malignancy. However, there are only few examples of such specific anomalies in human solid tumors. With the help of improved techniques, certain solid tumors have now been characterized with specific (unique) chromosomal rearrangements; for example, deletion 13q in retinoblastoma, deletion 11p in Wilms' tumor, deletion 6q in malignant melanoma, deletion 1p in neuroblastoma, deletion 3p in small-cell lung carcinoma, deletion 22q in meningioma, transloca-

Table 4
Wilm's Tumor Cells Showing Anomalies of Chromosome 11[a]

No. of cases		
With 11p—	Without 11p—	Reference
2	7	Slater and Bleeker-Wagemakers, 1980
1	—	Kaneko et al., 1981
1	—	Osada et al., 1981
2	—	Slater and Kraker, 1982
3	13	Slater et al., 1983
—	2	Kaneko et al., 1983
1	—	McGavran et al., 1983
3	1	Ferrell et al., 1983
1	—	Huerre et al., 1983
1[a]	—	Present report
Totals: 15 (65.1%)	23	

[a] In this tumor only one copy of chromosome 11 was present.

tion of 1q in breast tumors, translocation of 3p in renal cell carcinoma, translocation involving 1p in testicular tumors, to name only some (Pathak, 1983). Other solid tumors, when analyzed with further improved methodology, may also demonstrate specific chromosome anomalies. These specific anomalies may be responsible for tumor initiation and development. Such genetic alternations might be inherited from one parent having a balanced translocation or can develop *de novo* as constitutional anomalies. It can also be acquired in the target organs as tumor-specific anomalies. The "shared" chromosome anomalies, which are secondary in nature and observed in different tumors, are acquired during tumor progression and might be responsible for growth, proliferation, heterogeneity, and invasiveness of neoplasms.

Recently, LeBeau and Rowley (1984) have compiled data on human chromosomes specifically involved in alterations in certain tumors, location of fragile sites, and the localization of c-oncogenes on such chromosomes. A fragile site is a "hot spot" on certain human chromosomes that exhibits a high frequency of chromatid or isochromatid breakage. Such hot spots are inherited in a Mendelian fashion and can be demonstrated in increased frequency in culture medium deficient in folic acid residue (Sutherland, 1979a). Fragile sites in human chromosomes 1, 2, 3, 5, 6, 7, 8, 9, 10, 11, 12, 13, 16, 17, 20, and X have been well documented. Only the fragile site on the X chromosome has been associated with mental retardation in male carriers (Sutherland, 1979b). The functions of autosomal fragile sites are not known. However, in certain cancer

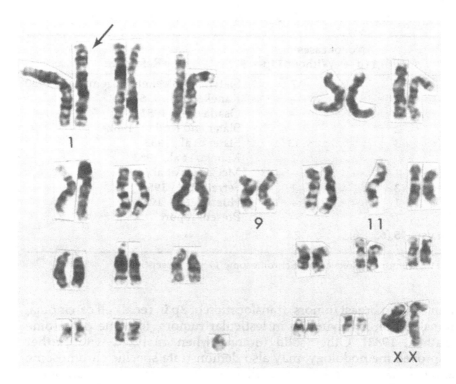

Fig. 13. A G-banded karyotype of a Wilms' tumor metaphase plate prepared after a short-term culture. Note the presence of pericentric inversion in the C-band region of one chromosome 9 (right side), single copy of chromosome 11, partial trisomy of the long arm of chromosome 1 (arrow showing translocation in the short arm), and 2–3 unidentified markers.

patients a particular fragile site may be expressed in higher frequency in peripheral blood cultures than in matched controls. One such case of a patient with hypercalcemia and papillary thyroid carcinoma has recently been reported (Pathak et al., 1982b), in which chromosome 11 showed both chromatid and isochromatid types of fragility in multiple blood samples. The break point in chromosome 11 appears in the proximal end of the long arm, which is also the fragile site. "Branched" morphology of this chromosome was also noted in 2–3% of metaphases. Data have been collected on the peripheral blood cultures of three patients with small-cell carcinoma of the lung. The fragile sites of both chromosomes 16 and 17 are expressed in higher frequency in these patients as compared to their normal relatives (our unpublished observation). More such effort is needed to generate extensive data on fragile sites and their relation to tumorigenesis.

It has been postulated that most human cancers result from genetic transposition, rather than mutations (Cairns, 1981). Such chromosomal rearrangements can activate certain genes that are normally inactive (regulated) because their products are not needed in that particular organ. Information recently available on oncogenes, alterations in gene physiology, some forms of gene amplification, and overproduction of a particular protein strongly indicate the importance of aberrant expression of certain genes in neoplastic transformation and tumor progression. To date, 21 oncogenes have been mapped on certain human chromosomes (Table 5). Of these, only a few have been shown to participate in the development of human tumors, although transformation activity has been demonstrated for most of the oncogenes in the rodent system (Pulciana et al., 1982). In Burkitt's lymphoma, for example, which has a specific 8;14 translocation, oncogene c-*myc* shows increased expression (Erikson et al., 1983). Another member of the *myc* gene family has been implicated in the development of neuroblastomas, a neurogenic tumor that usually occurs in childhood (Brodeur et al., 1984). The other genetic mechanism that involves oncogenes is deletion. A deletion may affect the human oncogene, c-*ras*, which has been localized to chromosome 11p14.1 (Jhanwar et al., 1983). A deletion of the chromosome region (11p13–14.1) containing this gene might lead to the development of AWTS, although, recently it was demonstrated that c-*Ha-ras1* is not deleted in aniridia–Wilms' tumor association (Huerre et al., 1983). The molecular evidence that human cancers are initiated by oncogenes has been reviewed recently (Weinberg, 1983).

7.2. Double Minutes and Homogeneously Staining Regions

Thus far, this discussion has included the involvements of constitutional chromosome abnormalities that could be inherited or originated *de novo*, and tumor-specific acquired chromosome abnormalities in certain human neoplasms. These chromosome abnormalities involved reciprocal translocations, inversions, and deletions. Two relatively new structural abnormalities, double minutes (DM) and homogeneously staining regions (HSR), found in a variety of human and animal neoplasms, should be added to this list. In addition, such novel entities can be induced artificially in tissue cultures by growing cells in the presence of increasing dosages of cytotoxic agents. Recent studies at both the cytological and molecular levels have indicated that DM and HSR represent alternative cytological forms of gene

Table 5
Summary of Human Oncogene Chromosome Locations and
Their Involvement in Specific Tumors

Oncogenes[a]	Chromosomes	Type of neoplasm
Blym-1, Nras	1	Neuroblastoma, breast tumors, testicular tumor, melanoma, and certain hematological tumors
fos, myc^N	2	Burkitt's lymphoma, cervical carcinoma
raf^{-1}	3	Renal cell carcinoma, small-cell lung carcinoma
$+ms$	5	Acute nonlymphocytic leukemia
myb, ras^{k-1}	6	Acute lymphocytic leukemia, ovarian carcinoma, malignant melanoma, retinoblastoma
erb^B	7	Acute nonlymphocytic leukemia
mos, myc	8	Acute lymphocytic leukemia, Burkitt's lymphoma
abl	9	Chronic myelogenous leukemia
ras^{H-1}, bcl-1	11	Wilm's tumor, non-Hodgkins' lymphoma
ras^{K-2}	12	Chronic lymphocytic leukemia
?	13	Retinoblastoma
?	14	Burkitt's lymphoma, nasopharyngeal carcinoma
fes	15	Acute promyelocytic leukemia
?	16	Acute myelomonocytic leukemia
erb^A	17	Acute crisis of chronic myelogenous leukemia
bcl-2, v-yes	18	Polycythemia vera, refractory anemia
src	20	Medullary carcinoma of the thyroid gland
?	21	Primary thrombocythemia, acute myeloid leukemia
sis	22	Chronic myeloid leukemia, meningioma, Burkitt's lymphoma
ras^{H-2}	X	One X chromosome disappears in most tumors of female origin
?	Y	Y chromosome disappears in most tumors of male origin

[a] ?, Oncogenes are not yet mapped on these chromosomes.

amplification, which raises the question of which gene sequences are amplified and what role(s) they play in neoplastic transformation, progression, and metastasis of cancer. Some of these questions and their possible answers have been discussed in recent reviews (Barker, 1982; Cowell, 1982; Biedler et al., 1983).

Biedler and Spengler (1976) observed unusually long and homogeneously stained chromosomal segments in G-banded metaphase cells of human neuroblastoma and Chinese hamster cell lines that were made resistant to methotrexate. Since then, such extended segments have been observed in other human and animal tumor cell lines. Double minutes and HSR have been reported only in tumor cells with cells taken directly from biopsy specimens (Pathak, 1980). The first detailed report on DM was presented by Cox et al. (1965) in tumor cells of neurogenic origin. Because most of the early reports of DM occurred in childhood tumors of neurgenic origin, many investigators suggested that DM played a role in such malignancy. Recent reports have shown that DM can be found in most, if not all, tumors in man and experimental animals (for review, see Barker, 1982). A metaphase plate showing typical DM from a malignant melanoma cell line is shown in Fig. 14.

Recent evidence indicates that both DM and HSR share many structural and functional properties. Both are found only in cancer cells, with a few exceptions; both stain lightly in G-banding; both contain "core" structure (unpublished data); and when present in the same cell population they are mutually exclusive in individual cells (Balaban-Malenbaum and Gilbert, 1977; 1980). Homogeneously staining regions and DM have been reported in cells of retinoblastoma (Reid et al., 1974; Balaban-Malenbaum et al., 1981; Gilbert et al., 1981; Balaban et al., 1982; Benedict et al., 1983a) and malignant melanoma (Pathak et al., 1983; Hubbell, 1983; de Salum et al., 1984). So far, DM and HSR have not been reported in Wilms' tumor and renal cell carcinoma cells; however, when more tumors are examined cytogenetically, DM and HSR will probably be demonstrated.

The presence of DM and HSR in tumor cells implies a direct relationship between gene amplification and tumorigenesis. This relationship may be secondary and DM and HSR may be formed in response to drug treatments or tumorigenesis. Recently, Pall (1981) proposed a model in which gene amplification is involved in the process of neoplastic transformation.

8. Concluding Remarks

Nonrandom chromosome anomalies that are specifically associated with certain human tumors can be inherited or acquired as

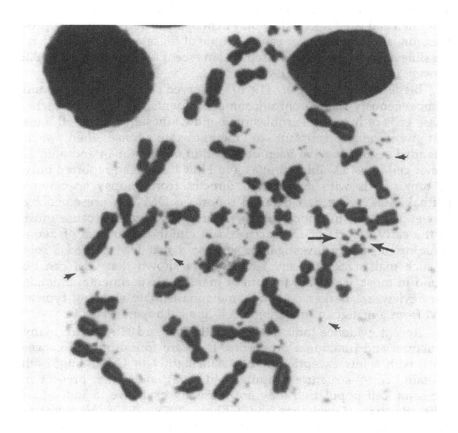

Fig. 14. A conventionally stained metaphase plate from a malignant melanoma cell line TCH 3116 showing regular chromosomes and small double bodies, called double minutes (DM). Darkly stained DM are marked by large arrows and some of the lightly stained DM by small arrows.

tumor-specific aberrations. These include deletion, translocation, and inversion. There are two types of chromosomal anomalies: (1) primary, which may be responsible for tumor initiation, and (2) secondary, which are shared by a variety of tumors and are responsible for tumor progression and invasiveness. There may also be two categories of oncogenes: (1) primary type responsible for tumor initiation, and (2) a secondary type, shared by very many tumors and responsible for tumor progression and metastasis.

Congenital chromosome anomalies observed in children should be interpreted not only in terms of their phenotypic abnormalities, but also in terms of predisposition to cancer development. Information concerning the incidence of cancer, if any, should be gathered in such families. Genetic instability observed in the normal blood and/or fibroblast cultures of certain individuals might serve as raw material and promote fixation of a particular type of chromosome anomaly in a target cell and thereby activate an oncogene responsible for tumor initiation.

Acknowledgments

It is a pleasure to acknowledge the assistance rendered by Dr. Uta Francke, Dr. L. C. Strong, Dr. N. Wang, and many others for contributing their microphotographs and supplying biopsy specimens from their patients. I also wish to thank Mrs. Angela Goodacre for her excellent technical assistance and Mrs. Ruby Kirkpatrick for her patience and superb secretarial assistance. This work was supported in part by research grant CA-32064 from the National Cancer Institute and a joint research project of The University of Texas M. D. Anderson Hospital and Tumor Institute at Houston and the John S. Dunn Research Foundation, Houston, Texas. My apology to all those "brave souls" whose papers have not been cited in this chapter. They were not omitted deliberately. Last, but not the least, my sincere thanks to Dr. T. C. Hsu for his constant encouragement and stimulating discussions during the course of this investigation.

References

American Cancer Society. (1983) *Cancer Facts and Figures,* pp. 17–18.

Anderson, D. E., L. Smith, Jr., and C. M. McBride (1967), Hereditary aspects of malignant melanoma. *JAMA* 200, 741–746.

Asal, N. R., R. S. Muneer, J. R. Geyer, L. M. Thompson, D. Riser, and O. M. Rennert (1983), Cytogenetic studies on renal cell carcinoma. *Am. J. Hum. Genet.* 35, 59a.

Atkin, N. B. and M. C. Baker (1981), A metastatic malignant melanoma with 24 chromosomes. *Hum. Genet.* 58, 217–219.

Bader, J. L., A. T. Meadows, L. E. Zimmerman, L. B. Rorke, P. A. Voute, L. A. Champion, and R. W. Miller (1982), Bilateral retinoblastoma with ectopic intracranial retinoblastoma: Trilateral retinoblastoma. *Cancer Genet. Cytogenet.* 5, 203–213.

Bader, J. L., R. W. Miller, A. T. Meadows, L. E. Zimmerman, L. A. A. Champion, and P. A. Voute (1980), Trilateral retinoblastoma. *Lancet* 2, 582–583.

Balaban, G., F. Gilbert, W. Nichols, A. Meadows, and J. Shields (1982), Abnormalities of chromosome #13 in retinoblastomas from individuals with normal constitutional karyotypes. *Cancer Genet. Cytogenet.* 6, 213–221.

Balaban, G., M. Herlyn, D. Guerry, IV, R. Bartolo, H. Koprowski, W. H. Clark, and P. C. Nowell (1984), Cytogenetics of human malignant melanoma and premalignant lesions. *Cancer Genet. cytogenet.* **11**, 429–439.

Balaban-Malenbaum, G. and F. Gilbert (1977), Double minute chromosomes and the homogeneously staining regions in chromosomes of human neuroblastoma cell lines. *Science* **198**, 739–741.

Balaban-Malendaum, G. and F. Gilbert (1980), Relationship Between Homogeneously Staining Regions and Double Minute Chromosomes in Human Neuroblastoma Cell Lines, in *Advances in Neuroblastoma Research* (Evans, A. E., ed.) New York, Raven Press.

Balaban-Malenbaum, G., F. Gilbert, W. W. Nichols, R. Hill, J. Shields, and A. T. Meadows (1981), A deleted chromosome no. 13 in human retinoblastoma cells: Relevance to tumorigenesis. *Cancer Genet. Cytogenet.* **3**, 243–250.

Balch, C. M., S. J. Soong, G. W. Milton, H. M. Shaw, V. J. McGovern, W. H. McCarthy, T. M. Murad, and W. A. Maddox (1983), Changing trends in cutaneous melanoma over a quarter century in Alabama, U. S. A., and New South Wales, Australia. *Cancer* **52**, 1748–1753.

Barker, P. E. (1982), Double minutes in human tumor cells. *Cancer Genet. Cytogenet.* **5**, 81–94.

Becher, R., Z. Gibas, and A. A. Sandberg (1983), Chromosome 6 in malignant melanoma. *Cancer Genet. Cytogenet.* **9**, 173–175.

Benedict, W. F., A. Banerjee, C. Mark, and A. L. Murphree (1983a), Nonrandom chromosomal changes in untreated retinoblastomas. *Cancer Genet. Cytogenet.* **10**, 311–333.

Benedict, W. F., A. L. Murphree, A. Banerjee, C. A. Spina, M. C. Sparkes, and R. S. Sparkes (1983b), Patient with 13 chromosome deletion: Evidence that the retinoblastoma gene is a recessive cancer gene. *Science* **219**, 973–975.

Biedler, J. L., P. W. Melera, and B. A. Spengler (1983), Chromosome Abnormalities and Gene Amplification: Comparison of Antifolate-Resistant and Human Neuroblastoma Cell Systems, in, *Chromosomes and Cancer from Molecules to Man*, Bristol-Meyers Cancer Symposia. (Rowley, J. D., and J. E. Ultman, eds.) New York, Academic Press.

Biedler, J. L. and B. A. Spengler (1976), Metaphase chromosome anomaly: Association with drug resistance and cell specific products. *Science* **191**, 185–187.

Bogenmann, E. and C. Mark (1983), Routine growth and differentiation of primary retinoblastoma cells in culture. *J. Natl. Cancer Inst.* **70**, 95–104.

Bove, K. E. and A. J. McAdams (1976), The nephroblastomatosis complex and its relationship to Wilms' tumor: A clinicopathologic treatist. *Perspect. Pediatr. Pathol.* **3**, 185–223.

Boveri, T. (1912), Beitrag zum studium des chromatins in den epithelzellen der carcinome. *Beitr. Path. Anat. Allg. Pathol.* **14**, 249.

Bowen, J. M., R. Cailleau, B. Giovanella, S. Pathak, and M. J. Siciliano (1983), A retrovirus-producing transformed mouse cell line derived from a human breast adenocarcinoma transplanted in a nude mouse. *In Vitro* **19**, 635–641.

Brodeur, G. M., R. C. Seeger, M. Schwab, H. E. Varmus, and J. M. Bishop (1984), Amplification of N-*myc* in untreated human neuroblastomas correlates with advanced disease stage. *Science* **224**, 1121–1124.

Cairns, J. (1981), The origin of human cancers. *Nature* **289**, 353–357.

Cavenee, W. K.; T. P. Dryja, R. A. Phillips, W. F. Benedict, R. Godbout, B. L. Gallie, A. L. Murphree, L. C. Strong, and R. L. White (1983), Expression of recessive alleles by chromosomal mechanisms in retinoblastoma. *Nature* **305**, 779–784.

Chaum, E., R. M. Ellsworth, D. H. Abramson, B. Haik, F. E. Kitchin, and R. S. K. Chaganti (1983), Cytogenetic analysis of 13 retinoblastoma tumors: Evidence of multifocal origin and in vivo gene amplification. *Am. J. Hum. Genet.* **35**, 61A.

Chen, T. R. and M. W. Shaw (1973), Stable chromosome changes in a human malignant melanoma. *Cancer Res.* **33**, 2042–2047.

Chen, T. R. and M. W. Shaw (1974), Studies of a cell line derived from a human malignant melanoma. *In Vitro* **10**, 216–224.

Cohen, A. J., F. P. Li, S. Berg, D. J. Marchetto, S. Tsai, S. E. Jacobs, and R. S. Brown (1979), Hereditary renal-cell carcinoma associated with a chromosomal translocation. *N. Engl. J. Med.* **301**, 592–595.

Cotlier, E., M. Rose, and S. A. Moel (1978), Aniridia, cataracts and Wilms' tumor in monozygous twins. *Am. J. Ophthalmol.* **86**, 129–132.

Courtenay, V. D., P. J. Selby, I. E. Smith, J. Mills, and M. J. Peckham (1978), Growth of human tumor cell colonies from biopsies using two soft-agar techniques. *Br. J. Cancer* **38**, 77–81.

Cowell, J. K. (1982), Double minutes and homogeneously staining regions: Gene amplification in mammalian cells. *Annu. Rev. Genet.* **16**, 21–59.

Cox, D., C. Yuncken, and A. I. Spriggs (1965), Minute chromatin bodies in malignant tumors of children. *Lancet* **2**, 55–58.

Cross, H. E., R. C. Hansen, G. Moorow, and J. R. Davis (1977), Retinoblastoma in a patient with a 13qXp translocation. *Am. J. Ophthalmol.* **84**, 548–554.

Cruciger, Q. V. J., S. Pathak, and R. Cailleau (1976), Human breast carcinomas: Marker chromosomes involving 1q in seven cases. *Cytogenet. Cell Genet.* **17**, 231–235.

Cutler, S. J. and J. L. Young, Jr., Eds. (1975), *Third National Cancer Survey: Incidence Data*, National Cancer Institute Monograph 41, DHEW Publication No. (NIH) 75-787.

Davidson, E. V., B. Gibbons, G. E. S. Aherne, and D. F. Roberts (1979), Chromosomes in retinoblastoma patients. *Clin. Genet.* **15**, 505–508.

de Salum, S. B., E. Slavutsky, S. Besuschio, and A. A. Pavlosky (1984), Homogeneously staining regions (HSR) in a human malignant melanoma. *Cancer Genet. Cytogenet.* **11**, 53–60.

Erikson, J., A. Ar-Rushdi, H. L. Drwinga, P. C. Nowell, and C. M. Croce (1983), Transcriptional activation of the translocated *C-myc* oncogene in Burkitt lymphoma. *Proc. Natl. Acad. Sci. USA* **80**, 820–824.

Ferrell, R. E., L. C. Strong, S. Pathak, and V. M. Riccardi (1983), Wilms' tumor (WT) cytogenetics: The variable presence of del(11p) in WT explants. *Am. J. Hum. Genet.* **35**, 63A.

Fraccaro, M., F. Lo Curto, and S. Scappaticci (1976), Chromosome Identification and Karyotypic Evolution in a Human Melanoma Cell Line (MEL-41), in *Chromosomes Today* (Pearson, P. L. and K. R. Lewis, eds.) New York, John Wiley & Sons.

Francke, U. (1976), Retinoblastoma and chromosome 13. *Cytogenet. Cell Genet.* **16**, 131–134.

Francke, U. (1983), Specific Chromosome Changes in the Human Heritable Tumors Retinoblastoma and Nephroblastoma, in *Chromosomes and Cancer from Molecules to Man* (Rowley, J. D. and J. E. Ultmann, eds.) New York, Academic Press.

Francke, U., D. L. George, M. G. Brown, and V. M. Riccardi (1977), Gene dose effect: Intraband mapping of the LDH-A locus using cells from four individuals with different interstitial deletions of 11p. *Cytogenet. Cell Genet.* **19**, 197–207.

Francke, U., L. B. Holmes, L. Atkins, and V. M. Riccardi (1979), Aniridia–Wilms' tumor association: Evidence for specific deletion of 11p13. *Cytogenet. Cell Genet.* **24**, 185–192.

Francke, U. and F. Kung (1976), Sporadic bilateral retinoblastoma and 13-chromosomal deletion. *Med. Pediatr. Oncol.* **2**, 379–385.

Gallie, B. L., D. M. Albert, J. J. Y. Wong, N. Buyukmihci, and C. A. Puliafito (1976), Heterotransplantation of retinoblastoma into the athymic "nude" mouse. *Invest. Ophthalmol.* **16**, 256–259.

Gallie, B. L., W. Holmes, and R. A. Phillips (1982), Reproducible growth in tissue culture of retinoblastoma tumor specimens. *Cancer Res.* **42**, 301–305.

Gardner, H. A., B. L. Gallie, L. A. Knight, and R. A. Phillips (1982), Multiple karyotypic changes in retinoblastoma tumor cells: Normal chromosome no. 13 in most tumors. *Cancer Genet. Cytogenet.* **6**, 201–211.

Gilbert, F., G. Balaban, W. Roy Breg, B. Gallie, T. Reid, and W. Nichols (1981), Homogeneously staining region in a retinoblastoma cell line: Relevance to tumor initiation and progression. *J. Natl. Cancer Inst.* **67**, 301–306.

Gilgenkrantz, S., C. Vigneron, M. J. Gregoire, C. Pernot, and A. Raspiller (1982), Association of del(11)(p15.1p12), aniridia, catalase deficiency, and cardiomyopathy. *Am. J. Med. Genet.* **13**, 39–49.

Godbout, R., T. P. Dryja, J. Squire, B. L. Gallie, and R. A. Phillips (1983a), Somatic inactivation of genes on chromosome 13 is a common event in retinoblastoma. *Nature* **304**, 451–453.

Godbout, R., B. L. Gallie, and T. P. Dryja (1983b), Lack of expression of one esterase D isoenzyme in retinoblastoma tumor cells. *Invest. Ophthalmol. Vis. Sci.* (Suppl.) **24**, 294.

Gödde-Salz, E. and H. Behnke (1981), Aniridia, mental retardation and an unbalanced reciprocal translocation of chromosome 8 and chromosome 11 with an interstitial deletion of 11p. *Eur. J. Pediatr.* **136**, 93–96.

Griffiths, M. H., D. P. Thomas, J. M. Xipell, and R. N. Hope (1977), Thorotrast-induced bilateral carcinoma of the kidney. *Pathology* **9**, 43–48.

Hagemeijer, A., W. Hoehn and E. M. E. Smit (1979), Cytogenetic analysis of human renal carcinoma cell lines of common origin (NC 65). *Cancer Res.* **39**, 4662–4665.

Hamburger, A. W. and S. E. Salmon (1977), Primary bioassay of human tumor stem cells. *Science* **197**, 461–463.

Hamburger, A. W., S. E. Salmon, M. B. Kim, J. M. Trent, B. Soehnlen, D. S. Alberts, and H. J. Schmidt (1978), Direct cloning of human ovarian carcinoma cells in agar. *Cancer Res.* **38**, 3438–3443.

Hansemann, D. von (1890), Uber asymmetrische Zellteilung in Epithelkrebsen und deren biologische Bedeutung. *Virchow's Arch. Path. Anat.* **119**, 299–326.

Hata, A., Y. Suzuki, Y. Fukushima, and Y. Kuroki (1982), A case of *de novo* reciprocal translocation, 46, XX, t(X;13) (P11;q11) with bilateral retinoblastoma, multiple malformations, and incontinentia pigmenti. *Japan. J. Hum. Genet* **27**, 168.

Hida, T., Y. Konishita, R. Matsumoto, N. Suzuki, and H. Tanaka (1980), Bilateral retinoblastoma with a 13qXp translocation. *J. Pediat. Ophthalmol. Strabismus* **17**, 144–146.

Hittner, H. M., V. M. Riccardi, and U. Francke (1979), Aniridia due to chromosome 11 deletion. *Ophthalmology* **86**, 1173–1183.

Hoegerman, S. F. (1979), Chromosome 13 long arm interstitial deletion may result from maternal inverted insertion. *Science* **205**, 1035–1036.

Horton, W. A., V. Wong and R. Eldridge (1976), Von Hippel-Lindau disease—clinical and pathological manifestations in nine families with 50 affected members. *Arch. Intern. Med.* **136**, 769–777.

Hossfeld, D. (1978), Chromosome 14q+ in a retinoblastoma. *Intern. J. Cancer* **21**, 720–723.

Hsu, T. C. (1974), Longitudinal differentiation of chromosomes. *Annu. Rev. Genet.* **7**, 153–176.

Hubbell, H. R. (1983), Gene amplification in neoplasia and chemotherapy. *Cancer Bull.* **35**, 132–137.

Heurre, C., S. Despoisse, S. Gilgenkrantz, G. M. Lenoir, and C. Junien (1983), c-Ha-ras1 is not deleted in aniridia-Wilms' tumor association. *Nature* **305**, 638–641.

Inoue, S., Y. Ravindranath, M. J. Ottenbreit, R. I. Thompson, and W. W. Zuelzer (1974), Chromosomal analysis of metastatic retinoblastoma cells. *Hum. Genet.* **25**, 111–118.

ISCN (1981), An international system for human cytogenetic nomenclature. *Cytogenet. Cell Genet.* **31**, 1–23.

Ishihara, T., Y. Kikuchi, and A. A. Sandberg (1963), Chromosomes of twenty cancer effusions: Correlation of karyotypic, clinical, and pathologic aspects. *J. Natl. Cancer Inst.* **30**, 1303–1361.

Jensen, R. D. and R. W. Miller (1971), Retinoblastoma: Epidemiological characteristics. *N. Engl. J. Med.* **285**, 307–311.

Jhanwar, S. C., B. G. Neel, W. S. Hayward, and R. S. K. Chaganti (1983), Localization of c-ras oncogene family on human germline chromosomes. *Proc. Natl. Acad. Sci. USA* **80**, 4794–4797.

Johnson, M. P., N. Ramsay, J. Cervenka, and N. Wang (1982), Retinoblastoma and its association with a deletion in chromosome #13: A survey using high-resolution chromosome techniques. *Cancer Genet. cytogenet.* **6**, 29–37.

Junien, C., S. Despoisse, C. Turleau, H. Nicolas, F. Picard, B. L. Marec, J. C. Kaplan, and J. de Grouchy (1982), Retinoblastoma, deletion 13q14, and esterase D: Application of gene dosage effect to prenatal diagnosis. *Cancer Genet. Cytogenet.* **6**, 281–287.

Junien, D., C. Turleau, J. de Grouchy, R. Said, M. O. Rethore, R. Tenconi, and J. L. Dufier (1980), Regional assignment of catalase (CAT) gene to band 11p13: Association with the aniridia–Wilms' tumor–gonadoblastoma (WAGR) complex. *Ann. Genet.* (Paris) **29**, 165–168.

Kakati, S., S. Y. Song, and A. A. Sandberg (1977), Chromosomes and causation of human cancer and leukemia XXII. Karyotypic changes in malignant melanoma. *Cancer* **40**, 1173–1181.

Kaneko, Y., M. C. Egues, and J. D. Rowley (1981), Interstitial deletion of short arm of chromosome 11 limited to Wilms' tumor cells in a patient without aniridia. *Cancer Res.* **41**, 4577–4578.

Kaneko, Y., K. Kondo, J. D. Rowley, J. W. Moohr, and H. S. Maurer (1983), Further chromosome studies on Wilms' tumor cells of patients without aniridia. *Cancer Genet. Cytogenet.* **10**, 191–197.

Kantor, A. F., W. A. Blattner, W. J. Blot, J. F. Fraumeni, J. K. McLaughlin, L. M. Schuman, L. L. Lindquist, N. Wang, and J. C. Hozier (1982), Hereditary renal carcinoma and chromosomal defects. *N. Eng. J. Med.* **307**, 1403–1404.

Kitchin, F. D. and R. M. Ellsworth (1974), Pleiotropic effects of the gene for retinoblastoma. *J. Med. Genet.* **11**, 244–246.

Klein, G. (1983), Specific chromosomal translocations and the genesis of B-cell-derived tumors in mice and men (minireivews). *Cell* **32**, 311–316.

Knudson, A G., Jr. (1971), Mutation and cancer: Statistical study of retinoblastoma. *Proc. Natl. Acad. Sci. USA* **68**, 820–823.

Knudson, A. G. and L. C. Strong (1972), Mutation and cancer: A model for Wilms' tumor of the kidney. *J. Natl. Cancer Inst.* **48**, 313–324.

Kusnetsova, L. E., E. L. Prigogina, H. E. Pogosianz, and B. M. Belkona (1982), Similar chromosomal abnormalities in several retinoblastoms. *Hum. Genet.* **61**, 201–204.

Kusyk, C. J., C. L. Edwards, F. E. Arrighi, and M. M. Romsdahl (1979), Improved method for cytogenetic studies of solid tumors. *J. Natl. Cancer Inst.* **63**, 1199–1203.

Ladda, R., L. Atkins, and J. Littlefield (1974), Computer-assisted analysis of chromosomal abnormalities: Detection of a deletion in aniridia/Wilms' tumor syndromes. *Science* **185**, 784–787.

LeBeau, M. M. and J. D. Rowley (1984), Heritable fragile sites in cancer. *Nature* **308**, 607–608.

Lele, K. P., L. S. Penrose, and H. B. Stallard (1963), Chromosome deletion in a case of retinoblastoma. *Ann. Hum. Genet.* **27**, 171–174.

Li, F. P., D. J. Marchetto, and R. S. Brown (1982), Familial renal carcinoma. *Cancer Genet. Cytogenet.* **7**, 271–275.

Little, J. H., J. Holt, and N. Davis (1980), Changing epidemiology of malignant melanoma in Queensland. *Med. J. Aust.* **1**, 66–69.

Machin, G. A. (1980), Persistent renal blastema (nephroblastomatosis) as a frequent precursor of Wilms' tumor: A pathological and clinical review. *Am. J. Pediatr. Hematol. Oncol.* **2**, 165–172; 253–261; 353–362.

Mark, J. (1970), Chromosomal analysis of a human retinoblastoma. *Acta Ophthalmol.* **48**, 124–135.

Matsuda, M., M. Osafune, E. Nakano, T. Kotake, T. Sonoda, S. Watanabe, T. Hada, T. Okochi, K. Higashino, Y. Yamamura, and T. Abe (1979), Characterization of an established cell line from human renal carcinoma. *Cancer Res.* **39**, 4694–4699.

Matsunaga, E. (1983), Retinoblastoma: A model for the study of carcinogenesis in humans (in Japanese). *Japan. J. Hum. Genet.* **28**, 57–71.

McCarthy, W. H., A. L. Black, and G. W. Milton (1980), Melanoma in New South Wales: An epidemiologic survey, 1970–1976. *Cancer* **45**, 427–432.

McCulloch, P. B., P. B. Dent, P. R. Hayes, and S. K. Liao (1976), Common and individually specific chromosomal characteristics of cultured human melanoma. *Cancer Res.* **36**, 398–404.

McFall, R. C., T. W. Sery, and M. Makadon (1977), Characterization of a new continuous cell line derived from a human retinoblastoma. *Cancer Res.* **37**, 1003–1010.

McGavran, L., R. Heideman, G. Waldstein, and P. Berry (1983), Interstitial deletion of 11p in renal nodule from a child with Wilms' tumor. *Am. J. Hum. Genet.* **35**, 67A.

Michalova, K., F. Kloucek, and J. Musilova (1982), Deletion of 13q in two patients with retinoblastoma, one probably due to 13q– mosaicism in the mother. *Hum. Genet.* **61**, 264–266.

Miller, R. W. (1969), Fifty-two forms of childhood cancer. United States mortality experience, 1960–1966. *J. Pediatr.* **75**, 685–689.

Miller, R. W., J. F. Fraumeni, Jr., and M. D. Manning (1964), Association of Wilms' tumor with aniridia, hemihypertrophy and other congenital malformations. *N. Engl. J. Med.* **270**, 922–927.

Mohandas, T., R. S. Sparkes, and L. J. Shapiro (1982), Genetic evidence for the inactivation of a human autosomal locus attached to an inactive X chromosome. *Am. J. Hum. Genet.* **34**, 811–817.

Motegi, T. (1981), Lymphocyte chromosome survey in 42 patients with retinoblastoma: Effort to detect 13q14 deletion mosaicism. *Hum. Genet.* **58**, 168–173.

Motegi, T. (1982), High rate of detection of 13q14 deletion mosaicism among retinoblastoma patients (using more extensive methods). *Hum. Genet.* **61**, 95–97.

Motegi, T., M. Komatsu, Y. Nakazato, M. Ohuchi, and K. Minoda (1982), Retinoblastoma in a boy with a *de novo* mutation of a 13/18 translocation: The assumption that the retinoblastoma locus is at 13q14, particularly at the distal portion of it. *Hum. Genet.* **60**, 193–195.

Muir, P. D. and F. W. Gunz (1979), A cytogenetic study of eight human melanoma cell lines. *Pathology* **11**, 597–606.

Murphree, A. L. and W. F. Benedict (1984), Retinoblastoma: Clues of human oncogenesis. *Science* **223**, 1028–1033.

Nichols, W. W., R. C. Miller, M. Sobel, E. Hoffman, R. S. Sparkes, T. Mohandas, I. Veomett, and J. R. Davis (1980), Further observations on a 13q Xp translocation associated with retinoblastoma. *Am. J. Ophthalmol.* **89**, 621–627.

Nöel, B., B. Quack, and M. O. Rethore (1976), Partial deletions and trisomies of chromosome 13; mapping of bands associated with particular malformations. *Clin. Genet.* **9**, 593–602.

Nowell, P. C. and D. A. Hungerford (1960), A minute chromosome in human chronic granulocytic leukemia. *Science* **132**, 1497.

Orye, E., M. J. Delbeke, and B. Vandenabeele (1971), Retinoblastoma and D-chromosome deletions. *Lancet* **ii**, 1376.

Osada, I., Y. Shiroko, Y. Miyamoto, M. Sekiguchi, G. Fujii, M. Ogata, H. Watanabe, and N. Kamada (1981), Establishment of a cell line (W-2) derived from human Wilms' tumor showing chromosome 11 short arm interstitial deletions. *Proc. Jap. Cancer Assoc.* Abstract of the 40th Annual Meeting, Sapporo, October, p. 181.

Pall, M. L. (1981), Gene-amplification model for carcinogenesis. *Proc. Natl. Acad. Sci. USA* **78**, 2465–2468.

Pathak, S. (1976), Chromosome banding techniques. *J. Reprod. Med.* **17**, 25–28.

Pathak, S. (1979), Cytogenetic research techniques in human and laboratory animals that can be most profitably applied to livestock. *J. Dairy Sci.* **62**, 836–843.

Pathak, S. (1980), Cytogenetic analysis in human breast tumors. *Cancer Genet. Cytogenet.* **1**, 281–289.

Pathak, S. (1983), Chromosome constitution of human solid tumors. *Cancer Bull.* **35**, 126–131.

Pathak, S. (1984), The role of tissue culture in cytogenetic oncology (abstract). *In Vitro* **20**, 265.

Pathak, S., H. L. Drwinga, and T. C. Hsu (1983), Involvement of chromosome 6 in rearrangements in human malignant melanoma cell lines. *Cytogenet. Cell Genet.* **36**, 573–579.

Pathak, S., L. C. Strong, R. E. Ferrell, and A. Trindade (1982a), Familial renal cell carcinoma with a 3;11 chromosome translocation limited to tumor cells. *Science* **217**, 939–941.

Pathak, S., T. C. Hsu, N. Samaan, R. C. Hickey (1982b), Cytogenetic abnormalities in a patient with hypercalcemia and papillary thyroid carcinoma. *Hum. Genet.* **60**, 291–293.

Pathak, S., M. J. Siciliano, R. Cailleau, C. L. Wiseman, and T. C. Hsu (1979), A human breast adenocarcinoma with chromosome and isoenzyme markers similar to those of the HeLa line. *J. Natl. Cancer Inst.* **62**, 263–271.

Phillips, R. A., B. L. Gallie, and H. A. Garner (1981), Cytogenetic studies on human retinoblastoma tumor cells growing in tissue culture. *Proc. Am. Assoc. Cancer Res. Am. Soc. Clin. Oncol.* **22**, 45.

Poole-Wilson, D. S. (1959), Occupational tumors of the bladder. *Proc. R. Soc. Med.* **53**, 801–814.

Pulciani, S., E. Santos, A. V. Lauver, L. K. Long, S. A. Aaronson, and M. Barbacid (1982), Oncogenes in solid human tumors. *Nature* **300**, 539–542.

Quinn, L. A., L. K. Woods, S. B. Merrick, N. M. Arabasz, and G. E. Moore (1977), Cytogenetic analysis of twelve human malignant melanoma cell lines. *J. Natl. Cancer Inst.* **59**, 301–307.

Rathert, P., H. Melchior, and W. Lutzeyer (1975), Phenacetin: A carcinogen for the urinary tract? *J. Urol.* **113**. 653–657.

Reid, T. W., D. M. Albert, A. S. Rabson, P. Russell, J. Craft, E. W. Chu, T. S. Tralka, and J. L. Wilcox (1974), Characteristics of an established cell line of retinoblastoma. *J. Natl. Cancer Inst.* **53**, 347–360.

Riccardi, V. M., H. M. Hittner, U. Francke, S. Pippin, G. P. Holmquist, F. L. Kretzer, and R. Ferrell (1979), Partial triplication and deletion of 13q; Study of a family presenting with bilateral retinoblastomas. *Clin. Genet.* **15**, 332–345.

Riccardi, V. M., E. Sujansky, A. C. Smith, and U. Francke (1978), Chromosomal imbalance in the aniridia Wilms' tumor association: 11p interstitial deletion. *Pediatrics* **61**, 604–610.

Rivera, H., C. Turleau, J. de Grouchy, C. Junien, S. Despoisse, and J. M. Zucker (1981), Retinoblastoma-del (13q14): Report of two patients, one with a trisomic sib due to maternal insertion. Gene-dosage effect for esterase. *D. Hum. Genet.* **59**, 211–214.

Rønne, M. (1984), An easy method for instant preparation of chromosome slides from solid tumors. *Anticancer Res.* **4**, 45–46.

Rowley, J. D. (1973), A new consistent chromosomal abnormality in chronic myelogenous leukemia identified by quinacrine fluorescence and Giemsa staining. *Nature* **243**, 290–293.

Rybak, J., A. Tharapel, S. Robinett, M. Garcia. C. Mankinen, and M. Freeman (1982), A simple reproducible method for prometaphase chromosome analysis. *Hum. Genet.* **60**, 328–333.

Seeger, R. C., S. A. Rayner, A. Banerjee, H. Chung, W. E. Laug, H. Neustein, and W. F. Benedict (1977), Morphology, growth, chromosomal pattern, and fibrinolytic activity of two new human neuroblastoma cell lines. *Cancer Res.* **37**, 1364–1371.

Semple, T. U., G. E. Moore, R. T. Morgan, L. K. Woods, and L. A. Quinn (1982), Multiple cell lines from patients with malignant melanoma: Morphology, karyology, and biochemical analysis. *J. Natl. Cancer Inst.* **68**, 365–380.

Slater, R. M. and E. M. Bleeker-Wagemakers (1980), Aniridia, Wilms' tumor and chromosome number 11. Abstract, 12th Annual Meeting of the International Society of Pediatric Oncology, Budapest, September, p. 88.

Slater, R. M. and Jan de Kraker (1982), Chromosome number 11 and Wilms' tumor. *Cancer Genet. Cytogenet.* **5**, 237–245.

Slater, R. M., J. de Kraker, P. A. Voute, and J. F. M. Delemarre (1983), A cytogenetic experience with 33 Wilms' tumors. (Abstract no. 8-22) 8th International Chromosome Conference, Lubeck, September 21–24.

Sparkes, R. S., H. Muller, and I. Klisak (1979), Retinoblastoma with 13q– chromosome deletion associated with maternal paracentric inversion of 13q. *Science* **203**, 1027–1029.

Strong, L. C. and A. G. Knudson (1973), Second cancers in retinoblastoma. *Lancet* **2**, 1086.

Strong, L. C., V. M. Riccardi, R. E. Ferrel, and R. S. Sparkes (1981), Familial retinoblastoma and chromosome 13 deletion transmitted *via* an insertional translocation. *Science* **213**, 1501–1503.

Sutherland, G. R. (1979a), Heritable fragile sites on human chromosomes. I. Factors affecting expression in lymphocyte culture. *Am. J. Hum. Genet.* **31**, 125–135.

Sutherland, G. R. (1979b), Heritable fragile sites on human chromosomes II. Distribution, phenotypic effects, and cytogenetics. *Am. J. Hum. Genet.* **31**, 136–148.

Sytkowski, A. J., J. P. Richie, and K. A. Bicknell (1983), New human renal carcinoma cell line established from a patient with erythrocytosis. *Cancer Res.* **43**, 1415–1419.

Trent, J. M., S. B. Rosenfeld, and F. L. Meyskens (1983), Chromosome 6q involvement in human malignant melanoma. *Cancer Genet. Cytogenet.* **9**, 177–180.

Turleau, C., C. Chavin-Colin, C. Junien, and J. de Grouchy (1983), Five patients with del(13)-retinoblastoma due to do novo and parental rearrangements. 8th International Chromosome Conference, Lubeck, September 21–24.

Vogel, F. (1979), Genetics of retinoblastoma. *Hum. Genet.* **52**, 1–54.

Wang, N. L. Soldat, S. Fan, S. Figemshau, R. Clayman, and E. Fraley (1983), The consistent involvement of chromosome 3 and 6 aberrations in renal cell carcinoma. *Am. J. Hum. Genet.* **35**, 73A.

Wang, N. and K. L. Perkins (1984), Involvement of band 3p14 in t(3;8) hereditary renal carcinoma. *Cancer Genet. Cytogenet.* **11**, 479–481.

Weinberg, R. A. (1983), A molecular basis of cancer. *Sci. Am.* **249**, 126–142.

Wilson, M. G., J. W. Towner, and A. Fujimoto (1973), Retinoblastoma and D-chromosome deletion. *Am. J. Hum. Genet.* **25**, 57–61.

Wolf, U. (1974), Theodor Boveri and His Book "On The Problem of the Origin of Malignant Tumors," in *Chromosomes and Cancer* (German, James, ed.) New York, Jon Wiley.

Yunis, J. J. (1982), Chromosomal Defects in Cancer, in *Gene Amplification* (Schimke, R. T., ed.) New York, Cold Spring Harbor Laboratory.

Yunis, J. J. and N. Ramsay (1978), Retinoblastoma and subband deletion of chromosome 13. *Am. J. Dis. Child.* **132**, 161–163.

Yunis, J. J. and N. K. C. Ramsay (1980), Familial occurrence of the aniridia Wilms' tumor syndrome with deletion 11p13–14.1. *J. Pediatr.* **96**, 1027–1030.

Elucidation of a Normal Function for a Human Proto-Oncogene

Keith C. Robbins and Stuart A. Aaronson

1. Introduction

Viruses have provided a means for the study of fundamental cellular mechanisms, such as DNA replication and gene regulation, in more readily dissectable ways than by studying the more complex cell. Thus, it was not without precedent that examination of processes leading to malignancy involved the study of RNA tumor viruses, designated type C retroviruses. These agents consist of two major groups: chronic and acute transforming retroviruses. The chronic viruses cause tumors—mostly leukemias—when inoculated into susceptible animals, but only after a latent period of several months. These viruses replicate without apparent transforming effect on known assay cells in tissue culture. In contrast, acute transforming viruses induce tumors within a very short period of days to weeks. They cause a variety of neoplastic diseases, including sarcomas, hematopoietic tumors, and even carcinomas. In tissue culture, these viruses generally induce foci of transformation in appropriate assay cells. This chapter documents how systematic investigation of one acute transforming retrovirus has led to identification of the normal function of a cellular gene that acquired the ability to induce malignant transformation when transduced by a chronic retrovirus genome.

2. A Primate Sarcoma Virus With Novel Properties

Simian sarcoma virus, SSV, was isolated from a naturally occurring woolly monkey fibrosarcoma (Thielen et al., 1971).

Although SSV, as well as other sarcoma viruses, possess the ability to transform fibroblasts in tissue culture and to induce solid tumors in vivo, this virus has the unique ability to induce glioblastomas in susceptible hosts (Wolfe et al., 1971; Wolfe et al., 1972). Biological characterization of SSV initially presented difficulties because of its association with an excess of nontransforming helper virus, designated simian sarcoma associated virus (SSAV) (Aaronson, 1973). Early investigations led to the isolation of cells nonproductively transformed by SSV (Aaronson, 1973). The ability to rescue the transforming virus by superinfection with a type C helper virus provided evidence of the replication defective nature of the SSV genome (Aaronson, 1973; Aaronson et al., 1975). Moreover, the development of clonal SSV transformants established the necessary biologic system for the subsequent molecular characterization of SSV structure and function.

An important feature of SSV, initially noted in biologic investigations, was the unusual morphology of cells transformed by the virus. Whereas transformed foci induced by most acute transforming viruses are composed of rounded or spindle-shaped, highly refractile cells, which often detach from the cell monolayer, SSV transformed foci were much more mounded in appearance and the transformed cells were fibroblastic in appearance (Fig. 1).

3. Molecular Cloning of the Biologically Active SSV Genome

The development of recombinant DNA technology made it possible to elucidate the molecular structure of the SSV genome. We constructed a λ phage library from cellular DNA containing the integrated SSV genome. Two clones were isolated, each of which were 5.8 kbp (kilobase pair) in length and scored as positive with our biochemical probe (Fig. 2). To determine whether our recombinant DNA clones possessed biological activity, they were analyzed by transfection of NIH/3T3 cells. Both clones possessed transforming activity of approximately 10^4 foci/pmol viral DNA (Robbins et al., 1981). Focus formation was a linear function of the amount of DNA added, indicating that a single DNA molecule was able to induce a transformed focus. When individual transformed foci were selected by the cloning cylinder technique, grown to mass culture, and superinfected with amphotropic mouse type C helper virus, focus-forming activity characteristic of SSV was rescued from each transformant tested. These and other findings con-

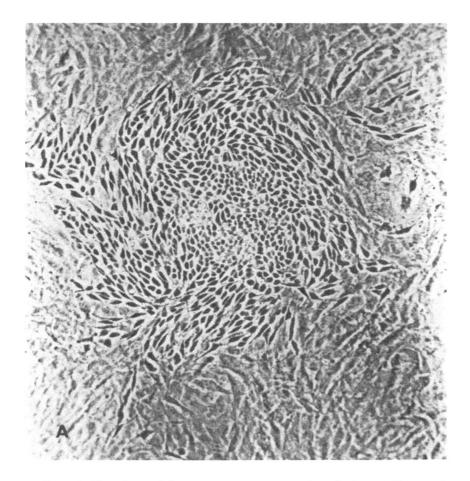

Fig. 1A. Transformed foci appearing in normal rat kidney cells at 7 d after infection with (A) Kirsten murine sarcoma virus or (B) simian sarcoma virus, 190×.

clusively demonstrated that our DNA clones contained the entire SSV genome.

4. Molecular Organization of the SSV Genome

In order to investigate the structure of the SSV genome, we constructed a physical map of one DNA clone, designated λ-SSV-

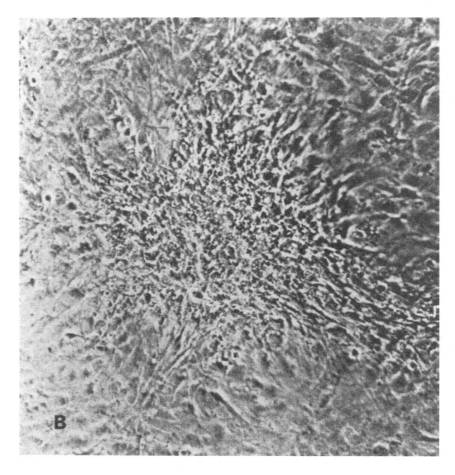

Fig. 1B.

11 clone 1. Restriction enzyme cleavage products were electrophoresed on agarose gels and visualized by ethidium bromide
staining. The relative location of cleavage sites on a linear map was
determined by appropriate double digestions. The results of these
studies, summarized in Fig. 3, served as a basis for further characterization of the DNA clone.

Other studies had shown that proviral DNAs of avian and
mammalian retroviruses contained long terminal repeats (LTR) that
possess signals for the initiation and termination of transcription
(Dhar et al., 1980l Shimotohno et al., 1980). We attempted to localize analogous regions on the λ-SSV-11 clone 1 physical map by
determining whether a specific constellation of restriction enzyme

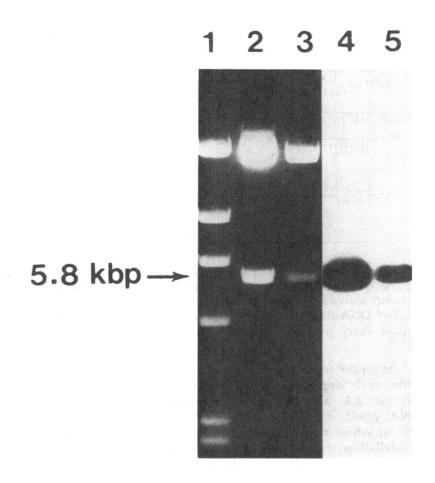

Fig. 2. Electrophoretic analysis of λ-SSV recombinant DNA clones. DNAs extracted from plaque-purified λ phages, λ-SSV-11 clone 1 and clone 2, were digested with Eco RI, electrophoresed on agarose gels, and stained with ethidium bromide (lanes 2 and 3, respectively). Fragments containing SSAV nucleotide sequences were identified by Southern blotting analysis using SSAV cDNA as a probe (lanes 4 and 5, respectively). Fragments of HindIII-digested λ DNA served as size standards (lane 1), arrowhead, 5.8 kbp.

sites was repeated within the molecule. As shown in Fig. 3, PstI and KpnI cleaved the molecule in identical locations with respect to two SacI sites located near either terminus at approximately 0.8 and 5.5 kbp on the restriction map. These regions, each approximately 0.5 kbp long, likely corresponded to the LTRs of SSV.

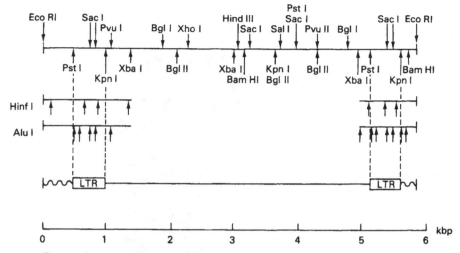

Fig. 3. Restriction map of λ-SSV-11 clone 1 DNA. Sites of restriction enzyme cleavage within the DNA insert were determined by double-digestion analysis. The sites of *Hinf*1 and *Alu*I cleavage within the terminal *Xba*I DNA fragments were determined by using the partial digestion method. Wavy lines, NRK cellular flanking sequences; LTR, long terminal repeat.

In order to establish more firmly the presence of LTRs and define their length, we constructed a detailed restriction map of the terminal 1.3- and 1.0-kbp *Xba*I fragments of λ-SSV-11 clone 1 DNA. *Hinf*I and *Alu*I were chosen for this purpose because the sites at which they cleave occur frequently in DNA. An identical constellation of two *Hinf*I and four *Alu*I sites was observed in each fragment within the regions defined by *Pst*I and *Kpn*I sites. Several unique *Hinf*I and *Alu*I sites were detected outside of these domains. These results demonstrated that terminal redundancies were present in the DNA clone and defined their length as 0.55 ± 0.02 kbp. From the location of the two LTRs, within λ-SSV-11 clone 1 DNA, it was possible to establish the length of the SSV genome as 5.1 kbp and the presence of flanking NRK cellular DNA sequences extending 0.45 and 0.25 kbp to the left and right ends, respectively, of the proviral DNA.

5. Detection and Localization of a Non-SSAV-Related Region of SSV

SSV transforms fibroblasts in tissue culture and induces solid tumors in susceptible hosts, whereas its parent SSAV possesses neither biologic activity. Thus, it was reasoned that comparison of their structures might help account for their different functions. In an effort to detect and localize such differences, we performed R-loop analysis of the SSV DNA clone with SSAV genomic RNA (Robbins et al., 1981). A representative of 30 R-loop structures analyzed is shown in Fig. 4. Two regions of DNA–RNA homology, 3.2 ± 0.2 and 0.7 ± 0.01 kbp, were detected. Within the larger region of homology, two loops of single-stranded RNA, representing SSAV sequences deleted from the SSV genome, were observed. Of particular note was the finding that the two regions of DNA–RNA homology were separated by 1.0 ± 0.1 kbp of λ-SSV-11 clone 1 DNA that lacked homology with SSAV RNA. These results demonstrated that λ-SSV-11 clone 1 contained a contiguous 1.0-kbp region that was unrelated to SSAV and was located within the transforming virus genome. This SSV-specific region was designated v-*sis*.

In order to orient the R-loop structure with respect to SSV genomic RNA and the λ-SSV-11 clone 1 DNA physical map, we took advantage of the fact that SSV codes for a *gag* gene product containing SSAV p12 and p30. Only the larger region of DNA–RNA homology possessed sufficient coding capacity for this gene product. Thus, the 3.2- and 0.7-kbp regions of DNA–RNA homology must be located 5′ and 3′, respectively, on SSV genomic RNA.

6.   v-*sis* Is Cell Derived and Required for SSV Transforming Activity

In an effort to identify the origin of the v-*sis* sequence, normal cellular DNAs were examined by the Southern technique using nick-translated v-*sis* DNA as a probe (Robbins et al., 1982a). As shown in Fig. 5, v-*sis*-related DNA fragments were detected at low copy numbers within cellular DNAs of species as diverse as human and quail. These results demonstrated that *sis* was derived from a well-conserved normal cellular gene.

It has been possible to demonstrate further that v-*sis* arose from within the woolly monkey genome. For these studies, we determined the extent to which a single-stranded v-*sis* DNA probe, prepared from cloned v-*sis*, could be hybridized by different normal cellular DNAs in solution (Robbins et al., 1982a). The highest extents of annealing were exhibited by DNAs of New World primates, with values ranging from 56 to 65%. Moreover, findings that the melting profile midpoint of woolly monkey cellular DNA-*sis* DNA hybrids was identical to that of homologous v-*sis* DNA

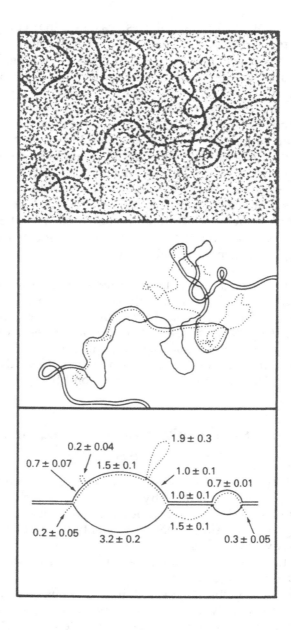

Fig. 4. R-loop analysis of λ-SSV-11 clone 1 DNA and SSAV RNA.
Solid line, λ-SSV-11 clone 1 DNA; dotted line, SSAV RNA. The contour
lengths indicated are expressed in kb and represent the mean ±SD
obtained from analysis of 30 separate molecules.

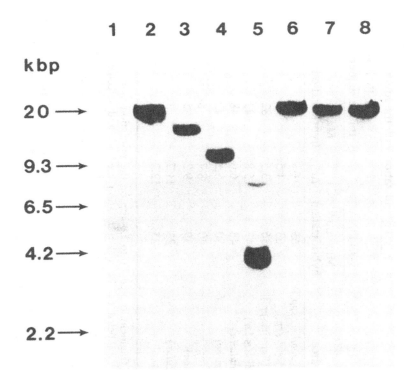

Fig. 5. Detection of *sis*-related sequences in DNAs of different vertebrate species. Eco RI-treated DNAs extracted from quail, mouse, rat, mink, cat, woolly monkey, gibbon ape spleen and human embryo lung fibroblasts, electrophoresed in lanes 1–8, respectively, were analyzed by hybridization with v-*sis* probe. Reference markers of *Hind*III-digested λ phage DNA were elctrophoresed in parallel.

hybrids (Table 1) demonstrated that v-*sis* arose from within the woolly monkey genome.

The region of SSV required for its transforming function was determined by analysis of deletion mutants constructed from a molecular clone of SSV DNA for their ability to transform NIH-3T3 cells in a transfection assay (Graham and van der Eb, 1973; Wigler et al., 1977). The intact viral genome (pSSV-11) exhibited a transforming activity of $10^{4.1}$ focus-forming units (FFU) per pmol of viral DNA (Fig. 6). A subgenomic clone, pSSV 3/1, from which the 3' long terminal repeat (LTR) was deleted, showed no reduction in biologic activity. In contrast, pSSV 3/2, a subclone that lacked the 3'

Table 1

V-sis Is Derived From the Genome of a New World Primate[a]

| | DNA source | Hybridization with the following: | | | |
| | | v-sis DNA | | Woolly monkey unique sequence DNA | |
		Maximum hybridization	Δt_m	Maximum hybridization	Δt_m
New World primate	Woolly monkey (Lagothrix spp.)	65	0	100	0
	Spider monkey (Ateles spp.)	63	1.5	97	1.1
	Squirrel monkey (Saimiri spp.)	56	3.5	82	3.8
Old World primate	Gibbon ape (Hylobates lar)	47	5.8	47	6.5
	Rhesus (Macaca mulatta)	48	6.0	48	6.2
	Human (Homo sapiens)	50	5.5	47	7.1
Carnivore	Cat (Felis catus)	40	8.7	5	ND[b]
	Mink (Mustela vison)	39	9.2	5	ND[b]
Rodent	Mouse (Mus musculus)	23	11.7	3	ND[b]
	Rat (Rattus rattus)	23	12.2	3	ND[b]

[a] The sis probe was prepared from a DNA fragment located 4.0 to 5.0 kbp on the restriction map of λ 1-SSV-11 clone 1 DNA. This DNA fragment was ^{32}P-labeled by the nick-translation method, and selected for single-stranded DNA complementary to SSV RNA, as described (Robbins et al., 1982b). Unique sequence cellular DNA was prepared from woolly monkey cells grown for 24 h in medium containing 10 μCi/mL[^{3}H] thymidine. Results are expressed as the final extent of hybridization at C_0t of 10^4 normalized to the extent of hybridization of sis or unique sequence DNA probes by λ-SSV-11 clone 1 and woolly monkey total cellular DNA, respectively. The temperatures at which 50% of hybrids were dissociated (t_m) were 89 and 90°C for the homologous sis probe hybrid, and self-associating unique sequence DNA, respectively. The Δt_m is the difference in t_m between the other DNA–DNA hybrids and the t_m of the homologous hybrid, expressed in degrees centigrade.
[b] ND = Not determined.

98

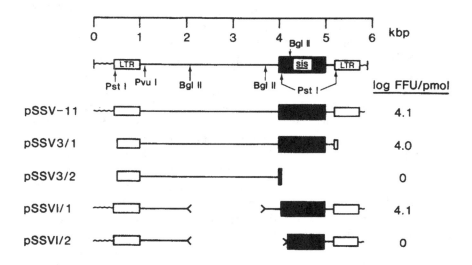

Fig. 6. Construction and biologic analysis of SSV deletion mutants. Deletion mutants were constructed from pSSV-11 DNA. Transfection of NIH/3T3 cells with plasmids containing SSV wild-type or mutant DNAs was performed by the calcium phosphate precipitation technique (Graham and van der Eb. 1973), as modified by Wigler et al. (1977). Transformed foci were scored at 14–21 d.

LTR, as well as all but 82 base pairs (bp) of v-*sis*, demonstrated no detectable transforming activity. These results indicated that v-*sis* was essential in SSV transformation. A mutant, pSSV I/1, which lacked an internal 1.8-kbp *Bgl*II fragment, transformed NIH/3T3 cells with an efficiency of $10^{4.1}$ FFU/pmol of viral DNA. However a subclone, pSSV I/2, which lacked an additional stretch of 345 bp of SSAV sequences, as well as the first 250 bp of v-*sis*, showed no transforming activity. These findings localized the SSV transforming gene to a region encompassing v-*sis*, along with 345 and 305 bp of flanking SSAV sequences, to the left and right of v-*sis*, respectively (Robbins et al., 1982b; Devare et al., 1983).

7. Predicted Coding Sequence of the SSV Transforming Gene

To precisely determine the structure of the SSV transforming gene, as well as to predict the structure of any protein it could encode, we established the primary nucleotide sequence of this gene (Devare et al., 1983). Examination of the region of SSV DNA to which its transforming gene had been localized indicated the presence of a long open reading frame. This reading frame initiated within SSAV sequences and terminated with an ochre codon within v-*sis* at position 4470 (Fig. 7). By sequence comparison with Moloney-MuLV, the open reading frame to the left of v-*sis* was identified as initiating from an internal stretch of the SSAV *env* gene. Moreover, sequence analysis of cloned SSAV DNA confirmed that this region codes for a portion of its *env* gene. The open reading frame of the SSAV *env* gene was identical from position 3657 to position 3810 at the 5′ end of the *sis* open reading frame (Devare et al., 1983). This stretch of sequences contained two more ATG codons in the same reading frame. One of these corresponded to the ATG codon that has been proposed as the initiator codon of the Moloney-MuLV *env* gene product (Shinnick et al., 1981). This initiator codon could be used for synthesis of the v-*sis* gene product from a spliced mRNA analogous to that used for the *env* gene products (Mellon and Duesberg, 1977; Rothenberg et al., 1978).

If the v-*sis* gene product were synthesized from the ATG at position 3657, a protein of approximtely 33,000 daltons containing 271 amino acids, would result. A v-*sis* gene product synthesized from the second or third ATG would result in proteins of around 30,000 or 26,000 daltons, respectively.

8. Detection of the SSV Transforming Gene Product

In order to confirm our sequence analysis of v-*sis*, as well as to develop antibodies capable of detecting the SSV transforming gene product, we synthesized peptides that represented amino and carboxy terminal regions of the putative v-*sis*-coded protein (Devare et al., 1983). Such peptides can be used as haptens to elicit antibodies capable of recognizing translational products in vivo (Walter et al., 1980; Sutcliffe et al., 1980). Serum against the amino terminal v-*sis* peptide, designated anti-*sis* N, as well as the carboxy terminal peptide, designated anti-*sis* C, were capable of recognizing a protein of 28,000 daltons specifically expressed in SSV transformed cells (Robbins et al., 1982a; Devare et al., 1983). These findings provided conclusive evidence that the SSV transforming gene directed the synthesis of a protein of 28,000 daltons (p28[sis]), which corresponded closely in size to the v-*sis* open reading frame.

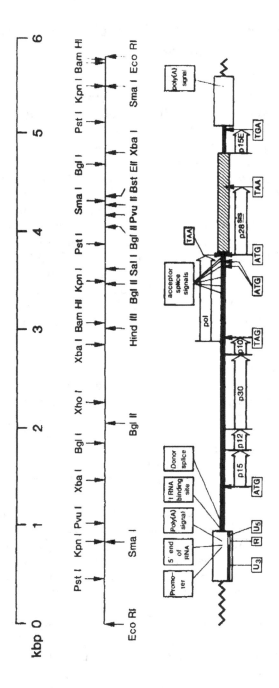

Fig. 7. Summary of the major structural features of the SSV genome. The v-*sis* long open reading frame, possible signals for promotion, and polyadenylation, as well as donor and acceptor splice signals, are illustrated.

9.   p28[sis] Is Related to Human Platelet-Derived Growth Factor

Independent investigations of the primary amino acid sequence of human platelet derived growth factor (PDGF) in combination with knowledge of the predicted amino acid sequence of p28[sis], have provided the first direct link between a transforming gene and a normal gene with known function (Antoniades and Hunkapiller, 1983; Doolittle et al., 1983; Waterfield et al., 1983).

Platelet-derived growth factor is a heat-stable (100°C), cationic (pI, 9.8) protein (Antoniades et al., 1979). It circulates in blood stored in the α granules of platelets and is released into serum during blood clotting (Kaplan et al., 1979). It represents the major protein growth factor of human serum and is a potent mitogen for connective tissue and glial cells in culture (Ross et al., 1974; Scher et al., 1979). Unreduced, biologically active PDGF exhibits multiple forms ranging in size from 28,000 to 35,000 daltons (Antoniades et al., 1979; Heldin et al., 1981; Deuel et al., 1981; Raines and Ross, 1982). Reduction of PDGF produces inactive, smaller peptides ranging in size from 12,000 to 18,000 daltons (Heldin et al., 1979).

Amino acid sequence analysis of the amino-terminal portions of both active human PDGF and its inactive reduced peptides revealed the presence of two related peptides (PDGF-1 and PDGF-2) in active PDGF preparations (Antoniades and Hunkapiller, 1983). These peptides were identical at eight of 19 positions near their amino termini, with no sequence gaps required for the homology alignment. Whether unreduced active PDGF is composed of homodimers, heterodimers, or a mixture of the two is not yet known.

A computer comparison of the PDGF amino trerminal sequences with the predicted amino acid sequence of p28[sis] revealed a striking similarity between these proteins (Doolittle et al., 1983). This similarity was discovered during a search for sequence homology between the PDGF amino-terminal sequences and other protein sequences in the Newat sequence database at the University of California, San Diego (Doolittle, 1981). Sequence comparisons with additional PDGF primary sequences obtained from peptide fragments generated by cyanogen promide cleavage of native PDGF further strengthened this relationship (Doolittle et al., 1983). Another group independently investigating PDGF structure has made similar conclusions (Waterfield et al., 1983).

The match between the 70 identified PDGF-2 residues and the corresponding segment of p28[sis] was 87.1%. Since v-sis arose from within the genome of a woolly monkey (Wong-Staal et al., 1981; Robbins et al., 1982a), a member of the family Cebidae (New World monkeys), and PDGF was isolated from human platelets, most, if not all, of the observed amino acid differences could represent species differences. This hypothesis is consistent with the known amino acid sequence similarity for myoglobin (90.8% identity) and fibrinopeptides A and B (70.0% identity) from humans and cebids (Doolittle, 1981). Moreover, seven of the nine observed differences can be derived from single base changes. This extensive sequence homology established that the v-*sis* transforming gene arose by viral recombination with a host-cell gene encoding PDGF or a very highly related protein.

10. Close Structural and Conformational Similarity Between the SSV Transforming Gene Product and Biologically Active PDGF

Utilizing antibodies against the amino and carboxy termini of the SSV transforming gene product, we were able to demonstrate that the primary translational product, p28^{sis}, of the SSV transforming gene undergoes cleavage to yield 11,000- and 20,000-dalton polypeptides, designated p11^{sis} and p20^{sis}, respectively (Robbins et al., 1983). The latter, which was shown to be derived from the carboxy terminus of p28^{sis}, is very similar in size to the inactive, reduced 18,000-dalton form of human PDGF-2. The sequence correspondence between PDGF-2 and the v-*sis* product beings at position 67. If cleavage of p28^{sis} were signaled by the two basic amino acids (lys:arg) at positions 65–66, a 160-residue protein, approximating p20^{sis} in its theoretical size, would result. Thus, p20^{sis} closely corresponds in size and amino acid sequence to that observed for PDGF-2.

Biologically active PDGF exhibits a dimeric structure that involves disulfide bonds. To determine whether v-*sis* translational products possessed a similar structure, we examined the electrophoretic mobility of p28^{sis} under nonreducing conditions. In the absence of reducing agents, p28^{sis} exhibited a molecular mass of 56,000 daltons (Fig. 8). Our observations that this polypeptide was detectable with antibodies to both N and C termini of p28^{sis} are most consistent with the possibility that p56^{sis} is a disulfide linked dimer of p28^{sis}. Evidence that the C but not N terminal *sis* antibodies also bound discretre *sis*-related polypeptides ranging in size

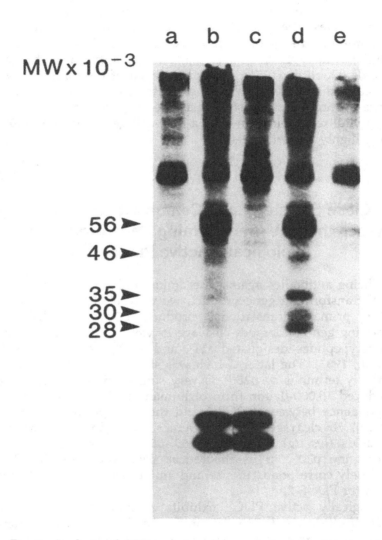

Fig. 8. Analysis of SSV transforming gene products in nonreducing conditions. Lysates of metabolically labeled SSV-transformed cells were immunoprecipitated with preimmune (lane a), anti-*sis*-N (lanes b, c) or anti-*sis* C (lanes d, e) serum. In some cases, antibodies were incubated before immunoprecipitation with 5 μg of *sis*-N (lane c) or *sis*-C (lane e) peptide. Immunoprecipitates were analyzed by SDS-PAGE in the absence of reducing agent.

from 28,000 to 46,000 daltons implied further processing of p56^{sis} to smaller forms, some of which closely resembled the sizes of unreduced PDGF.

11. Anti-PDGF Serum Recognizes SSV Transforming Gene Products

Additional evidence of the close conformational similarity between the v-sis-coded proteins and PDGF has derived from immunological studies. Anti-PDGF serum was shown to recognize p28^{sis}, as well as the processed unreduced forms of the protein recognized by the anti-sis-C peptide serum (Robbins et al., 1983). In addition, anti-PDGF recognized a 24,000-dalton protein not detected with either anti-sis N or C peptide sera. Pulse chase analysis using anti-PDGF serum established p56^{sis} as a rapidly formed dimer of p28^{sis}. It was possible to demonstrate further processing in which p24^{sis} emerged as the most stable product of the SSV transforming gene detectable with the available antisera. Figure 9 summarizes our present knowledge concerning processing of the SSV transforming gene product. The dimeric nature of the SSV transforming gene product, as well as its rapid proteolytic processing, are consistent with the known dimeric structure and susceptibility to proteolysis of PDGF. Such structural homologies imply that SSV transformation involves constitutive expression of a protein possessing striking similarities to PDGF.

12. The Human c-sis Locus

In the human, the c-sis proto-oncogene is located on chromosome 22 (Swan et al., 1982; Dalla Favera et al., 1982) and is expressed in a majority of fibrosarcomas and glioblastomas, but not normal fibroblasts (Eva et al., 1982). We have isolated DNA clones that comprise all of the human sequences homologous to v-sis. In an effort to better understand the structural relationship between this human proto-oncogene and the gene(s) encoding PDGF, we determined the nucleotide sequence of the v-sis-related regions present in these clones. The results of these studies revealed a coding sequence comprising five exons which, if contiguous, would correspond to the complete v-sis coding sequence (Devare et al., 1983). Moreover, the predicted amino acid sequen-

p28$^{\underline{sis}}$ PROCESSING

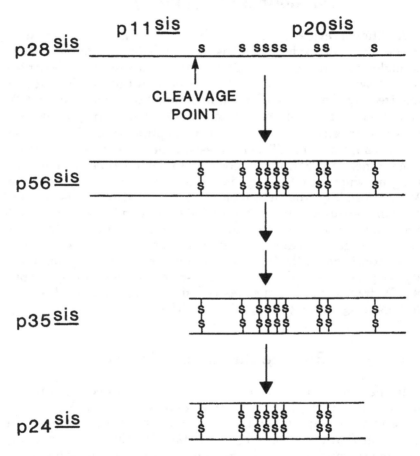

Fig. 9. Pulse chase analysis of v-*sis* translational products. SSV-transformed cells were pulsed labeled for 15 min with [^{35}S]-methionine and cysteine and chased for periods of 0–105 min. Immediately after the chase period, cells were washed in ice-cold PBS and disrupted. Cell lysates were immunoprecipitated with anti-PDGF or normal rabbit serum and immunoprecipitates were analyzed by SDS-PAGE in the absence of reducing agent. A representation of the results from this experiment is shown.

ceof the human c-*sis* gene product corresponded in 102 of the 104 positions determined for PDGF polypeptide chain 2 (Fig. 10). These findings demonstrated that human c-*sis* is the structural gene for one of the two polypeptides of this potent mitogen, and define, for the first time, a normal biologic function for a proto-oncogene.

13.   Mechanism of SSV Transformation

The profound alterations in normal growth regulation induced by the cell-derived transforming genes of retroviruses have many

```
                  ┌►(v-sis-helper virus junction)    ┌►(exon 2)            60
p28sis            MTLTWQGDPI PEELYKMLSG HSIRSFDDLQ RLLQGDSGKE DGAELDLNMT RSHSGGELES
c-sis             ***** *****E***D ********** ***H**P*E* ********** **********


                    ┌►(exon 3)                                            120
p28sis            LARGKRSLGS LSVAEPAMIA ECKTRTEVFE ISRRLIDRTN ANFLVWPPCV EVQRCSGCCN
c-sis             ****R***** *TI******* ********** ********** ********** **********
PDGF-2                 **** *TI******* *****E***C *C***?**?? ??????**** **K**T****
PDGF-1                      SI*E*VP* V****IVIY* ****EL*??? ****
Peptide I              **** *TI******* ********** *******
Peptide II                  SI*E*VP* V*****VIY* *P*SQV*P*S ********** *
Peptide III                                     *S ********** **********
Peptide IV                                      *T ********** **********


                       ┌►(exon 4)                                         180
p28sis            NRNVQCRPTQ VQLRPVQVRK IEIVRKKPIF KKATVTLEDH LACKCEIVAA ARAVTRSPGT
c-sis             ********** ********** ********** ********** ******T*** **P*****G
PDGF-2            ****K***S* *****?**** ******
Peptide III       ********** ***?***
Peptide IV        ********** ********** **
Peptide V                             ***** ***?*?**** *****?**** *


                    ┌►(exon 5)                       226
p28sis            SQEQRAKTTQ SRVTIRTVRV RRPPKGKHRK CKHTHDKTAL KETLGAtrm
c-sis             ********P* T********* ********** F********* ******trm
```

Fig. 10. Comparison of the predicted amino acid sequences of v-*sis* with that of human c-*sis* and with the protein sequence data of PDGF peptides. The amino acid sequences of PDGF-1 and -2 are from Antoniades and Hunkapiller (1983) and those of peptides I–V are from Waterfield et al. (1983). The locations of c-*sis* exons are indicated by arrows. Amino acid numbers start from the first methionine of v-*sis*. Asterisks indicate identity with p28[sis].

similarities to the growth promoting actions of certain hormones and growth factors. Each exerts pleiotropic effects on cellular metabolism and possesses the ability to induce sustained cell replication. Our studies have revealed a high degree of relatedness between the transforming gene product of a primate sarcoma virus and a potent growth factor for human fibroblasts, smooth muscle cells, and glial cells. Thus, as depicted in Fig. 11, the mechanism by which this *onc* gene transforms cells may involve the constitutive expression of a protein with functions very similar to those of PDGF.

Recent studies have provided an additional link between growth factors and oncogenes. Purification of the cellular receptor for epidermal growth factor (EGF) has led to the elucidation of a portion of its amino acid sequence. A computer search has revealed a very close similarity between the EGF receptor and the product of the *erb-B onc* gene (Downward et al., 1984). Thus, transformation by another acute transforming retrovirus may also involve pathways through which growth factors exert their proliferative effects.

A major family of *onc* genes codes for protein kinases with specificity for phosphorylation of tyrosine residues (Weiss et al., 1982); another has an associated GTP-binding (guanosine triphosphate) activity (Shih et al., 1979). Moreover, previous computer searches have revealed distant homology between the *src* gene product and cyclic adenosine monophosphate kinase (Barker and Dayhoff, 1982) and possibly between the *Blym* gene product and transferrin (Goubin et al., 1983). Although these relationships are very distant, it is possible that other proteins with growth regulatory functions may be found to correspond to the products of known or as yet uncharacterized *onc* genes. The continued search for relationships of this kind will be of obvious interest and importance.

There have been reports of human osteosarcoma and blioblastoma cell lines that release PDGF-like ppolypeptides (Heldin et al., 1980; Nister et al., 1982; Graves et al., 1983). Moreover, *sis*-related transcripts have been detected frequently in human tumors of connective tissue origin, but not in normal fibroblasts (Eva et al., 1982). Thus, it is possible that activation of *sis* transcription alone or in combination with other genetic alterations affecting the *sis* structural locus may cause the sustained abnormal proliferation of human cells responsive to the growth stimulatory effects of a PDGF-like molecule. If so, *sis* activation may be a step in the processes leading normal human cells of certain tissue types toward malignancy.

NORMAL WOUND HEALING

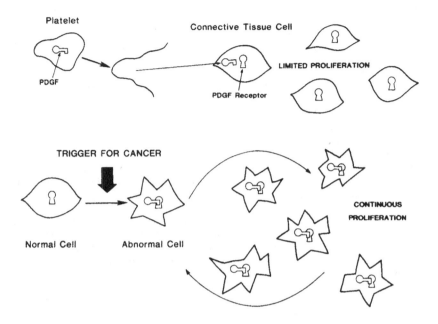

Fig. 11. Possible mechanism of SSV-induced transformation compared to normal PDGF function.

References

Aaronson, S. A. (1973), Biologic characterization of mammalian cells transformed by a primate sarcoma virus. *Virology* 52, 562–567.

Aaronson, S. A., J. R. Stephenson, S. Hino, and S. R. Tronick (1975), Differential expression of helper viral structural polypeptides in cells transformed by clonal isolates of woolly monkey sarcoma virus. *J. Virol.* 16, 1117–1123.

Antoniades, H. N., C. D. Scher, and C. D. Stiles (1979), Purification of human platelet-derived growth factor. *Proc. Natl. Acad. Sci. USA* 76, 1809–1813.

Antoniades, H. N. and M. W. Hunkapiller (1983), Human platelet-derived growth factor (PDGF): Amino terminal amino acid sequence. *Science* 220, 963–965.

Barker, W. C. and M. O. Dayhoff (1982), Viral *src* gene products are related to the catalytic chain of mammalian cAMP-dependent protein kinase. *Proc. Natl. Acad. Sci. USA* 79, 2836–2839.

Dalla Favera R., R. C. Gallo, A. Giallongo, and C. M. Croce (1982), Chromosomal localization of the human homolog (c-*sis*) of the simian sarcoma virus *onc* gene. *Science* 218, 686–688.

Deuel, T. F., J. S. Huang, R. T. Proffit, U. U. Baenziger, D. Chang, and B. B. Kennedey (1981), Human platelet-derived growth factor. Purification and resolution into two active protein fractions.*J. Biol. Chem.* 256, 8896–8899.

Devare, S. G., E. P. Reddy, J. D. Law, K. C. Robbins, and S. A. Aaronson (1983), Nucleotide sequence of the simian sarcoma virus genome: Demonstration that its acquired cellular sequences encode the transforming gene product, p28^{sis}. *Proc. Natl. Acad. Sci. USA* **80**, 731–735.

Dhar, R., W. L. McClements, L. W. Enquist, and G. W. Vande Woude (1980), Nucleotide sequences of integrated Moloney sarcoma provirus long terminal repeats and their host and viral junctions. *Proc. Natl. Acad. Sci. USA* **77**, 3937–3941.

Doolittle, R. F. (1981), Similar amino acid sequences: Chance or common ancestry. *Science* **214**, 149–159.

Doolittle, R. F., M. W. Hunkapiller, L. E. Hood, S. G. Devare, K. C. Robbins, S. A. Aaronson, and H. N. Antoniades (1983), Simian sarcoma virus *onc* gene, v-*sis*, is derived from the gene (or genes) encoding a platelet-derived growth factor. *Science* **221**, 275–277.

Downward, J., Y. Yarden, E. Mayes, G. Scrace, P.Totty, P. Stockwell, A. Ullrich, J. Schlessinger, and M. D. Waterfield (1984), Close similarity of epidermal growth factor receptor and v-*erb-B* oncogene protein sequences. *Nature* **307**, 521–527.

Eva, A. K. C. Robbins, P. R. Andersen, A. Srinivasan, S. R. Tronick, E. P. Reddy, N. W. Ellmore, A. T. Galen, J. A. Lautenberger, T. S. Papas, E. H. Westin, F. Wong-Staal, R. C. Gallo, and S. A. Aaronson (1982), Cellular genes analogous to retroviral *onc* genes are transcribed in human tumor cells. *Nature* (Lond.) **295**, 116–119.

Goubin, G., D. F. Goldman, J. Luce, P. E. Neiman, and G. M. Cooper (1983), Molecular cloning and nucleotide sequence of a transforming gene detected by transfection of chicken B-cell lymphoma DNA. *Nature* (Lond.) **302**, 114–119.

Graham, F. L. and A. J. van der Eb (1973), A new technique for the assay of infectivity of human adenovirus 5 DNA. *Virology* **52**, 456–467.

Graves, D. T., A. J. Owen, and H. N. Antoniades (1983), Evidence that a human osteosarcoma cell line which secretes a mitogen similar to platelet-derived growth factor requires growth factors present in platelet-poor plasma. *Cancer Res.* **43**, 83–87.

Heldin, C. H., B. Westermark, and A. Wasteson (1979), Platelet-derived growth factor: Purification and partial characterization. *Proc. Natl. Acad. Sci. USA* **76**, 3722–3726.

Heldin, C. H., B. Westermark, and A. Wasteson (1980), Chemical and biological properties of a growth factor from human-cultured osteosarcoma cells: Resemblance with platelet-derived growth factor. *J. Cell. Phys.* **105**, 235–246.

Heldin, C. H., B. Westermark, and A. Wasteson (1981), Demonstration of antibody against platelet-derived growth factor. *Exp. Cell. Res.* **136**, 255–261.

Kaplan, D. R., F. C. Chao, C. D. Stiles, H. N. Antoniades, and C. D. Sher (1979), Platelet alpha-granules contain a growth factor for fibroblasts. *Blood* **53**, 1043–1052.

Mellon, P. and P. H. Duesberg (1977), Subgenomic, cellular Rous sarcoma virus RNAS contain oligonucleotides from the 3' half and the 5' terminus of virion RNA. *Nature* **270**, 631–634.

Nister, M., C. H. Heldin, A. Wateson, and B. Westermark (1982), A platelet-derived growth factor analog produced by a human clonal glioma cell line. *Ann. NY Acad. Sci.* **397**, 25–33.

Raines, E. W., and R. Ross (1982), Platelet-derived growth factor I. High yield purification and evidence for multiple forms. *J. Biol. Chem.* **257**, 5154–5160.

Robbins, K. C., S. G. Devare and S. A. Aaronson (1981), Molecular cloning of integrated simian sarcoma virus: Genome organization of infectious DNA clones. *Proc. Natl. Acad. Sci. USA* **78**, 2918–2922.

Robbins, K. C., H. N. Antoniades, S. G. Devare, M. W. Hunkapiller, and S. A. Aaronson (1983), Structural and immunological similarities between simian sarcoma virus gene product(s) and human platelet-derived growth factor. *Nature* (Lond.) **305**, 605–608.

Robbins, K. C., S. G. Devare, E. P. Reddy, and S. A. Aaronson (1982a), In vivo identification of the transforming gene product of simian sarcoma virus. *Science* **218**, 1131–1133.

Robbins, K. C., R. L. Hill, and S. A. Aaronson (1982b), Primate origin of the cell-derived sequences of simian sarcoma virus. *J. Virol.* **41**, 721–725.

Ross, R. J. Glomset, B. Kariya, and L. Harker (1974), A platelet-dependent serum factor that stimulates the proliferation of arterial smooth muscle cells in vitro. *Proc. Natl. Acad. Sci. USA* **71**, 1207–1210.

Rothenberg, E., D. J. Donoghue, and D. Baltimore (1978), Analysis of a 5' leader sequence on murine leukemia virus 21S RNA: Heteroduplex mapping with long reverse transcriptase products. *Cell* **13**, 435–451.

Scher, C. D., R. C. Shepard, H. N. Antoniades, and C. D. Stiles (1979), Platelet-derived growth factor and the regulation of the mammalian fibroblast cell cycle. *Biochim. Biophys. Acta* **560**, 217–241.

Shih, T. Y., M. O. Weeks, H. A. Young, and E. M. Scolnick (1979), Identification of a sarcoma virus-coded phosphoprotein in nonproducer cells transformed by Kirsten or Harvey murine sarcoma virus. *Virology* **96**, 64–79.

Shimotohno, K., S. Mizutani, and H. M. Temin (1980) Sequence of retrovirus provirus resembles that of bacterial transposable elements. *Nature (Lond.)* **285**, 550–554.

Shinnick, T. M., R. A. Lerner and J. G. Sutcliffe (1981) Nucleotide sequence of Moloney murine leukemia virus. *Nature* (Lond.) **293**, 543–548.

Sutcliffe, J. G., T. M. Shinnick, N. Green, F. T. Liu, H. L. Niman, and R. A. Lerner (1980), Chemical synthesis of a polypeptide predicted from nucleotide sequence allows detection of a new retroviral gene product. *Nature* (Lond.) **287**, 801–805.

Swan, D., O. W. McBride, K. C. Robbins, D. A. Keithley, E. P. Reddy, and S. A. Aaronson (1982), Chromosomal mapping of the simian sarcoma virus *onc* gene analog in human cells. *Proc. Natl. Acad. Sci. USA* **79**, 4691–4695.

Theilen, G. H., D. Gould, M. Fowler, and D. L. Dungworth (1971), C-type cirus in tumor tissue of a woolly monkey *(Lagothrix spp.)* with fibrosarcoma. *J. Natl. Cancer Inst.* **47**, 881–899.

Walter, G., K. H. Scheidtmann, A. Carbone, A. P. Laudano, and R. F. Doolittle (1980), Antibodies specific for the carboxy- and amino-terminal regions of simian virus 40 large tumor antigen. *Proc. Natl. Acad. Sci. USA* **77**, 5197–5200.

Waterfield, M. D., G. T. Scrace, N. Whittle, P. Stroobant, A. Johnsson, A. Wasteson, B. Westermark, C. H. Heldin, J. S. Huang, and T. F. Deuel (1983), Platelet-derived growth factor is structurally related to the putative transforming protein p28[sis] of simiansarcoma virus. *Nature* **304**, 35–39.

Weiss, R., N. Teich, H. Varmus, and J. Coffin, Eds. (1982), *RNA Tumor Viruses* (2nd ed.). Cold Spring Harbor Laboratory, Cold Spring Harbor, NY.

Wigler, M., S. Silverstein, L. S. Lee, A. Pellicer, Y. Cheng, and R. Axel (1977), Transferof purified herpes virus thymidine kinase gene to cultured mouse cells. *Cell* **11**, 223–232.

Wolfe, L. G., F. Deinhardt, G. J. Theilen, H. Rabin, T. Kawakami, and L. K. Bustad (1971), Induction of tumors in marmoset monkeys by simiansarcoma virus, Type 1 (*Lagothrix*): A preliminary report. *J. Natl. Cancer Inst.* **47**, 1115–1120.

Wolfe, L. G., R. K. Smith, and F. Deinhardt (1972), Simian sarcoma virus type 1 (*Lagothrix*): Focus assay and demonstration of nontransforming associated virus. *J. Natl. Cancer Inst.* **48**, 1905–1907.

Wong-Staal, F., R. Dalla Favera, E. P. Gelmann, V. Manzari, S. Szala, S. F. Josephs, and R. C. Gallo (1981), The v-*sis* transforming gene of simian sarcoma virus is a new *onc* gene or primate origin. *Nature* (Lond.) **294**, 273–275.

Detection of HSV-2 Genes and Gene Products in Cervical Neoplasia

Cecilia M. Fenoglio-Preiser and
James K. McDougall

1. Introduction

In considering the etiology of cervical cancer, it is wise to keep in mind that it is probably not sufficient that one be exposed to a single oncogenic agent. Rather, it appears that there may be interaction between a potential oncogenic agent(s) and other predisposing factors. Cervical neoplasia may be the result of long-standing interactions between numerous factors that we can dissect to determine the role of putative oncogenic agents or other factors that may modify the ability of oncogenic agents to induce neoplasms. When one considers any of the potential oncogenic agents, either alone or in combination, one must account for the observation that the majority of cervical cancers arise within the transformation zone (Richart, 1973), despite the fact that the entire cervix is presumably exposed to these oncogenic agent(s) (Fenoglio and Ferenczy, 1982). There appears to be a unique sensitivity of the epithelium within the transformation zone for the subsequent development of neoplasms, relative to the rest of the cervix. We will come back to this observation when we discuss postulated mechanisms for the induction of cervical cancers, after surveying the epidemiology of cervical neoplasia. herpes genital infections in general, cervical neoplasia in general, and studies linking HSV-2 to cervical neoplasia.

2. Etiologic Factors

2.1. Sexual Factors

The etiologic factors have recently been surveyed (Fenoglio and Ferenczy, 1982), and they include epidemiologic factors (socioeconomic status, age, sexual factors, age at first marriage, age at first pregnancy, age at first intercourse, marital instability), hereditary factors, the influence of the male, chemical factors, radiation, infectious agents, immunologic factors, and other, undefined factors.

2.2. Epidemiologic Factors

A number of epidemiologic factors have been postulated to play a role in the induction of cervical neoplasia (Table 1).

Patients with a low socioeconomic status have a higher prevalence of cervical neoplasia than individuals in higher income groups (Clemmesen and Nielsen, 1951; Graham et al., 1960; DeVessa and Diamond, 1980). In addition, people in low-income brackets tend to have a higher mortality than those in the high-income brackets (Wakefield et al., 1973; Beral, 1974).

With respect to race, religion, and culture, the Third National Cancer Survey performed in the United States found a higher incidence rate of carcinoma *in situ* and invasive carcinoma of the cervix in blacks than in whites (DeVessa and Diamond, 1980; Henson and Tarone, 1977). Waki et al. (1969) compared a Hindu and Moslem population and found a lower incidence of cervical cancer among the Moslems than the Hindus. It was postulated that this

Table 1
Epidemiologic Factors in Cervical Neoplasia

Low socioeconomic status
Circumcisional status of male patient
Race, religion, culture
Association with "high risk" male
Early age of first pregnancy
Marital instability
Multiple sexual partners
Early sexual activity
Promiscuity
Smoking

might be related to the circumcisional status of the Moslems (Hindus are uncircumcised). Jordan and Key (1981) studied the incidence of cervical neoplasia in the Southwest part of the United States and found that in patients under 35 yr of age, cervical carcinoma was more frequent among American Indians and Spanish American whites than among other women. In patients who were 60 and older, the Indian cervical cancer rate was much higher than in the non-Indian population.

Of all postulated factors, sexual activity has the strongest association with the subsequent development of cervical carcinoma. Age at first intercourse, number of pregnancies, marital stability, circumcisional status of the male, frequency of intercourse, and exposure to "high risk" males are all correlated with an increased incidence of cervical neoplasia.

Attention was brought to the importance of sexual factors in the genesis of this disorder by Gagnon (1950), who studied 13,000 Canadian nuns and found no cases of cervical cancer. Other studies have subsequently demonstrated that fewer cases of cervical cancer are found among unmarried than married women (Doll et al., 1966; Terris, 1967).

Early age at first marriage and first pregnancy, both of which have been associated with an increased incidence of cervical neoplasia (Terris et al., 1967; Boyd and Doll, 1964; Beral, 1974; Christopherson and Parker, 1965; Barron and Richart, 1971), are essentially related to age at first intercourse, which appears to be the single most important factor in the genesis of cervical neoplasia (Martin, 1967). This risk is enhanced by increased numbers of pregnancies (Barron and Richart, 1971; Maliphant, 1949; Singer, 1976).

Marital instability, including separation, divorce, widowhood, extramarital sexual activity, and numerous marriages, is also associated with an increased risk of cervical neoplasia (Fasal et al., 1981; Martin, 1967; Kessler, 1976). All of the above-mentioned studies suggest that there is a positive correlation between sexual activity and the subsequent development of cervical neoplasia (Fenoglio and Ferenczy, 1982; Rotkin, 1973; Swan and Brown, 1981).

2.3. Male Role

Rotkin (1973) viewed the female at risk as the host, the male coital partner as the donor, and the intervening vector as his "contribution." The nature of the contribution is poorly understood. In 1936, Handley studied the incidence of cervical cancer among Fijians who were circumcised and lived side-by-side with an uncircumcised Indian population and found that the uncircumcised Indians had more cervical cancer than the Fijians, suggesting that circumcisional status was important. It was postulated that smegma, which accumulates in the uncircumcised male, is responsible for transmitting an "oncogenic" agent.

More recently, it has been demonstrated that there is a strong association of cervical cancer in women whose sexual partners have genital cancers, particularly of the penis (Graham et al., 1979; Graham and Schotz, 1979; Martinez, 1969). In 1976, Kessler demonstrated that the incidence of cervical cancer in second (or third) wives of males whose first or second wife had had cervical cancer was increased over that occurring in the control population, suggesting that the husbands might be transmitting an infectious agent from the first or second wife to the second or third wife. Thus, the recommendation that condoms be used in sexually active couples (Richardson and Lyon, 1981) to help control or prevent cervical neoplasia is based on the belief that an oncogenic agent is venereally transmitted from the male to the female.

2.4. Hereditary Factors

Stern et al. (1967) suggested that there was a hereditary predisposition for the development of cervical cancer, but subsequent twin studies have not been able to confirm these results (Nielsen and Clemmesen, 1957; Harvald and Hauge, 1963).

If genetic influences are involved in carcinogenesis of the cervix, they are undoubtedly subtle and involve factors such as immune response genes with potentially increased susceptibility to certain infections or an inability to combat them once acquired. Alternatively, there may be a failure to effectively eliminate neoplastic cells caused by a localized immunosuppression or faulty immune responses (Fenoglio and Ferenczy, 1982).

2.5. Chemical Factors

In many systems, chemicals are known to be carcinogenic. It is, therefore, not surprising that numerous chemical compounds have been studied with respect to their oncogenic properties in the cervix. These studies usually utilize a variety of laboratory animals with the application of the potential carcinogen to cervical epithelium. This results in the production of a variety of lesions that range from cervical atypias to invasive carcinomas. The most commonly utilized agents involve methylcholanthrene or 3,4-benzypyrene. Other substances that have been studied include oral contraceptive hormones, which have led to conflicting conclusions.

These studies are summarized in a previous publication (Fenoglio and Ferenczy, 1982).

2.6. Radiation

Dysplasias following irradiation for cervical carcinoma were originally described in 1963 by Patten et al. (1963). Dysplasia occurs in approximately a quarter of the cases and does not usually follow pelvic irradiation for other diseases. The pathogenesis of the epithelial abnormality in this setting is unclear, but the dysplasia that is produced is histologically similar to that present in the nonirradiated cervix (Patten et al., 1963; Wentz and Reagan, 1970).

2.7. Infectious Agents

Given that the epidemiologic observations indicate that cervical neoplasia has many attributes of a communicable disease, the most serious contenders for an etiologic agent have been infectious agents. Numerous viruses, bacteria, chlamydiae, mycoplasmas, parasites, and fungi are known to be venereally transmitted. Of these, certain organisms have had their period in the investigational limelight. *Trichomonas vaginalis* produces epithelial atypia upon repeated intravaginal inoculations (Patten et al., 1963; Frost, 1961). Syphilis and chlamydiae have also been incriminated as potential etiologic agents since an increased incidence of these infections has been found in patients with cervical neoplasias as compared to control populations (Clemmesen, 1965; Rojel, 1953; Schachter et al., 1975).

However, viruses are the leading contenders for a major role in the induction of neoplasia since they have a documented ability to cause tumors in animals. The viruses most seriously considered to play a role as potential carcinogens in the induction of cervical cancer are HSV-2 and human papillomavirus (HPV). Recent epidemiologic, colposcopic, and cytopathologic studies have focused attention on the high prevalence of condylomatous lesions of the cervix in sexually active women. It is known that condylomas are associated with the presence of human papillomavirus, and the sudden increase of cervical condylomata appears to be related to an increase in the clinical and pathological awareness of this lesion, rahter than an increase in incidence (Fenoglio and Ferenczy, 1982). In fact, many cervical lesions that had been previously interpreted as intraepithelial neoplasia grade 1 (mild dysplasia) have been reinterpreted as flat variants of cervical condyloma acuminatum. The flat condyloma, which is also known as condyloma planum or non-condylomatous cervical wart virus infection, cannot be seen with the naked eye, but can be detected by exfoliative cytology or colposcopy (Fenoglio and Ferenczy, 1982). These lesions contain evidence of viral antigens and viral particles as seen by electron microscopy (Woodruff et al., 1980; Kurman et al., 1981; Della Torre et al., 1978; Hills and Laverty, 1979). HPV viral infections and their ability to cause cancer are the subject of another chapter in this book. The role of herpesviruses and cervical neoplasia is discussed below.

3. Herpes Genitalis Infections

The relationship of herpes simplex virus (HSV) infections and cervical neoplasia has been recently summarized (Fenoglio et al., 1982). HSV infections have been known for centuries, but it was only in the 1960s that Schneweis and Brandes (1961) and Nahmias et al. (1967) confirmed that infections of the genital region are predominantly herpesvirus type 2 (HSV-2) and primarily involve postpubertal individuals, are venereally transmitted, and are usually seen in sexually active adults of either sex. HSV-2 causes approximately 32% of all human herpetic infections and 85% of venereal herpetic infections (Solontis and Jeansson, 1977). In recent years there has been an increase in incidence of female genital herpes, requiring much more emphasis on the importance of these lesions in a gynecologic practice. A recent national survey evaluating data from a random sample of patient consultations with physicians in an office-based practice in the United States indicates that patient consultation for genital herpes increased from 3.4/100,000 in 1960 to 29.7/100,000 in 1979 (Centers for Disease Control, 1982). In some patient populations, herpes infections are the most commonly encountered sexually transmitted disease (Sumaya et al., 1980).

It is likely that genital herpes infections will develop in females who have had sexual contact with males with active genital herpes infections. Deardourff et al. (1974) recovered HSV from 15% of 273 randomly selected males without a past history of herpes infection. The male may act as a reservoir for HSV infections, and recovery of the virus from prostatic fluid or vas deferens is possible (Deardourff et al., 1974). Furthermore, it is possible to demonstrate HSV-2 viral RNA within the epithelium of prostatic tissues (Fenoglio et al., 1982).

In the western world, HSV is now the most common cause for isolated genital ulcerations, accounting for 20–50% of such lesions in patients attending a sexually transmitted disease clinic (Chappel et al., 1978; Friedrich et al., 1979; Corey and Holmes, 1983). During the acute viral infection, a variety of clinical manifestations may be evident, including fever, headache, malaise, and myalgias. The predominant local symptoms include pain, itching, dysuria, vaginal or uretheral discharge, and tender inguinal adenopathy. The genital lesions are usually painful, with the severity of local symptoms increasing during the first week of the illness and gradually receding during the second week (Corey et al., 1983).

Following the acute infection, cervical vaginal shedding of HSV occurs and continues even after the genital symptoms regress. The quantity of virus shed during the primary genital infection appears to be higher than that during subsequent asymptomatic viral shedding in the same individual (Vontver et al., 1979). Herpes simplex virus can be isolated from the cervix, often in the absence of genital symptoms, from between 2–8% of women attending sexually transmitted disease clinics (Nahmias et al., 1967; Wentworth et al., 1973). The duration of the pain and lesions, and the length of time of viral shedding is significantly longer in the initial, rather than the recurrent, genital infections. Symptomatic primary infections usually occur within 3–7 d following exposure (Centifanto et al., 1972).

3.1. Productive Infections

Herpesvirus infections normally result in the production of live replicating virus particles that are released from the cell (Fig. 1). Productive infections are cytopathic to cells and are recognizable clinically or cytologically by virtue of characteristic features. Acute productive infections are highly cytopathic, result in the symptoms noted above, and are associated with the development of vesicles and ulcers.

The individual's antibody status is an important determinant of the risk of recurrence and the clinical severity of the acute disease (Sabin, 1975). Previous exposure to either HSV-1 or -2 results in the generation of herpes-specific antibodies that may modify the clinical response to HSV-2 infections. The neutralizing antibodies are produced in response to viral structural or nonstructural antigens and result in more efficient modulation of the disease if present (Anderson et al., 1974). In some individuals, recurrent lesions develop even in the presence of specific neutralizing antibo-

HSV
INFECTIONS

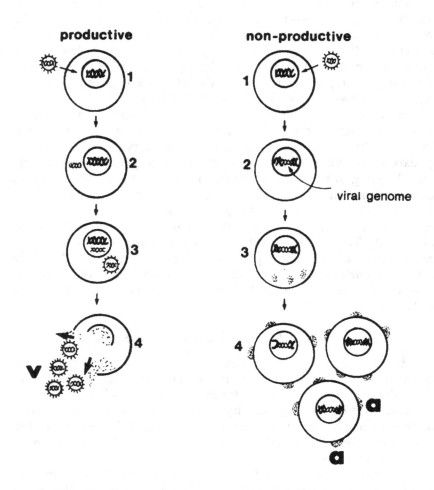

Fig. 1. Diagrammatic representation of productive and nonproductive HSV infections. Productive infections result in the release of viral progeny (v). Nonproductive infections do not result in the release of viruses, but viral antigens (a) may be detected in or on the cells.

dies (Sabin, 1975). These recurrences can be the result of either a reinfection or the activation of the latent state (Underwood and Weed, 1974).

Acute infections are usually associated with cytolysis from the severe cytopathic effects induced by the virus. Cytologic examination is routinely used in many laboratories for diagnosing acute herpes infections, but this is not as sensitive as isolating the virus from the lesions or the use of immunohistological techniques (Corey and Holmes, 1983).

The cytological manifestations of an acute infection progress in a sequential manner, with the first visible change being marked cytoplasmic and nuclear hypertrophy, followed by nuclear and cytoplasmic edema and the appearance of a perinuclear halo. The nucleoli enlarge and the nucleoplasm becomes granular with ribonucleoprotein bodies within the nucleoplasm. At this time, the nucleoli degenerate. Simultaneously, the cytoplasmic ground substance becomes denser, opaque, and appears purple or bluish-green with the Papanicolau stain. These changes are related to altered protein and RNA synthesis in the cells. As the nucleoli disappear, there is progressive increase in the number of ribonucleoprotein bodies (B bodies) (Kotcher et al., 1972).

The cytologic diagnosis of genital herpes infections is facilitated by the recognition of multinucleated giant cells in the pap smears. They were first described in 1963 by Stern and Long who realized their potential value as markers of a viral infection (Frost, 1961). These giant cells form as a result of cell fusion, with resulting large syncytial epithelial cell masses that may contain up to 30 nuclei. The enlarged nuclei appear to be packed with small acidophilic bodies so that a distinct homogeneous ground glass texture is seen under low magnification. When these granules coalesce and move toward the center of the nuclei, they form the typical single, coarsely granular acidophilic intranuclear inclusion known as the Cowdry A inclusion (Fig. 2) (Naib, 1976; Ng et al., 1970).

According to Ng et al. (1970), about 80% of infected cells in acute HSV infections display the characteristic ground glass nuclei. This contrasts with recurrent disease, in which ground glass nuclei are found in only approximately 50% of the cases.

The histological features of acute HSV infections include the presence of pronounced ulcerated lesions and intact vesicles. The histological criteria for making the diagnosis are similar to those used cytologically (Tobin et al., 1979).

3.2. Latent Infections

Herpesviruses are the prototype of viruses that may exist in a latent form and then become activated to produce recurrent infections. Indeed, recurrence is the clinical hallmark of these infections.

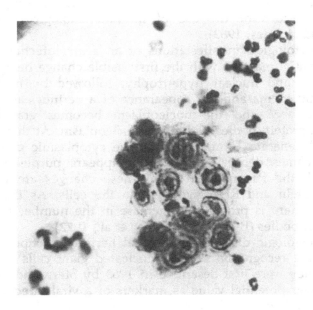

Fig. 2. Cervical smear with cells containing typical HSV inclusions.

After the primary infection, the virus may remain in cells in the latent state. The exact site of this latency is controversial, but is thought to be sensory ganglia or epithelium (Fenoglio et al., 1982; Galloway et al., 1979, 1982). Stevens defined a *latent infection* as a persistent infection in which the infectious agent is not present, or is present only intermittently, in tissues harboring the viral genome in a "reactivatable" state (Stevens, 1978a, b; Stevens et al., 1976). This contrasts with *persistent infections*, which are defined as those in which the virus, or at least the viral genome, is retained in the asymptomatic host for a long time, and *chronic infections*, in which the persistent infection is present but infectious virus can be recovered utilizing conventional virologic methods from the appropriate tissues at any given time.

4. Pathologic Features of Cervical Neoplasia

Cervical neoplasia constitutes a spectrum of malignancy ranging from cervical intraepithelial neoplasia through microinvasive
carcinoma to invasive carcinoma and metastatic cancer. The first
step in transformation of cervical cells to the neoplastic state
involves the formation of cervical intraepithelial neoplasia. This is
a generic term used to describe the changes previously diagnosed
as dysplasia through carcinoma *in situ*. Cervical intraepithelial neoplasia is characterized by an intraepithelial proliferation of neoplastic cells that are confined to the area above the plane of the basement membrane of the cervical epithelium. Immature neoplastic
cells of the intraepithelial neoplasias are distinguishable from the
immature cells of squamous metaplasia by virtue of the cellular
pleomorphism, irregular and atypical mitotic figures, poorly
developed cellular boundaries, and irregular distribution of the
cells in the neoplastic (Fig. 3), as compared to the metaplastic state
(Fig. 4).

Microinvasive carcinoma occurs when the neoplastic cells
transgress the plane of the basement membrane of either the surface epithelium or the underlying glandular epithelium. It includes
invasive foci with extension into the underlying stroma up to, and
including, a depth of 3 mm. Invasive carcinoma consists of any
neoplastic epithelial squamous cell population that extends more
than 3 mm into the underlying cervical stroma and can invade
widely into surrounding tissues, such as rectum, urinary bladder,
and so on. Metastatic disease occurs when the neoplastic cells are
present at noncontiguous sites, such as regional lymph nodes, liver,
and so on.

Traditionally, cervical intraepithelial neoplasia was considered
to be a two-disease system, consisting of carcinoma *in situ*, in
which the entire thickness of the cervical epithelium was involved
with neoplastic cells, and dysplasia, which included those situations in which the epithelium was involved to a lesser extent. Dysplasia was considered to be a cancer precursor and was subdivided
into mild, moderate, and severe. Many of the assumptions on
which this two-disease system were based have been reexamined,
and the data currently suggests that the precursor lesions form a
continuum that begins with the equivalent of mild dysplasia (CIN
1) and ends with, but does not include, microinvasive carcinoma.
These studies include ultrastructural examination, investigations on
cell contact inhibition and tissue culture, cellular kinetic studies
utilizing tritiated thymidine, chromosomal analysis, nuclear DNA

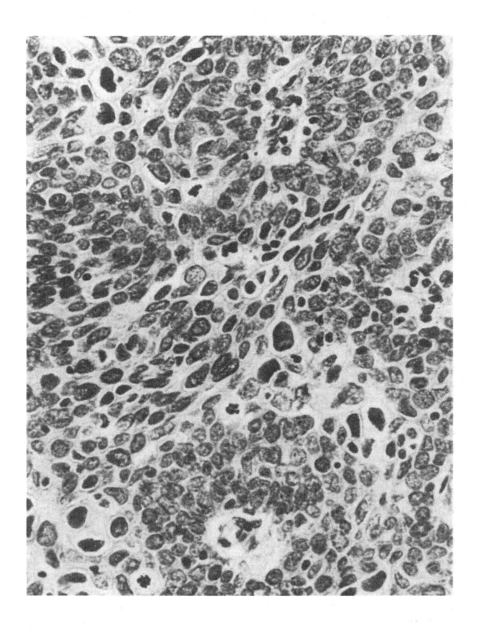

Fig. 3. Light micrograph of CIN 3. Cells are characterized by marked pleomorphism and a disorderly array.

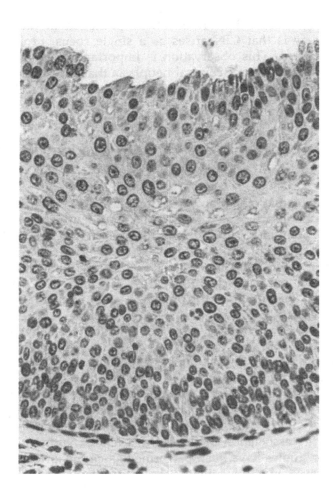

Fig. 4. Light micrograph of immature squamous metaplasia. The cells are relatively uniform in size, increasing somewhat as one goes from the basal layer to the surface. The marked pleomorphism present in Fig. 3 is not evident in the squamous metaplasia.

distribution patterns, cellular metabolic studies, long-term clinical followup studies of individual patients, and mathematical modeling of cytology-screened populations (Barron and Richart, 1968, 1969; Richart, 1973). These studies support the fact that cervical cancer precursors are part of a single disease process. The most important piece of information that arises from a pathogenetic and etiologic point of view is that CIN arises as a single focus, probably as a single-cell event. This observation is important in considering the possible viral etiology of cervical neoplasia that may take place as a hit-and-run event, as postulated by Galloway and McDougall (1983).

5. Seroepidemiologic Studies Linking HSV-2 to Cervical Neoplasia

The epidemiology of cervical neoplasia has been extensively studied and appears related to a number of identifiable risk factors (Table 1) (Adam et al., 1973, 1974; Anzai et al., 1975; Aurelian and Strnad, 1976; Centifanto et al., 1972; Choi et al., 1977; Gagnon, 1950; Heise et al., 1979; Ito et al., 1976; Kaufman and Rawls, 1974; Kawana et al., 1976; Kessler, 1974, 1976; Nahmias et al., 1970; Naib et al., 1966; Nealon and Christophersen, 1979; Nehama, 1973; Ory et al., 1974, 1975; Pasca et al., 1975; Rawls et al., 1971, 1970, 1968a,b, 1969; Royston and Aurelian, 1970; Singer and Reid, 1979; Smith et al., 1972a,b; Tarro et al., 1976a,b; Thiry et al., 1977; Thomas and Rawls, 1978; Tobin et al., 1978, 1979; Vontver et al., 1979; Wakefield et al., 1973).

Since Naib et al. (1966) observed that there was an increased rate of cervical neoplasia in patients who had cytologically detectable herpetic cervicitis, there has been a continuing controversy regarding the association of these two events. Numerous seroepidemiologic studies have been performed since this original description and have generally validated the association (Table 2).

Most of these seroepidemiologic studies have taken the form of case-control groups in which the prevalence of HSV-2 apntibodies and/or antigens among women with cervical neoplasia are compared with women without such lesions in a control group. The cases are selected from all socioeconomic classes and a wide range of ages are represented. Usually, invasive cancer and all grades of CIN are analyzed separately, with only a rare attempt to control for the effect of variation of the duration of the disease or therapeutic intervention. In some studies, the cases are matched to controls

Table 2
Seroepidemiology of HSV Ab and Cervical Neoplasia[a]

---

1. HSV Ab more frequent Ca Cx than controls (Adam et al., 1974)
2. HSV NA 52% Ca Cx, 31% CIN, 22% controls (Adam et al., 1973)
3. Ab to AG4   Ab to whole HSV

0%	10%	Controls
67%	100%	CIS
90%	100%	Untreated Ca Cx
8%	100%	RT Rx Ca Cx

   (Aurelian et al., 1973)
4. Ab to AG 4 by microcomplement fixation 9% controls, 35% ox atypia, 58% CIS, 91% Ca Cx (Aurelian and Strnad, 1976)
5. Ig M Ab to AG 4 in Ca Cx higher than controls (Aurelian et al., 1977)
6. HSV Ab Ca Cx higher than controls (Choi et al., 1977)
7. CF HSV Ab to AG4 higher Ca Cx than controls (Heise et al., 1979)
8. Relative risk cervical Ca in women with HSV Ab 10.4 (Ory et al., 1975)
9. HSV 2 Ab 17% controls, 58% atypia, 73% CIS (Pasca et al., 1976)
10. HSV Ab 9% controls, high SEC 22% controls, low SEC 33%, CIN 83% Ca Cx (Rawls et al., 1970)
11. HSV 2 Ab 36.7% controls, 80% Ca Cx (Seth et al., 1978)

---

[a] Abbreviations: HSV, herpes simplex virus; SEC, Socioeconomic class; Ab, antibody; NA, neutralizing antibody; Ca Cx, carcinoma cervix; CIS, carcinoma *in situ*; CF, complement fixing.

with respect to age, race, and socioeconomic status. In others, they are selected in an undefined fashion from essentially healthy volunteers. Usually, however, the controls are not examined to exclude the presence of abnormal cervical cytology and/or active herpetic infections. Also, usually the marital status and coital practices are not considered in selection of patients (Kessler, 1976). Choi et al. (1977) studied a cohort of 23,146 pregnant women for 37–56 mo subsequent to the collection of prenatal serum, and found 57 cases of carcinoma of the cervix. Controls were selected for each of these cases with respect to age, residence, number of prior cytologic smears, and date of entry into the study. HSV-1 and HSV-2 antibody activity was then assessed by indirect hemagglutination tests. The proportion of cancer cases that were positive for HSV infections was greater than that of the control group (Choi et al., 1977).

Rawls et al. (1970) found antibodies to HSV-2 among 83% of women with invasive cancer and 33% of women with carcinoma *in situ*. Antibodies were found in 22 and 9% of control groups of women from lower and higher socioeconomic groups, respectively.

Seth et al. (1978) found that patients with squamous cell carcinomas of the cervix had a higher incidence and titer or HSV-2 antibodies when compared to matched controls. The mean antibody titer to HSV-1 was also significantly higher among patients with cervical cancer than among women with other cancers or in patients without cancer. Ory et al. (1975) examined the association between cervical dysplasia and HSV-2 antibodies in a low-income housing project and found that the prevalence of HSV-2 antibodies rose sharply with advancing age. They found a significant absence of antibodies in young nulliparous women. There was a tendency of CIN to be related to age, age at first pregnancy, and total number of pregnancies. The major finding in this study was that 15- to 24-yr-old women with HSV-2 infections had a relative risk of 5.44 of having cervical dysplasia compared to women without HSV antibodies. These data are consistent with the concept that HSV infections may be associated with the initiation of cervical neoplasias.

Thomas and Rawls (1978) studied the serum from 75 women with cervical carcinoma *in situ*, 84 with squamous dysplasia, and 130 controls, all of whom had been previously interviewed and tested for antibodies against a number of organisms. These patients were also analyzed for HSV-2 antibodies. Carcinoma *in situ* and severe dysplasia were usually associated with HSV-2 antibodies. An association was also found between mild dysplasia and infections by *Trichomonas vaginalis*, adenovirus, and *Mycoplasma pneumoniae*. Severe dysplasia was less frequently related to these variables. The relative risk of dysplasia increased with the number of different pathogens that could be detected. These investigators concluded that HSV-2 may be a cause of carcinoma *in situ*, but that dysplasia is a nonspecific reaction of the cervical epithelium to chronic inflammation. Furthermore, dysplastic lesions might be a precursor to carcinoma *in situ*, but are distinguished from it by their reduced severity.

Graham et al. (1982) examined the interaction of exposure to various numbers of sexual partners and the presence of antibodies to herpes simplex virus type 2 in 181 cases of cervical dysplasia, carcinoma *in situ*, carcinoma of the cervix, and 130 control patients in Los Angeles county. They found that the risk of cancer of the cervix was enhanced with the number of sexual partners, frequency and duration of using a vaginal douche, early age at first pregnancy, and antibodies to HSV-2 as meaured by radioimmunoassay. It was also found that for women with only one or no sexual partner, the risk for developing cervical neoplasia was elevated if evidence of antibodies to HSV-2 were present. The same was true for women with two or more sexual partners.

6. Herpes-Specific Antigens in Cervical Neoplasia

Concomitant with an ordered morphologic sequence of events in herpes infected cells, there is a definable sequence of biochemical events following viral infection. Three phases of protein synthesis have been identified. The first occurs early after infection when there is a rapid decrease in host protein synthesis with only a minor production of viral proteins. In the second phase, protein synthesis increases rapidly with incorporation of amino acids into viral proteins. The proteins can be divided into two classes, one of which requires the onset of viral DNA replication and one of which does not. After most of the viral DNA has been made, the third phase occurs and is identified by a steady decline in viral protein synthesis followed by virus assembly.

Three major groups of viral polypeptides have thus been described (alpha, beta, and gamma) with their synthesis coordinately regulated and proceeding in an ordered cascading sequence. Alpha polypeptides are those made early in infection and can be detected experimentally after withdrawal of cycloheximide or puromycin from the culture medium of infected cells. The beta polypeptides require functioning alpha polypeptides, and the gamma group require both alpha and beta functioning polypeptides to be present. The structural viral polypeptides are in the gamma group and are made late in infection. Cells that are infected with HSV-2 synthesize at least 50 infected cell polypeptides (ICSP) (Cassai, 1980; Honess and Roizman, 1974; Killington et al., 1978; Roizman and Morse, 1978; Spear and Roizman, 1980). Killington et al. (1978) have shown that virus-specific ICSPs of HSV-2 share antigenic sites with HSV-1.

The presence of viral proteins (viral antigens) can be identified on infected cells utilizing one of the following techniques: ferritin labeling (Metcalf and Helmsen, 1977; Hanse et al., 1979), complement fixation (Adam et al., 1972, 1973), indirect hemagglutination (Choi et al., 1977), and immunohistology (Fenoglio, et al., 1982;

Cho and Feng, 1978; Hilgers and Hilgers, 1976; Marttila and Kalimo, 1977; Benjamin and Ray, 1975; Crum and Fenoglio, 1980; Fenoglio, 1980; Leary et al., 1976; McDougall et al., 1980a, 1981, 1982).

New proteins frequently appear on the surfaces and in the nucleus and/or cytoplasm of virally transformed neoplastic cells (Kutinova et al., 1973; Hollinshead and Tarno 1973; Hollinshead et al., 1973, 1974; Tarro et al., 1981). Some of these proteins are related to the structural proteins of the transforming herpesvirus and others are nonstructural and synthesized shortly after infection of susceptible cells, even when the synthesis of new DNA is prevented and they are in the alpha and beta classes of HSV-induced polypeptides (ICSP). Early proteins of DNA viruses, which are expressed in cells during the infective cycle, can persist in transformed cells, as in the case of the T-antigen of papovaviruses (Black et al., 1963), adenoviruses, and EBV-determined nuclear antigen (EBNA) (Henle and Henle, 1973, 1978).

Since the knowledge that the patient with cancer has been infected with HSV-2 is not sufficient to implicate the virus in the pathogenesis of the carcinoma, attempts have been made to demonstrate that antigenic markers, other than viral structural proteins, are present. Powell and Purifoy (1976) isolated and characterized proteins that bind DNA from cells infectd with HSV-2. They characterized two HSV-2-specific proteins that they termed ICSP-11/12 and ICSP-34/35. These were considered to be early nonstructural viral proteins (Powell and Purifoy, 1976). Using rabbit monospecific antisera to these antigens, clinical material obtained from patients with genital neoplasias have been examined (Dreesman et al., 1980; Kaufman et al., 1981; McDougall et al., 1980a, 1982; Fenoglio et al., 1982). Dreesman et al. (1980) found that anti-ICSP 34/35 gave a staining pattern that was perinuclear and cytoplasmic in location. This staining pattern was similar to that described by Flannery et al. (1977) utilizing an antiserum designated as anti-VP 143. We now know that VP 143 is identical to ICSP 34/35. Four percent of patients with normal, inflamed, metaplastic, or mildly or moderately dysplastic epithelium was positive, utilizing the ICSP 34/35 antiserum, whereas patients with carcinoma *in situ* or invasive carcinomas had a positive reaction in 38% of cases. Similar, but weaker, patterns were observed when tissues were studied with an antiserum to ICSP 11/12. However, no reactivity was seen using an antiserum to whole HSV virions. The specificity of the reaction is confirmed by absorbing the anti-ICSP 34/35 serum with HSV-2-infected cell lysates.

Melnick et al. (1979) established five epithelial cell lines from biopsies of an invasive cervical carcinoma and examined them for the presence of HSV antigens or virus-induced changes. Immunofluorescent studies utilizing serum to VP 143 detected this antigen in the perinuclear region of three of the 21 cell lines examined (Melnick et al., 1979). These results were similar to those for hamster cells transformed by the virus and then stained with this antibody (Flannery et al., 1977).

Our results localizing HSV-2 antigens, using these antisera, closely parallel those reported by Dreesman et al. (1980). When nonneoplastic cervical tissues were examined, HSV antigens were occasionally seen in isolated mature squamous epithelial cells near the surface in the epithelium of the portio or transformation zone, in a pattern suggesting an acute infection. Approximately 30% of patients with CIN grade 1–2 lesions had detectable antigens. Patients with CIN 3 had 12% incidence of detectable antigens. HSV antigens were demonstrable in 20% of invasive squamous cell carcinomas (McDougall et al., 1980a,b; Fenoglio et al., 1982).

Gilman et al. (1980) recently demonstrated the presence of two HSV-2 related proteins having molecular weights of 38,000 and 118,000 in the serum of patients with cancer of the cervix that appeared to be tumor-specific and independent of past herpes infections or known risk factors for cervical cancer. This was determined by screening the serum of patients and controls for a large number of HSV-1- and HSV-2-related proteins. Radiolabeled proteins were immunoprecipitated with the patient's sera. The presence of these two proteins was compared in the two populations, and was studied with respect to social, economic, and sexual history.

More recently, monoclonal antibodies were prepared according to the method of Köhler and Milstein (1975) against HSV-2 (Goldstein et al., 1983). Three HSV-2 specific monoclonal antibodies produced were utilized to study cervical biopsy material. One of these (6-A6) reacted primarily with a 140,000-dalton protein. Another (6-H11) reacted primarily with a 38,000-dalton protein. None of the three HSV-2 specific monoclonal antisera gave positive staining reactions on transformed cells or on neoplastic cervical tissues, although they reacted with HSV-2 infected cells. However, the monospecific antisera ICSP 11/12 and VP 143 obtained from Drs. Powell and Courtney, respectively, were positive both on virus-infected cells and transformed cells, as well as on neoplastic cells of some patients with CIN or cervical carcinoma (McDougall et al., 1982). That the two antisera ICSP 11/12 and VP 143 detect the same protein was demonstrated by immunoprecipitation studies with extracts of HSV-2 infected cells in which the two antisera precipitated a single band of HSV-2 protein with identical electrophoretic mobilities with an estimated molecular weight of 118,000.

As noted above, Gilman et al. (1980) demonstrated antibodies to two HSV proteins of 38,000 and 118,000 molecular weights. Presumably, the 118,000 molecular weight protein is similar to that described by Gilman. The 28,000 molecular weight protein is also of interest because it has been shown that a protein of this size is encoded within the BGL II fragment N of HSV-2 DNA (Docherty et al., 1981). This region has been shown to have transforming ability in rodent cells (Galloway and McDougall, 1981). The data concerning localization of herpes-associated antigens on cervical neoplastic cells is summarized in Table 3.

Table 3
HSV Antigens and Cervical Neoplasia[a]

1. AG 4 found in tumor biopsies (Aurelian et al., 1971)
2. HSV Ag shown by anticomplement IF (Christenson, 1982)
3. ISCP 34, 35 4% SM, mild dysplasia 3%, moderate dysplasia 10%, severe dysplasia 31%, CIS and Ca Cx 40% (Dreesman et al., 1980)
4. 38,000 and 118,000 MW HSV 2 proteins in serum of Ca Cx pts but not controls (Gilman et al., 1980)
5. HSV NV Ag in Ca Cx cell membrane sonicates (Hollinshead and Tarro, 1973)
6. HSV NV Ag in tissue extract Ca Cx (Hollinshead et al., 1973)
7. ICSP 11/12 33% CIN, 20% Ca Cx (McDougall et al., 1980)
8. VP 143 and ICSP 11/12 in CIN and Ca Cx (McDougall et al., 1982)
9. V 143 on Ca Cx Cul liners (Melnick et al., 1979)
10. Ag isolated from HSV reacted with 94% Ca Cx (Notter and Docherty, 1976)
11. HSV Ag on cytology: Nl 9%, inflamed 41%, CIN 61%, Ca Cx 94% (Pasca et al., 1975)
12. NV Ag by PAGE analysis Ca Cx (Tarro et al., 1976b)
13. HSV Chromium release assay controls 74.2%, CIN I 83.8%, CIN II 95% (Thomas and Rawls, 1978)

[a] Abbreviations: NV, nonvirion; HSV, herpes simplex virus; AG, antigen; SM, squamous metaplasia; Ca, carcinoma; Cx, cervix; MW, molecular weight; CIN, cervical intraepithelial neoplasia; Nl, normal; PAGE, polyacrylamide gel electrophoresis.

It is tempting to speculate that the presence of viral-related antigens are consistent with the concept that HSV-2 is involved in the initiation and/or maintenance of the transformed state of cells in CIN and cervical carcinoma. However, this evidence is very indirect. A more direct approach is to find the presence of putative transforming sequences of the HSV-2 genome in neoplastic cervical cells (Fig. 5).

7. HSV Genetic Sequences in Cervical Neoplasia

In 1972, it was first reported that genetic sequences homologous to a portion of the HSV-2 genome were present in the neoplastic cells of a patient with an invasive squamous cell carcinoma of the cervix (Frenkel et al., 1972). However, not all laboratories were able to confirm these findings (zur Hausen et al., 1974; Pagano, 1975). One of the major problems at the molecular level was that the molecular probes used in the hybridization techniques were not sufficiently sensitive to allow negative results to be conclusive (McDougall et al., 1981). By analogy with the results from viruses such as SV40 and adenovirus, it is necessary to exclude the presence of as small a region as 1–2% of the HSV-2 genome per cell since an equivalent amount of a specific region of each of the smaller ongocenic viruses is capable of initiating and maintaining the transformed cellular phenotype (Sambrook et al., 1977).

One approach subsequently used for demonstrating the presence of herpes genetic sequences in cervical tissues is the *in situ* hybridization reaction. This method allows the examination of the tumor tissue directly without the dilution of nucleic acid sequences that might occur during extraction of DNA or RNA from tumor samples that consist of a mixture of cell types.

Cervical tissues obtained during colposcopic examination and biopsy were frozen, the diagnoses confirmed, then used for *in situ* hybridization studies. Control cervical tissues were obtained from the transformation zone of hysterectomy specimens in patients with nonneoplastic disorders. The cervical tissues were then studied for evidence of the presence of herpes-specific RNA (Jones et al., 1978; McDougall et al., 1980a,b, 1981, 1982; Eglinet al., 1981). The probes for our studies were prepared by extracting HSV-2 DNA from virions banded in sucrose gradients or directly from infected cells, as described by Walboomers and Schegget (1976). This was then purified by centrifugation in sodium iodide equilibrium density gradients and labeled with tritium using the nick-

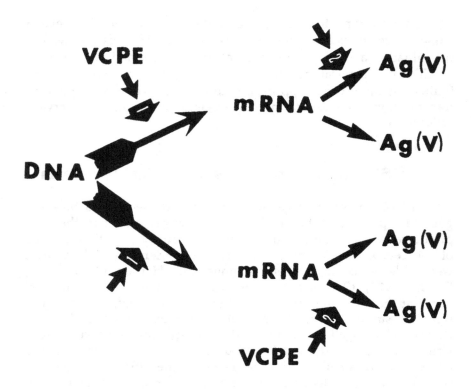

Fig. 5. Diagrammatic representation of amplification of genetic products. The nucleus contains DNA. From this, messenger RNA is made that contains complementary viral sequences. The messenger RNA represents an amplified cell product. Proteins that may be recognizable as viral antigens (Ag)(v) may be made from the virus-specific mRNA. Viral cytopathic effects (VCPE) may block the synthesis of message from DNA (arrow 1) or the synthesis of protein from RNA (arrow 2).

translation method of Maniatas et al. (1976). The specific activity of the probe was approximately 10^7 count/min/µg HSV-2-infected and -transformed cells grown on glass slides and frozen sections of tumors induced in hamsters by inoculation of the transformed cells were fixed in absolute ethanol at −20°C. These slides were dried and 10 µL of denatured probe in 6× SSC containing 5×10^5 count/min was applied, covered with a glass coverslip, and incubated at 68°C for 18 h. After extensive washing in 2× SSC at 4°C, the slides were dehydrated through graded ethanols, dried, and dipped in photographic emulsion. Examination of these cytologic hybridization preparations demonstrated the ability to detect HSV-2 RNA in cells containing less than 5% of the viral genome in a few copies (Galloway et al., 1980).

The cervical tissues were divided into three categories: (1) benign, including squamous metaplasia and reserve cell hyperplasia; (2) cervical intraepithelial neoplasia; and (3) invasive carcinoma. Tissues obtained that did not include the transformation zone were also subjected to *in situ* hybridization analysis, despite the fact that cervical neoplasias do not arise in this region. Biopsies were interpreted as benign if the squamous epithelium matured in a normal fashion, or if they contained immature cells of squamous metaplasia or reserve cell hyperplasia, either at the surface or in the underlying endocervical glands. The CIN lesions were classified according to the criteria by Richart (1973). Additionally, tissues were obtained from patients with condylomata and vulvar and vaginal intraepithelial neoplasias. After *in situ* hybridization with nick-translated HSV-2 DNA, in a method similar to that used on infected and transformed cells, the biopsies were stained with 10% Giemsa and examined for evidence of silver grains over the epithelia, indicating the presence of HSV RNA.

Specificity of the reaction was controlled by two methods: Unrelated radioactive probes were hybridized to serial sections from the same biopsies. Nick-translated DNA from adenovirus type 2, SV40, and bacteriophage lambda hybridized under the same conditions as the tritiated HSV-2 DNA gave negative results. Pretreatment of the sections with $0.07M$ NaOH or ribonuclease resulted in a 90% reduction in the autoradiographic grains detected after hybridization with HSV-2 DNA, confirming that the complementary sequences detected were RNA.

By the *in situ* hybridization reaction, HSV RNA was found mainly in the areas in which there was increased replication of cells in the transformation zone, either as the result of basal cell hyperplasia or CIN (Fig. 6). It was also present in invasive carcinoma cells. HSV RNA was detected in 42% of CIN lesions, 13% of nonneoplastic squamous proliferations, and 30% of invasive lesions.

The results of these findings were, at the very least, suggestive that there is an association between the presence of the RNA transcripts complementary to HSV-2 nucleic acid sequences and the cells undergoing the neoplastic alterations in the cervix. However, these results must be viewed with caution since it is well known that HSV-2 can infect the genital area and remain latent in women (Baringer, 1974). the results of the *in situ* hybridization, using whole virus probes, would allow the detection of both primary infections as well as reinfections of tissue following activation of virus. However, by employing a battery of restriction endonuclease-derived and cloned subgenomic fragments, one can distinguish

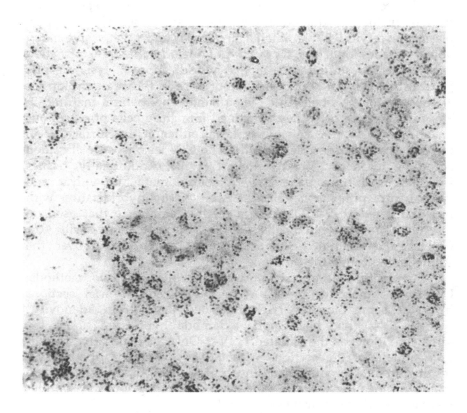

Fig. 6. *In situ* hybridization of neoplastic squamous epithelium showing
the localization of radioautographic grains over the neoplastic cells.

between permissive and nonpermissive HSV infections in tissue
sections. This is achieved by nick translating these fragments and
then utilizing the *in situ* hybridization reactions on serial sections.
The results of such studies indicate that the viral RNA detected in
neoplastic cervical cells is preferentially associated with specific
subsets of HSV fragments (McDougall et al., 1981, 1982) and that
the RNA species detected in the neoplastic cervical tissues are limited to three regions of the viral genome: positions 0.7 to 0.4, 0.58
to 0.63, and 0.82 to 0.85. Two of these regions have been implicated
in transformation in vitro. However, no one sequence was invariably expressed in all of the HSV positive specimens. Thus, it has
not been possible to identify a tumor-specific gene in this setting
(Galloway and McDougall, 1983).

Of particular interest is the fact that in some cases of cervical, vulvar, or vaginal neoplasia positive for HSV viral genetic sequences, using either the whole viral probe or the endonuclease-derived subgenomic probes, the distribution of cells positive by *in situ* hybridization was similar to the distribution of cells positive for ICSP 11/12. Of additional interest is the fact in that patients with nonneoplastic hyperplasias of the basal cell layer in the cervical transformation zone one is also able to detect HSV-specific RNA in approximately 13% of the cases. The positive cells in the hyperplasias or neoplasias are always confined to the basal layers orneoplastic cells and are always confined to the transformation zone.

Occasionally, viral RNA is detected in superficial portions of the squamous epithelium, not only in the cervical transformation zone but also in the portio. Under these circumstances, further investigation utilizing the full battery of endonuclease-derived subgenomic HSV-2 probes shows that all are positive, indicating that the superficial layers of the squamous epithelium are productively infected. We have also encountered situations in which condylomatous lesions, a condition known to be associated with infection by HPV, may have superficial cells infected with HSV (Fig. 7). This superficial location in acute infections contrasts markedly with the more basal localization of HSV-2 in the early CIN lesions and reserve cell hyperplasias, as noted above.

8. Postulated Mechanisms of Oncogenesis for Cervical Neoplasia

An understanding of the etiology of cervical neoplastic disorders is essential if one is to attempt to control or prevent them. The mere exposure of cells to a potential oncogenic agent is probably insufficient o induce cancer without the presence or addition of other predisposing factors. Thus, cervical cancer may represent the end product of a chronically infected state in which there has been a long latent period and extended clinical course. Despite these considerations, there is considerable evidence supporting the hypothesis that herpesviruses can cause both human, as well as animal, tumors.

By combining the results of the antigen and *in situ* hybridization studies with epidemiologic observations and histological analysis, one could postulate the following series of events: In the patient who has an acute HSV infection, the virus randomly infects

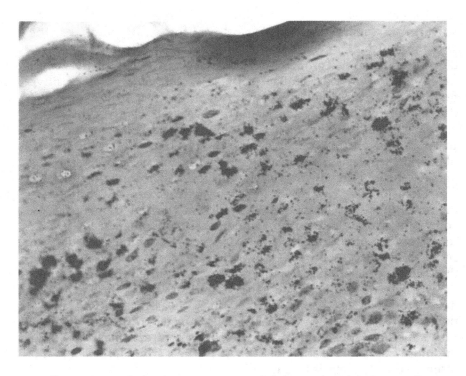

Fig. 7. *In situ* hybridization of a condyloma caused by the papilloma-virus. Superficial regions of this lesion contain evidence of an acute her-pesvirus infection.

the superficial nondividing squamous epithelium either in the por-tio or in the transformation zone (Fig. 8). It may also involve the superficial epithelium of other squamous lesions, such as condylo-mas. However, because such acute infections are generally cyto-pathic, the cells undergo cytolysis and die. Alternatively, they are shed as part of the physiologic desquamative process that accom-panies squamous cell maturation. The end result is that the acutely infected cells are no longer present to undergo subsequent transformation into a neoplasm.

A second type of HSV infections might occur at specific times in the reproductive periods of a woman's life. This could be an infection of the replicating immature squamous cells in the basal layers of the transformation zone, which is forming at the time of the menarche or is remodeled following each pregnancy (Oster-gard, 1979). This is consistent with the findings of Naib et al. (1966), who showed that herpetic infections of the cervix have a

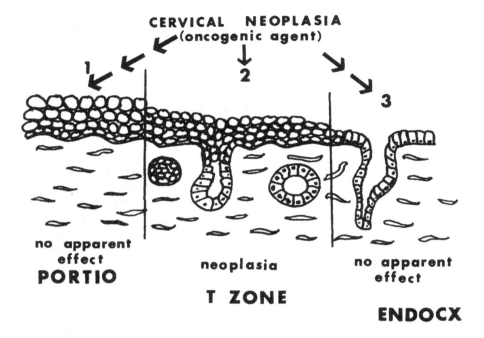

Fig. 8. Diagrammatic representation of the clinical observation that cervical neoplasia arises in a restricted area of the cervix. The cervix is divided into three discrete areas: the portio, T-zone, and endocervix.

predilection for involving the area of the squamocolumnar junction in the transformation zone.

In order to explain the apparently unique sensitivity of immature squamous epithelium in the transformation zone to HSV infections, one can postulate that HSV-specific receptors might be present on the squamous cell surfaces (Fig. 9). Certainly, in experimental cell systems, adsorption of HSV to cell surfaces in the initial phases of cellular attachment varies with different viral strains and with different host cells, suggesting that there is a differential affinity between the cellular and viral structures involved in the attachment process. This suggests the presence of HSV-specific membrane receptors on the cell surface. The nature of the cellular receptor and the virus envelope structure essential for the initiation of the infection has not been defined, although it appears that cell surface glycopeptides are involved (Vahlne et al., 1978, 1979).

If one examines the surfaces of squamous cells as they differentiate in the cervical transformation zones using the scanning electron microscope, one finds that the immature squamous cell is covered by microvili (Ferenczy and Richart, 1974; Ferenczy and Fenoglio, 1979). With cellular maturation, these are lost and microridges appear. Large areas of the mature squamous cell surface are flat and devoid of any surface protrusions. It is easy to imagine that with this morphological rearrangement of the squamous cell membrane there is a biochemical rearrangement of the intrinsic proteins within these plasma membranes such that previously exposed intrinsic proteins may become internalized. It is attractive to postulate that some of these proteins may act as viral receptors or receptors for other potentially oncogenic agents (Fig. 9). Hyperplastic or neoplastic squamous epithelial cells also have surface features resembling those of immature squamous epithelia, in that microvilli rather than microridges are present. Such cells might continue to express viral receptors if they in fact exist. Thus, it may be that glycopeptide differences in the squamous membrane of the immature transformation zone or remodeling transformation zone may play a critical pathogenic role in the preferential affinity of this epithelium for herpesvirus infections.

It is quite likely that once herpesvirus infection occurs, the virus need not persist to induce or maintain the transformed state. There is no indication that continued expression of herpesvirus genes is necessary to maintain the transformed state or that certain sequences of the HSV DNA are always retained or expressed (Galloway and McDougall, 1983). Rather, there is increasing evidence to suggest that cells can remain transformed in the absence of detectable herpesvirus sequences, suggesting the hypothesis that the virus acts in a "hit-and-run" manner (Skinner, 1976; Hampar et al., 1976; zur Hausen, 1980) to induce changes in cells that cause them to be tumorigenic (Galloway and McDougall, 1983).

It is also conceivable that HSV, which represents a potent mutagen (Schlehofer and zur Hausen, 1982), can cause the partial inactivation of certain host cell genomes or selective gene amplification. It would be attractive to postulate that one of the genes switched on is in the family of genes known as oncogenes. These represent genetic sequences that are important in normal cellular growth and development and are involved in cellular differentiation (Bishop, 1982). Oncogene-specified proteins have "transforming" abilities with the capacity to markedly alter cell function by modulating gene expression, affecting cell structural components such as the microfilaments of plasma membrane. There may also be protein kinases involved in phosphorylation reactions (Fenoglio and Lefkowitch, 1983). Certainly, these cellular oncogenes might be induced following either the expression or

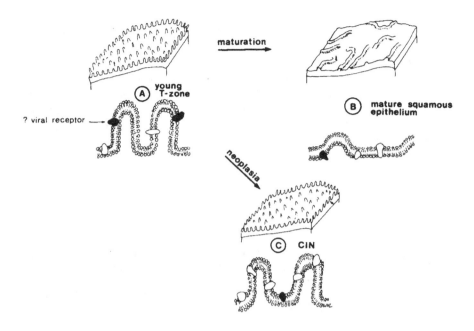

Fig. 9. Diagrammatic representation of possible role of viral receptors (see text).

insertion of HSV sequences. It has already been shown that transformation by HSV stimulates the production of c-type viruses (Hampar et al., 1976; Duff and Rapp, 1975).

It is unlikely that HSV acts alone, and it may be that a synergism exists between HSV and HPV, both of which commonly affect the cervix. Initiation by HSV and promotion by HPV is a hypothesis proposed by zur Hausen (1982) based on (1) the demonstration of DNA of different types of HPVs in cervical cancer biopsy samples, as well as in CINs, (2) studies revealing the initiator-like functions of HSV infections, and (3) analogous interactions of papillomavirus infections with initiators in the induction of certain animal and human cancers, It would also be in keeping with a hit-and-run hypothesis for the action of HSV, as proposed by Galloway and McDougall (1983), and the inconsistent detection of HSV DNA in cancer of the cervix.

Many questions remain unanswered. Are squamous cell neoplasms of the lower female genital tract associated with altered expression of cellular oncogenes,and if so, are these oncogenes activated by mutagenic agents such as HSV? Is it necessary to have the continued presence of HSV genetic sequences to maintain an initiated state? Is infection with human papillomavirus a *sine qua non* of the neoplastic process? Is there a local immunodeficiency associated with the presence of numerous infecting organisms that allows for the establishment of a latent infection of the basal compartment of the cervical transformation zone by one or more of these viruses? Are there herpesvirus receptors on the immature squamous cells of the forming or remodeling transformation zones? Current methodologies will hopefully provide some of the answers to these questions.

References

Adam, E., R. H. Kaufman, J. L. Melnick, A. H. Levy, and W. E. Rawls (1972), Seroepidemiologic studies of herpesvirus type 2 and carcinoma of the cervix. *Am. J. Epidemiol.* **96**, 427–42.

Adam, E., R. H. Kaufman, J. L. Melnick, A. H. Levy, and W. E. Rawls (1973), Seroepidemiologic studies of herpesvirus type 2 and carcinoma of the cervix IV dysplasia and carcinoma in situ. *Am. J. Epidemiol.* **98**, 77–87.

Adam, E., E. K. Sanders, J. L. Melnick, A. H. Levy, and W. E. Rawls (1974), Antibodies to herpesvirus type 2 in breast cancer and cervical cancer patients. *Cancer* **33**, 147–152.

Anderson, F. D., R. N. Ushijima, and C. Larson (1974), Recurrent herpes genitalis. Treatment with Mycobacterium bovis (BCG). *Obstet. Gynecol.* **43**, 797–805.

Anzai, T., G. R. Dreesman, R. J. Courtney, E. Adam, W. Rawls (1975), Antibody to herpes simplex virus 2-induced nonstructural proteins in women with cervical cancer and in control groups. *J. Natl. Cancer Inst.* **54(5)**, 1051–1959.

Aurelian, L., J. D. Standberg, L. V. Melendez, and L. A. Johnson (1971), Herpesvirus type 2 isolated from cervical tumor cells grown in tissue culture. *Science* **174**, 704–707.

Aurelian, L., B. Schumann, R. L. Marcus, and H. J. Davis (1973), Antibody to HSV-2 inuced tumor specific antigens in serums from patients with cervical carcinoma. *Science* **181**, 161–164.

Aurelian, L. and B. S. Strnad (1976), Herpesvirus type 2-related antigens and their relevance to hymoral and cell mediated immunity in patients with cervical cancer. *Cancer Res.* **36**, 810–820.

Aurelian, L., B. S. Strnad, and M. F. Smith (1977), Immunodiagnostic potential of a virus-coded tumor-associated antigen (AG-4) in cervical cancer. *Cancer* **39**, 1834–1849.

Baringer, J. R. (1974), Recovery of herpes simplex virus from human sacral ganglions. *N. Engl. J. Med.* **291**, 828–830.

Barron, B. A. and R. M. Richart (1969), Follow-up study of patients with cervical dysplasia. *Am. J. Obstet. Gynecol.* **105**, 386–393.

Barron, B. A. and R. M. Richart (1968), A statistical model of the natural history of cervical carcinoma based on a prospctive study of 557 cases. *J. Natl. Cancer Inst.* **41**, 1343–1353.

Barron, B. A. and R. M. Richart (1971), An epidemiologic study of cervical neoplastic disease. Based on a self-selected sample of 7000 women in Barbados, West Indies. *Cancer* **27**, 978–986.

Benjamin, D. R. and C. G. Ray (1975), Use of immunoperoxidase on brain tissue for the rapid diagnosis of herpes encephalitis. *Am. J. Clin. Pathol.* **64(4)**, 472–476.

Beral, V. (1974), Cancer of the cervix: A sexually transmitted disease. *Lancet* **1**, 1037–1040.

Bishop, J. M. (1982), Oncogenes. *Sci. Am.* **246(3)**, 80–92.

Black, P. H., W. P. Rowe, H. C. Turner, and R. T. A. Huebner (1963), A specific complement-fixing antigen present in SV 40 tumor and transformed cells. *Proc. Natl. Acad. Sci. USA* **50**, 1148–1156.

Boyd, J. T. and R. Doll (1964), A study of the aetiology of carcinoma of the cervix uteri. *Br. J. Cancer* **13**, 419–434.

Cassai, E., D. DiLuca, R. Manservigi, M. Tognon, and A. Rotola (1980), Comparative analysis of the virion polypeptides specified by Herpes simplex virus type 2 stains. *Arch. Virol.* **64(1)**, 35–45.

Centers for Disease Control (1982), *Morbid. Mortal. Weekly Rep.* **31**, 137–139.

Centifanto, W. M., D. M. Drylie, S. L. Deardourff, and H. E. Kaufman (1972), Herpesvirus type 2 in the male genitourinary tract. *Science* **178**, 318–319.

Chappel, T., W. J. Brown, C. Jeffries, and J. A. Stewart (1978), The microbiological flora of penila ulcerations. *J. Infect. Dis.* **137(1)**, 50–56.

Cho, C. T. and K. K. Feng (1978), Sensitivity of the virus isolation and immunofluorescent staining methods in diagnosis of infections with herpes simplex virus. *J. Infect. Dis.* **138(4)**, 536–540.

Choi, N. W., P. T. Shettigara, H. A. H. Abu-Zeld, and N. A. Nelson (1977), Herpesvirus infection and cervical anaplasia—A seroepidemiological study. *Int. J. Cancer* **19(2)**, 167–171.

Christenson, B. (1982), Herpes virus-related antigens in herpes simplex virus type 2-transformed cells in the course of cervical carcinoma. *Eur. J. Cancer Clin. Oncol.* **18(12)**, 1345–1352.

Christopherson, W. M., and J. E. Parker (1965), Relation of cervical cancer to early marriage and childbearing. *N. Engl. J. Med.* **273**, 235–239.

Clemmesen, J. (1965), *Statistical Studies in the Aetiology of Malignant Neoplasms*, Kobenhaun, Munksgaard.

Clemmesen, J., and A. Nielsen (1951), The social distribution of cancer in Copenhagen 1943 to 1947. *Br. J. Cancer* **5**, 159–171.

Corey, L., H. G. Adams, Z. A. Brown, and K. K. Holmes (1983), Genital herpes simplex virus infections: Clinical manifestations, course, and complications. *Ann. Intern. Med.* **98(6)**, 958–972.

Corey, L., and K. K. Holmes (1983), Genital herpes simplex virus infections: Current concepts in diagnosis, therapy, and prevention. *Ann. Intern. Med.* **98(6)**, 973–983.

Crum, C. P. and C. M. Fenoglio (1980), The immunoperoxidase technique. A review of its application to diseases of the female genital tract. *Diag. Gynec. Obstet.* **2(2)**, 103–115.

Deardourff, S. L., F. A. Deture, and D. M. Deylie (1974), Association between herpes hominis type 2 and the male genitourinary tract. *J. Urol.* **112**, 126–127.

Della Torre, G., S. Pilotti, G. de Pabo, and F. Rilke (1978), Viral particles in cervical condylomatous lesions. *Tumori* **64(5)**, 549–553.

DeVessa, S. S. and E. L. Diamond (1980), Association of breast cancer and cervical cancer incidences with income and education among whites and blacks. *J. Natl. Cancer Inst.* **65(3)**, 515–528.

Docherty, J. J., J. H. Subak-Sharpe, and C. M. Preston (1981), Identification of a virus-specific polypeptide associated with a transforming fragment (BglII-N) of herpes simplex virus type 2 DNA. *J. Virol.* **40(1)**, 126–132.

Doll, R., P. Payne, and J. Waterhouse (1966), *Cancer Incidence in Five Continents UICC, Springer, Berliner.*

Dreesman, G. R., J. Burek, E. Adam, R. H. Kaufman, and J. L. Melnick (1980), Expression of herpesvirus-induced antigens in human cervical cancer. *Nature* **283**, 591–593.

Duff, R. and F. Rapp (1975), Quantitative assay for transformation of 3T3 cells by herpes simplex virus type 2. *J. Virol.* **15(3)**, 490–496.

Eglin, R. P., F. Sharp, A. B. MacLean, J. C. M. Macnab, J. B. Clements, and N. M. Wilkie (1981), Detection of RNA complementary to herpes simplex virus DNA in human cervical squamous cell neoplasms. *Cancer Res.* **41**, 3597–3603.

Fasal E., M. E. Simmons, and J. B. Kampert (1981), Factors associated with high and low risk of cervical neoplasia. *J. Natl. Cancer Inst.* **66(4)**, 631–636.

Fenoglio, C. M. (1980), Antigens, enzymes and hormones. Their roles as tumor markers in gynecologic neoplasia. *Diag. Gynecol. Obstet.* **2(1)**, 33–42.

Fenoglio, C. M. and A. Ferenczy (1982), Etiologic factors in cervical neoplasms. *Semin. Oncol.* **9**, 349–372.

Fenoglio, C. M., D. A. Galloway, C. P. Crum, R. U. Levine, R. M. Richart and J. T. McDougal (1982), Herpes simplex virus and cervical neoplasia. *Prog. Surg. Pathol.* **4**, 45–82.

Fenoglio, C. M. and J. H. Lefkowitch (1983), Viruses and cancer. *Med. Clin. North Am.* **67**, 1105–1127.

Ferenczy, A. and C. M. Fenoglio (1979), Female Genital Tract, in, *Electron Microscopy,* (Johannessen, J., ed.) McGraw Hill, New York.

Ferenczy, A. and R. M. Richart (1974), *Female Reproductive System. Dynamics of Scan and Transmission Electron Microscopy,* Wiley, NY.

Flannery, V. L., R. J. Courtney, and P. A. Schaffer (1977), Expression of an early, nonstructural antigen of herpes simplex virus in cells transformed in vitro by herpes simplex virus. *J. Virol.* **21(1)**, 284–291.

Frenkel, N., B. Roizman, E. Cassai, and A. Nahmias (1972), DNA fragment of herpes simplex 2 and its transcription in human cervical cancer tissue. *Proc. Natl. Acad. Sci. USA* **69**, 3784–3789.

Friedrich, E. G., K. Burch, and J. P. Bahr (1979), The vulvar clinic: An eight-year appraisal. *Am. J. Obstet. Gynecol.* **135(8)**, 1036–1040.

Frost, J. K. (1961), Cytology of benign conditions. *Clin. Obstet. Gynecol.* **4**, 1075–1096.

Gagnon, F. (1950), Contribution to study of etiology and prevention of cancer of cervix of uterus. *Am. J. Obstet. Gynecol.* **60**, 516–522.

Galloway, D. A., C. D. Copple, and J. K. McDougall (1980), Analysis of viral DNA sequences in hamster cells transformed by herpes simplex virus type 2. *Proc. Natl. Acad. Sci. USA* **77(2)**, 880–884.

Galloway, D. A., C. M. Fenoglio, and J. K. McDougall (1982), Limited transcription of the herpes simplex virus genome when latent in human sensory ganglia. *J. Virol.* **41(2)**, 686–691.

Galloway, D. A., C. M. Fenoglio, M. Shevchuk, and J. K. McDougall (1979), Detection of herpes simplex RNA in human sensory ganglia. *Virology* **95(1)**, 265–268.

Galloway, D. A., and J. K. McDougall (1981), Transformation of rodent cells by a cloned DNA fragment of herpes simplex virus type 2. *J. Virol.* **38(2)**, 749–760.

Galloway, D. A. and J. K. McDougall (1983), The oncogenic potential of herpes simplex viruses: Evidence for a "hit-and-run" mechanism. *Nature* **302**, 21–24.

Gilman, S. C., J. J. Docherty, A. Clarke, and W. E. Rawls (1980), Reaction patterns of herpes simplex virus type 1 and type 2 proteins with sera of patients with uterine cervical carcinoma and matched controls. *Cancer Res.* **40(12)**, 4640–4647.

Goldstein, L. C., L. Corey, J. K. McDougall, E. Tolentio, and R. C. Nowinski (1983), Monoclonal antibodies to herpes simplex viruses: Use in antigenic typing and rapid diagnosis. *J. Infect. Dis.* **147(5)**, 829–837.

Graham, S., M. Levin, and A. M. Lillienfield (1960), The socioeconomic distribution of cancer of various sites in Buffalo, N.Y. *Cancer* **13**, 180–191.

Graham, S., R. Priore, M. Graham, R. Browne, W. Burnett, and D. West (1979), Genital cancer in wives of penile cancer patients. *Cancer* **44**, 1870–1874.

Graham, S., W. Rawls, M. Swanson, and J. McCurtis (1982), Sex partners and herpes simplex virus type 2 in the epidemiology of cancer of the cervix. *Am. J. Epidemiol.* **115(5)**, 729–735.

Graham, S. and W. Schotz (1979), Epidemiology of cancer of the cervix in Buffalo, New York. *J. Natl. Cancer Inst.* **63(1)**, 23–27.

Hampar, B., S. A. Aaronson, J. G. Derge, M. Chakrabarty, S. D. Showalter, and C. Y. Dunn (1976), Activation of an endogenous mouse type C virus by ultraviolet-irradiated herpes simplex virus type 1 and 2. *Proc. Natl. Acad. Sci. USA* **73(2)**, 646–650.

Handley, W. S. (1936), The prevention of cancer. *Lancet* **1**, 987–991.

Hansen, B. L., G. N. Hansen, and B. F. Vestergaard (1979), Immunoelectron microscopic localization of herpes simplex virus antigens in infected cells using the unlabelled antibody-enzyme method. *J. Histochem. Cytochem.* **27**, 1455–1461.

Harvald, B. and M. Hauge (1963), Heredity of cancer elucidated by a study of unselected twins. *JAMA* **186**, 749–753.

Heise, E. R., L. S. Kucera, M. Raben, and H. Homesley (1979), Serological response patterns to herpesvirus type 2 early and late antigens in cervical carcinoma patients. *Cancer Res.* **39(10)**, 4022–4026.

Henle, W. and G. Henle (1973), Evidence for an oncogenic potential of the Epstein-Barr virus. *Cancer Res.* **33**, 1419–1423.

Henle, W. and G. Henle (1978), Comparison of Immune Responses and Viral Markers in Herpesviruses-Associated Carcinomas, in *Oncogenesis and Herpesviruses*, (de The, G., W. Henle, and F. Rapp, eds.), International Agency for Research on Cancer, IARC Scientific Publications No. 24, Lyon.

Henson, D. and R. Tarone (1977), An epidemiologic study of cancer of the cervix, vagina, and vulva based on the third National Cancer Survey in the United States. *Am. J. Obstet. Gynecol.* **129(5)**, 525–532.

Hilgers, F. and J. Hilgers (1976), An immunofluorescent technique with counterstain on fixed cells for the detection of antibodies to human herpesviruses; antibody patterns in patients with Hodgkin's diseases and nasopharyngel carcinoma. *Intervirology* **7(6)**, 309–327.

Hills, E., and C. R. Laverty (1979), Electron microscopic detection of papillomavirus particles in selected koilocytotic cells in a routine cervical smear. *Acta Cytol.* **23(1)**, 53–56.

Hollinshead, A. C. and G. Tarro (1973), Soluble membrane antigens of lip and cervical carcinomas: reactivity with antibody for herpesvirus nonvirion antigens. *Science* **179**, 698–700.

Hollinshead, A. C., O. Lee, P. B. Chretien, J. L. Tarpley, W. E. Rawls, and E. Adam (1973), Antibodies to herpesvirus nonvirion antigens in squamous carcinomas. *Science* **182**, 713–715.

Hollinshead, A. C., G. Tarro, W. A. Foster, Jr., L. J. Seigel, and W. Jaffurs (1974), Studies of tumor-specific and herpesvirus nonvirion antigens. *Cancer* **34**, 1122–1125.

Honess, R. W. and B. Roizman (1974), Regulation of herpesvirus macromolecular synthesis: I. Cascade regulation of the synthesis of three groups of viral proteins. *J. Virol.* **14**, 8–19.

Ito, H., F. Tsutsui, S. Kurhihara, T. Akabayashi, T. Tobi, and C. Nichimura (1976), Serum antibodies to herpesvirus early antigens in patients with cervical carcinoma determined by anti-complement immunofluorescent technique. *Int. J. Cancer* **18**(5), 557–563.

Jones, K. W., C. M. Fenoglio, M. Shevchuk-Chaban, N. J. Maitland, and J. K. McDougall (1978), Detection of Herpesvirus-2mRNA in Human Cervical Biopsies by In Situ Cytological Hybridization, in *Oncogenesis and Herpesviruses*, (de Thé, G., W. Henle, and F. Rapp, eds.), International Agency for Research on Cancer (IARC), Lyon.

Jordan, S. W. and C. R. Key (1981), Carcinoma of the cervix in Southwestern American Indians: Results of a cytologic detection program. *Cancer* **47**(10), 2523–2532.

Kaufman, R. H. and W. E. Rawls (1974), Herpes genitalis and its relationship to cervical cancer. *Am. Cancer Soc.* **24**(5), 258–265.

Kaufman, R. H., G. R. Dreesman, J. Burek, M. O. Korhonen, D. O. Matson, J. L. Melnick, K. L. Powell, D. J. Purifoy, R. J. Courtney, and E. Adam (1981), Herpesvirus induced antigens in squamous-cell carcinoma in situ of the vulva. *N. Engl. J. Med.* **305**(a), 483–488.

Kawana, T., J. D. Cornish, M. F. Smith, and L. Aurelian (1976), Frequency of antibody to a virus-induced tumor-associated antigen (AG-4) in Japanese sera from patients with cervical cancer and controls. *Cancer Res.* **36**(6), 1910–1914.

Kessler, I. I. (1974), Perspectives on the epidemiology of cervical cancer with special reference to the herpesvirus hypothesis. *Cancer Res.* **34**, 1091–1110.

Kessler, I. (1976), Human cervical cancer as a venereal disease. *Cancer Res.* **36**, 783–791.

Killington, R. A., R. E. Randall, J. Yeo, R. W. Honess, I. W. Halliburton, and D. H. Watson (1978), Observations on Antigenic Relatedness Between Viruses of the Herpes Simplex "Neutroseron" in, *Oncogenesis and Herpesviruses* (de Thé, G., W. Henle, and F. Rapp, eds.), International Agency for Research Cancer (IARC), Lyons. *I RC Sci. Pub.* **24**, 185 194.

Köhler, G. and C. Milstein (1975), Continuous cultures of fused cells secreting antibody of predefined specificity. *Nature* **256**, 495–497.

Kotcher, E., L. A. Gray, Q. C. James, C. A. Frick, and D. W. Bottorff (1962), Cervical cell inclusion bodies and viral infection of the cervix. *Ann. NY Acad. Sci.* **97**, 571–589.

Kurman, R. J., K. H. Shah, W. D. Lancaster, and A. B. Jenson (1981), Immunoperoxidase localization of papillomavirus antigens in cervical dysplasia and vulvar condylomas. *Am. J. Obstet. Gynecol.* **140**(8), 931–935.

Kutinova, L., V. Vonka, and M. Broucek (1973), Increased oncogenicity and synthesis of herpesvirus antigens in hamster cells exposed to herpes simplex type 2 virus. *J. Natl. Cancer Inst.* 50, 759–766.

Leary, J. F., M. F. D. Notter, and P. Todd (1976), Laser flow cytophotometric immunoperoxidase detection of herpes simplex virus type 2 antigens in infected cultured human cells. *J. Histochem. Cytochem.* 24(17), 1249–1257.

Maliphant, R. G. (1949), Incidence of cancer of uterine cervix. *Br. Med. J.* 2, 978–982.

Maniatis, T., S. G. Kee, A. Efstratiadis, and F. C. Kafatos (1976), Amplification and characterization of a globin gene synthesized in vitro. *Cell* 8(2), 163–182.

Martin, C. E. (1967), Marital and coital factors in cervical cancer. *Am. J. Public Health* 57, 803–814.

Martinez, I. (1969), Relationship of squamous cell carcinoma of the cervix uteri to squamous cell carcinoma of the penis among Puerto Rican women married to men with penile carcinoma. *Cancer* 24, 77–780.

Marttila, R. J. and K. O. K. Kalimo (1977), Indirect immunofluorescence detection of human IgGM and IgG antibodies against herpes simplex virus type 1 induced cell surface antigens. *Acta. Pathol. Microbiol. Scan.* 85(3), 195–200.

McDougall, J. K., C. P. Crum, C. M. Fenoglio, L. C. Goldstein, and D. A. Galloway (1982), Herpesvirus-specific RNA and protein in carcinoma of the uterine cervix. *Proc. Natl. Acad. Sci. USA* 79(12), 3853–3857.

McDougall, J. K., D. A. Galloway, C. Crum, R. Levine, R. Richart, and C. M. Fenoglio (1981), Detection of nucleic acid sequences in cervical tumors. *Gynecol. Oncol.* 12(2pt.2), S42–S55.

McDougall, J. K., D. A. Galloway, and C. M. Fenoglio (1980a), Cervical carcinoma detection of herpes simplex virus RNA in cells undergoig neoplastic change. *Int. J. Cancer* 25(1), 1–8.

McDougall, J. K., D. A. Galloway, D. J. M. Purifoy, K. L. Powell, R. M. Richart, and C. M. Fenoglio (1980b), Herpes Simplex Virus Expression in Latently Infected Ganglion Cells and in Cervical Neoplasia in, *Viruses in Naturally Occurring Cancers* (Essex, M., G. Todaro, and H. zur Hausen, eds.), Cold Spring Harbor Laboratory, Cold Spring Harbor.

Melnick, J. L., E. Adam, R. Lewis, and R. H. Kaufman (1979), Cervical cancer cell lines containing herpesvirus markers. *Intervirology* 12(2), 111–114.

Metcalf, J. F. and R. Helmsen (1977), Immunoelectron microscopic localization of herpes simplex virus antigens in rabbit cornea with antihuman IgG antiferritin hybrid antibodies. *Invest. Ophthalmol. Vis. Sci.* 19, 779–786.

Nahmias, A. J., W. E. Josey, Z. M. Naib, C. F. Luce, and B. J. A. Guest (1970), Antibodies to herpesvirus hominis types 1 and 2 in humans. II. Women with cervical cancer. *Am. J. Epidemiol.* 91, 547–552.

Nahmias, A. J., Z. M. Naib, W. Josey, and A. C. Clepper (1967), Genital herpes simplex infection. Virologic and cytologic studies. *Obstet. Gynecol.* 29, 395–400.

Naib, Z. M. (1976) *Exfoliative Cytopathology* (2nd Ed.) Little Brown, Boston.

Naib, Z. M., A. J. Nahmias, and W. E. Josey (1966), Cytology and histopathology of cervical herpes simplex infection. *Cancer* 19, 1026–1031.

Nealon, N. A. and W. M. Christopherson (1979), Cervix cancer precursors in young offspring of low-income families. *Obstet. Gynecol.* 54(2), 135–139.

Nehama, S. (1973), Workshop on the treatment and prevention of herpes simplex virus infections. *J. Infect. Dis.* 127, 117–119.

Ng, A. B. P., J. W. Reagan, and E. Lindner (1970), The cellular manifestations of primary and recurrent herpes genitalis. *Acta. Cytol.* **14,** 124–129.

Nielsen, A. and J. Clemmesen (1957), Twin studies in the Danish Cancer Registry. *Br. J. Cancer* **11(3),** 327–336.

Notter, M. F. and J. J. Docherty (1976), Reaction of antigens isolated from herpes simplex virus-transformed cells with sera of squamous cell carcinoma in patients. *Cancer Res.* **36(12),** 4399–4401.

Ory, H. W., R. Jenkins, J. Y. Byrd, A. J. Nahmias, C. W. Tyler, D. Allen, and S. B. Conger (1975), The epidemiology and interrelationship of cervical dysplasia and type 2 herpesvirus in a low-income housing project. *Am. J. Obstet. Gynecol.* **123(3),** 269–274.

Ory, H., Conger, B., Richart, R., and Barron, B. (1974), Relation of type 2 herpesvirus antibodies to cervical neoplasia. *Am. J. Obstet. Gynecol.* **43,** 901–904.

Ostergard, D. R. (1979), The effect of pregnancy on the cervical squamocolumnar junction in patients with abnormal cervical cytology. *Am. J. Obstet. Gynecol.* **134(7),** 759–760.

Pagano, J. S. (1975), Disease and mechanisms of persistent DNA virus infection: latency and cellular transformation. *J. Infect. Dis.* **132(2),** 209–223.

Pacsa, A. S., L. Kummerländer, B. Pejtsik, and K. Pali (1975), Herpesvirus antibodies and antigens in patients with cervical anaplasia and controls. *J. Natl. Cancer Inst.* **55,** 775–780.

Pacsa, A. S., Kummerländer, B. Pejtsik, K. Krommer, and K. Pali (1976), Herpes simplex virus-specific antigens in exfoliated cervical cells from women with and without cervical anaplasia. *Cancer Res.* **36,** 2130–2132.

Patten, S. F., Jr., J. W. Reagan, M. Oberauf, and L. A. Ballard (1963), Postirradiation dysplasia of uterine cervix and vagina: An analytical study of the cells. *Cancer* **16,** 173–182.

Powell, K. L. and D. J. M. Purifoy (1976), DNA-binding proteins of cells infected by Herpes simplex virus type 1 and type 2. *Intervirology* **7,** 225–239.

Rawls, W. E., H. L. Gardner, R. W. Flanders, S. P. Kowry, R. H. Kaufman, and J. L. Melnick (1971), Genital herpes in two social groups. *Am. J. Obstet. Gynecol.* **110,** 682–689.

Rawls, W. E., H. L. Gardner, and R. L. Kaufman (1970), Antibodies to genital herpesvirus in patients with carcinoma of the cervix. *Am. J. Obstet. Gynecol.* **107,** 710–716.

Rawls, W. E., D. Laurel, J. L. Melnick, J. M. Glicksman, and R. H. Kaufman (1968a), A search for viruses in smegma, premalignant and early malignant cervical tissues. The isolation of herpesviruses with distinct antigenic properties. *Am. J. Epidemiol.* **87,** 647–655.

Rawls, W. E., W. A. F. Tompkins, M. Figueroa, and J. L. Melnick (1968b), Herpes virus type 2: association with carcinoma of the cervix. *Science* **161,** 1255–1256.

Rawls, W. E., W. A. F. Tompkins, and J. L. Melnick (1969), The association of herpesvirus type 2 and carcinoma of the uterine cervix. *Am. J. Epidemiol.* **89,** 547–554.

Richardson, A. C. and J. B. Lyon (1981), The effect of condom use on squamous cell cervical intraepithelial neoplasia. *Am. J. Obstet. Gynecol.* **140(8),** 909–913.

Richart, R. M. (1973), Cervical Intraepithelial Neoplasia, in *Pathology Annual* (Sommers, S. C., ed.) Appleton-Crofts, New York.

Roizman, B. and L. S. Morse (1978), Human Herpesvirus 1 as a Model of Regulation of Herpesvirus Macromolecular Metabolism: A Review, in *Oncogenesis and Herpesviruses,* (de Thé, G., W. Henle, and F. Rapp, eds.), International

Agency for Research on Cancer, Scientific Publications, Lyon.

Rojel, J. (1953), The interrelation between uterine cancer and syphilis. *Acta. Pathol. Microbiol. Scand.* (B) (Suppl.) **97**, 1–82.

Rotkin, I. D. (1973), A comparison review of key epidemiological studies in cervical cancer related to current searches for transmissible agents. *Cancer Res.* **33**, 1353–1367.

Royston, I. and L. Aurelian (1970), Immunofluorescent detection of herpesvirus antigens in exfoliated cells from human cervical carcinoma. *Proc. Natl. Acad. Sci. USA* **67**, 204–212.

Sabin, A. B. (1975), Misery of recurrent herpes: What to do? *N. Engl. J. Med.* **293(19)**, 986–968.

Sambrook, J., D. A. Galloway, W. Topp, and M. Botcham (1977), in *International Cell Biology*, 1976–1977) Viral gene function and cell transformation. The arrangement of viral DNA sequences in the geno of cells transformed by SV40 or adenovirus. (B. R. Brinkley, K. R. Porter, eds.) Rockefeller University Press, N.Y. 539–552.

Schachter, J., E. C. Hill, E. B. King, V. R. Coleman, P. Jones, and K. F. Meyer (1975), Chlamydial infection in women with cervical dysplasia. *Am. J. Obstet. Gynecol.* **123(7)**, 753–757.

Schlehofer, J. R. and J. zur Hausen (1982), Induction of mutations within the host cell genome by partially inactivated herpes simplex virus type 1. *Virology* **122(2)**, 471–475.

Schneweis, K. E. and H. Brandes (1961), Typendifferenzen beim herpes simplex virus. *Zentralbl Bakteriol.* **183**, 556–558.

Seth, P., S. E. Prakash, and D. Ghosh (1978), Antibodies to herpes simplex virus types 1 and 2 in patients with squamous-cell carcinoma of uterine cervix in India. *Int. J. Cancer* **22(6)**, 708–714.

Singer, A. (1976), The Cervical Epithelium During Pregnancy and the Puerperium, in *The Cervix* (Jordon, J. A., H. Singer, eds.) Saunders, London.

Singer, A. and B. L. Reid (1979), Does the male transmit cervical cancer? *Contemp. Obstet. Gynecol.* **13**, 173–175.

Skinner, G. R. (1976), Transformation of primary hamster embryo fibroblasts by type 2 simplex virus: Evidence for a "hit-and-run" mechanism. *Br. J. Exp. Path.* **57(4)**, 361–376.

Smith, J. W., E. Adam, J. L. Melnick, and W. E. Rawls (1972), Use of the chromium release test to demonstrate patterns of antibody response in humans to herpesvirus types 1 and 2. *J. Immunol.* **109**, 554–564.

Smith, J. W., S. P. Lowry, J. L. Melnick, and W. E. Rawls (1972b), Antibodies to surface antigens of herpesvirus type 1- and 2-infected cells among women with cervical cancer and control women. *Infect. Immun.* **5**, 305–310.

Spear, P. G. and B. Roizman (1980), Herpes Simplex Viruses in DNA Tumor Viruses, in *Molecular Biology of Tumor Viruses* (2nd Ed.) (Tooze, J., ed.) Cold Spring Habor Laboratory, Cold Spring Harbor.

Stern, E., P. A. Lachenbruch, and W. J. Dixon (1967), Cancer of the uterine cervix II. A biometric approach to etiology. *Cancer* **20**, 190–201.

Stevens, J. G. (1978a), Persistent, Chronic, and Latent Infections by Herpesviruses: A Review, in *Oncogenesis and Herpesviruses* (de Thé, G., W. Henle, and F. Rapp, eds.), International Agency for Research on Cancer (IARC), Scientific Publications No. 24, Lyon.

Stevens, J. G. (1978b), Latent characteristics of selected herpesviruses. *Adv. Cancer Res.* **26**, 227–256.

Stevens, J. G., M. L. Cook, and M. C. Jordan (1976), Reactivation of latent herpes simplex virus after pneumococcal pneumonia in mice. *Infect. Immun.* **11**, 635–639.

Sumaya, C. V., J. Marx, and K. Ullis (1980), Genital infections with herpes simplex virus in a university student population. *Sex. Transm. Dis.* **7**(1), 16–20.

Swan, S. H. and W. L. Brown (1981), Oral contraceptive use, sexual activity, and cervical carcinoma. *Am. J. Obstet. Gynecol.* **139**)1), 52–57.

Tarro, G., G. G. Giordano, A. Tripodi, R. Cerra, M. DiGioia, A. Battista, and R. Smeraglia (1976a), Herpes simplex virus nuclear nonvirion antigens detected by anti-complement immunofluorescence. *Tumori* **62**(6), 609–614.

Tarro, G., G. G. Giordano, M. DiGioia, R. Cocchiara, R. Smeraglia, and A. Tripodi (1976b), Herpes simplex virus tumor-associated antigens in cancer patients. *Tumori* **62**(6), 615–622.

Tarro, G., G. D'Alessandro, A. Mascolo, L. Bossa, S. Maturo, G. Flamino, and C. Esposito (1981), Perspectives and limits of an immunoenzymatic assay (ELISA) for herpes simplex virus (HSV) tumor associated antigens (TAA). *Cancer Detect. Prev.* **4**, 47–51.

Terris, M., F. Wilson, H. Smith, E. Spring, and J. H. Nelson (1967), Epidemiology of the cancer of the cervix. V. The relationship of coitus to carcinoma of the cervix. *Am. J. Public Health* **57**, 840–847.

Thiry, L., S. Sprecher-Goldberger, E. Hanecart-Pokorni, I. Gould, and M. Bossens (1977), Specific non-immunoglobulin G antibodies and cell-mediated response to herpes simplex virus antigens in women with cervical carcinoma. *Cancer Res.* **37**(5), 1301–1306.

Thomas, D. B. and W. E. Rawls (1978), Relationship of herpes simplex virus type 2 antibodies and squamous dysplasia to cervical carcinoma in situ. *Cancer* **42**, 2716–2725.

Tobin, S. M., W. D. Wilson, E. N. Fish, and F. R. Papsin (1978), Relation of herpesvirus hominis type 2 to carcinoma of the cervix. An animal model for the induction of long-term latency of herpesvirus hominis type 2. *Obstet. Gynecol.* **51**(6), 707–712.

Tobin, S. M., E. N. Fish, M. V. V. S. Cooter, and F. R. Papsin (1979), Relation of HSV-II to carcinoma of the cervix. *Obstet. Gynecol.* **53**(5), 553–558.

Underwood, G. E. and S. D. Weed (1974), Recurrent cutaneous herpes simplex in hairless mice. *Infect. Immun.* **10**(3), 471–474.

Vahlne, A., B. Nyström, M. Sandberg, A. Hamberger, and E. Lycke (1978), Attachment of herpes simplex virus to neurons and glial cells. *Gen. Virol.* **40**(2), 359–371.

Vahlne, A., B. Svennerholm, and E. Lycke (1979), Evidence for herpes simplex virus type-selective receptors on cellular plasma membranes. *J. Gen. Virol.* **44**(1), 217–225.

Vontver, L. A., W. C. Reeves, M. Rattray, L. Corey, M. A. Remington, E. Tolentino, A. Schweid, and K. K. Holmes (1979), Clinical course and diagnosis of genital herpes simplex virus infection and evaluation of topical surfactant therapy. *Am. J. Obstet. Gynecol.* **133**(5), 548–554.

Wahi, P. N., S. Mali, and U. K. Luthra (1969), Factors influencing cancer of the cervix in North India. *Cancer* **23**, 1221–1226.

Wakefield, J., R. Yule, and A. Smith (1973), Relation of abnormal cytological smears and carcinoma of the cervix uteri to husband's occupation. *Br. Med. J.* **2**, 142–143.

Walboomers, J. M. M. and J. T. Schegget (1976), A new method for the isolation of herpes simplex virus type 2 DNA. *Virology* **74**(1), 256–258.

Wentworth, B. B., P. Bonin, K. K. Holmes, and E. R. Alexander (1973), Isolation of viruses, bacteria and other organisms from veneral disease clinic patients: Methodology and problems associated with multiple isolations. *Health Lab. Sci.* **10**, 75–81.

Wentz, W. B. and J. W. Reagan (1970), Clinical significance of postirradiation dysplasia of the uterine cervix. *Am. J. Obstet. Gynec.* **106**, 812–817.

Wolontis, S. and S. Jeansson (1977), Correlation of herpes simplex virus types 1 and 2 with clinical features of infection. *J. Infect. Dis.* **135**(1), 28–33.

Woodruff, J. D., L. Braun, R. Cavalieri, P. Gupta, F. Pass, and K. V. Shah (1980), Immunologic identification of papillomavirus antigen in condyloma tissue from the female genital tract. *Obstet. Gynecol.* **56**(6), 727–732.

zur Hausen, H. (1980), The role of viruses in human tumors. *Adv. Cancer Res.* **33**, 77–107.

zur Hausen, H. (1982), Human genital cancer: Synergism between two virus infections or synergism between a virus infection and initiating events? *Lancet* **2**(8312), 1370–1372.

zur Hausen, H., H. Schulte-Holthauser, H. Wolf, K. Dorries, and H. Egger (1974), Attempts to detect virus-specific DNA in human tumors. II. Nucleic acid hybridization with complementary RNA of human herpes group tissues. *Int. J. Cancer* **13**, 657–664.

Papillomaviruses in Anogenital Neoplasms

Wayne D. Lancaster, Robert J. Kurman, and A. Bennett Jenson

1. Introduction

In the past, the search for a virus involved in the induction of human cancer has been frustrating. With the advent of more sophisticated techniques in molecular biology, a number of viruses have gained renewed interest as possible human cancer viruses; one such virus is the human papillomavirus (HPV). Although HPV was one of the first viruses to be visualized by the electron microscope, little information was available on the biology of the virus until recently. In early studies (reviewed by Rowson and Mahy, 1967), there was little indication that HPV may be associated with malignancy. As early as the 1930's, however, experimental evidence indicated that the cottontail rabbit papillomavirus (CRPV) was oncogenic in its host species (Rous and Beard, 1935). Other animal papillomaviruses were subsequently shown to produce tumors in laboratory animals and some were capable of morphologic transformation of cells in culture (Olson et al., 1969). Unfortunately, neither experimental transmission of HPV to laboratory animals nor a tissue culture system permissive for virus replication or expression of biological activity has been successful. For these reasons, research on HPV has been limited for the most part to physical and chemical characterization of virions obtained from papillomas.

Two recent developments that render HPV attractive from the standpoint of viral oncogenesis is the discovery of multiple, minimally related virus types with anatomic site preference, and the detection of HPV antigens and DNA in lesions with malignant

153

potential that were previously thought to be caused by other infectious agents or were of unknown etiology. The inability to define a system permissive for the replication of these viruses in culture has been circumvented to some extent by molecular cloning of virus DNA sequences that permits detailed molecular analysis.* This review will describe the methods used to detect papillomaviral antigens and DNA sequences in premalignant and malignant lesions of the anogenital tract, and to briefly review new information available on HPV. Recent, more detailed descriptions of animal and human papillomaviruses and their biology can be found in Lancaster and Olson (1982), Pfister (1984), and Jenson et al., 1984).

2. Papillomavirus Properties

2.1. Chemical Composition

Members of the papillomavirus genus are small (50–55 nm diameter), unenveloped viruses with an icosahedral symmetry. Their genome consists of a circular, double-stranded DNA molecule containing about 8000 base pairs (8 kb). Virions can be easily isolated from papillomas that are virus-positive with use of electron microscopy, by mechanically disrupting the epithelium followed by a series of differential centrifugation steps and banding in CsCl. In most preparations, two bands can be visualized—one band at 1.33 gm/mL representing "full" virions that contain DNA, and another band at 1.29 gm/mL that is composed of "empty" virus shells. After removal of CsCl by dialysis, DNA is isolated by rupture of virions with ionic detergent and removal of protein by organic extraction. The resultant DNA preparation generally contains two forms of DNA; a supercoiled fraction (Fo I) and a nicked-circular form (Fo II). If a nick occurs at the same site on both DNA strands, a unit length linear molecule (Fo III) is generated. These three virus DNA forms have different migration patterns in agarose gels.

The papillomavirus genome is capable of coding for only a limited number of polypeptides. Polypeptides of "full" virions consist of a major component of approximately 50,000 D and two or three minor components. Host cell-derived histones are associated with virion DNA and are absent in "empty" virions. Because it is difficult to obtain large quantities of virus, structural polypeptide analysis is incomplete.

2.2. Papillomavirus Plurality

One of the more interesting features of the papillomavirus genus is the multiplicity of virus types infecting a given host. To date, five different viruses have been identified that infect cattle. These viruses have different degrees of DNA sequence homology, antigenic relatedness, and tissue specificity (cutaneous or mucosal surfaces), and induce different types of lesions (fibropapillomas or papillomas).

The HPVs show even greater diversity. Eighteen different HPV types have now been described and it is anticipated that as detection techniques become more sophisticated, additional types will be discovered. To be classified as a new virus type, there may be no more than 50% DNA sequence homology under standard conditions of hybridization to previously typed viruses; a virus DNA that hybridizes to greater than 50% to a given virus type is considered a subtype (Coggin and zur Hausen, 1979). Standard hybridizations are run at 25°C below the melting temperature of the DNAs (T_m, 25°C), which allows for about 17% base mismatch (Laird et al., 1969).

As the list of HPV types grows, it appears that the viruses can be grouped with respect to sequence homology and site of infection (Table 1). Viruses infecting cutaneous surfaces are more likely to have some degree of homology to other HPVs infecting the skin than those infecting mucosal surfaces. Although a particular virus type is preferentially associated with a given lesion, it can, on occasion, be found in other lesions. For example, HPV-1 is associated with approximately 85% of plantar warts, but HPV-2 has also been detected in a small percentage of plantar warts, and vice versa (Jenson et al., 1982b).

Of interest is the group of HPVs (types 3, 5, 8–10, 12–15, and 17) found associated with individuals with epidermodysplasia verruciformis (EV), a rare recessive disorder characterized by generalized pityriasis-like lesions or flat warts (Jablonska et al., 1972). These virus types (except for types 3 and 10) have not been detected in warts from healthy individuals, but have been identified in lesions from immunosuppressed renal allograft recipients (Lutzner et al., 1980) and HPV-5 sequences have been detected in skin cancers from these patients (Lutzner et al., 1983). Lesions containing HPV-5 and HPV-8 frequently undergo malignant conversion when present on sun-exposed areas, and hybridization analysis of primary and metastatic cancers have shown the presence of HPV type 5 or type 8 DNA sequences within these tumors (Orth et al., 1980; Ostrow et al., 1982; Pfister et al., 1983a).

Table 1
The Human Papillomaviruses

Site	Lesion	Homology within group, %
CUTANEOUS		
HPV-1	Plantar wart (Favre et al., 1975)	<1% (Heilman et al., 1980; Ostrow et al., 1981)
HPV-2	Common wart (Orth et al., 1977)	
HPV-4	Plantar wart (Gissmann et al., 1977)	
HPV-7	Butchers' common wart (Orth et al., 1981; Ostrow et al., 1981)	
HPV-3	Flat wart (Orth et al., 1978)	35% (Kremsdorf et al., 1983)
HPV-10	Flat wart (Green et al., 1982)	
HPV-5	EV[a] (Orth et al., 1980)	5–39% (Kremsdorf et al., 1983; Kremsdorf et al., 1984)
HPV-8	EV (Orth et al., 1980	
HPV-12	EV (Kremsdorf et al., 1983)	
HPV-14	EV (Kremsdorf et al., 1984)	
HPV-9	EV (Orth et al., 1980)	5–19% (Kremsdorf et al., 1984)
HPV-15	EV (Kremsdorf et al., 1984)	
HPV-17	EV (Kremsdorf et al., 1984)	
MUCOCUTANEOUS/MUCOSAL		
HPV-6	Genital wart (Gissmann and zur Hausen, 1980)	3–25% (Pfister et al., 1983b)
HPV-11	Laryngeal papilloma (Gissmann et al., 1982)	
HPV-13	Focal epithelial Hyperplasia (Pfister et al., 1983b)	
HPV-16	Cervical carcinoma (Dürst et al., 1983)	<1% (Boshart et al., 1984)
HPV-18	Cervical carcinoma (Boshart et al., 1984)	

[a] Pityriasis-like lesions of epidermodysplasia verruciformis.

2.3. Evolutionary Relatedness

2.3.1. DNA Sequence Homology

Analysis of papillomavirus genomes has been difficult because the lack of a suitable tissue culture system permissive for their replication. Because many of the genomes of these viruses have now been molecularly cloned, DNA sequence analysis has provided new insights into possible functions of the virus genome. The entire nucleotide sequence for bovine papillomavirus type 1 (BPV-1) (Chen et al., 1982), HPV-1a (Danos et al., 1982), and HPV-6b (Schwarz et al., 1983) has been determined. Two striking similarities exist between the viral sequences—the presence of a number of open reading frames within only one strand of virus DNA that are roughly colinear between the viral genomes, and the high degree of nucleotide sequence homology exhibited in two noncontiguous regions of the viral DNAs.

These two regions of sequence homology were previously detected by molecular hybridization under conditions in which heteroduplexes with approximately 75% sequence homology would remain stable. Under normal conditions of hybridization, in which >80% base matching is required for stability, these regions of homology could not be detected (Law et al., 1979). Subsequently, Heilman et al. (1980) demonstrated by nonstringent hybridization that some of the HPV DNAs that were tested (HPV-1, HPV-2, and HPV-4) were as related to each other as to BPV-1, thus indicating the extent of divergence of these viruses. A number of investigators have used nonstringent hybridization techniques to detect new papillomavirus DNA sequences in human neoplasms employing a variety of human and animal papillomavirus DNAs as probes (Krzyzek et al., 1980; Lancaster and Jenson, 1981; Lancaster et al., 1983; Okagaki et al., 1983).

2.3.2. Common Antigens

The papillomaviruses are also related antigenically. Orth et al. (1978a) observed that sera from domestic rabbits bearing transplantable CRPV-induced carcinomas reacted not only with virions in CRPV-induced papillomas, but also with virions in nuclei of human warts. Expanding on this, Jenson et al. (1980) showed that an antiserum prepared against detergent-disrupted HPV (but not intact virions) purified from a pool of plantar warts reacted with a variety of human and animal papillomas. The reaction was limited to nuclei in the upper layers of the epithelium and failed to react with virus-negative (by electron microscopy) papillomas. The antiserum was not cross-reactive with normal epithelium or cells infected with viruses from other virus families. Such antisera have been used to detect papillomavirus structural antigens in a number of human lesions from the skin and mucous membranes. In addition, these antisera have been shown to be reactive with virus-containing, formalin-fixed, paraffin-embedded tissues (reviewed by Kurman et al., 1983).

The common antigenic determinants being detected with these antisera are unknown. However, the predicted amino acid sequence deduced from the nucleotide sequence of the putative open reading frame encoding the major structural component of BPV-1, HPV-1a, and HPV-6b indicates a high degree of amino acid identity within discrete regions. This suggests that these areas are highly conserved and are not normally exposed to the immune system of the host and may represent the cross-reactive determinants. Cross-reactive sera from CRPV-induced, tumor-bearing rabbits may be the result of exposure of the immune system of rabbits to viral structural polypeptides that are not assembled into mature virions. In early studies (Mellors, 1960; Osato and Ito, 1967), antigens cross-reactive with antibody to intact CRPV could frequently be detected in transplantable carcinomas, but no infectious virions were present.

2.4. Papillomavirus Genome Function

Functional aspects of HPV genomes are unknown; however, information is available from animal papillomavirus systems. Because the genomic organization is highly conserved among the papillomaviruses, it is reasonable to assume similar relationships with respect to genome structure and function between animal and human papillomaviruses. Since some of the animal papillomaviruses are highly oncogenic, it is likely that all or a portion of this function may be a property of some of the HPVs.

Lowy et al. (1980) demonstrated that cloned BPV-1 sequences were capable of transforming mouse cells. In addition, a 69% fragment of the BPV-1 genome was capable of cell transformation, but with a somewhat reduced efficiency. Studies confirmed that RNA was transcribed only from this region in cells transformed by intact DNA or the 69% transforming fragment (Heilman et al., 1982). In BPV-1-induced bovine fibropapillomas, RNA was detected that was derived exclusively from within this 69% transforming region in the nonproductive fibromatous area of the fibropapilloma, whereas the entire viral genome was represented in the epithelial (papillomatous) portion in which virus structural antigens are expressed (Amtmann and Sauer, 1982; Engel et al., 1983). It is unknown whether RNA derived from the 69% transforming region is translated; however, Barthold and Olson (1978) were able to detect a faint membrane fluorescence on cells derived from BPV-induced fibromas using sera from tumor-bearing horses and cattle. Other investigators have been unsuccessful in demonstrating virus-specific antigens associated with BPV-transformed cells, and no evidence exists for such antigens in human papillomas.

Examination of the viral genome in transformed cells, nonproductive portions of fibropapillomas, and tumors induced in laboratory animals reveals one of the more interesting aspects of papillomavirus biology; apparent lack of integration of the viral genome for maintenance of the transformed state. For BPV, this lack of integration has been documented in a variety of tumors and cell lines and to a level of sensitivity of 0.1 genome equivalent per cell in cloned, virus-transformed mouse cells (Lancaster and Olson, 1980; Lancaster, 1981; Law et al., 1981). In some CPRV-induced tumors, however, about 1% of the viral sequences present in a number of tumor DNA preparations yielded patterns after restriction enzyme digestion that would be consistent with viral–cellular DNA junction pieces. This would suggest that CRPV sequences can integrate into the host-cell genome in tumors induced by the virus (Wettstein and Stevens, 1982). Analysis of HPV DNA sequences in EV carcinomas has not shown evidence for integration; however, in some tumors there were deletions in the viral genome (Orth et al., 1980; Ostrow et al., 1982; Pfister et al., 1983a).

2.5. Virus Host–Cell Interactions

Productive papillomavirus infection of epithelial cells results in hyperplasia of cells in the spinous layer (acanthosis). These cells show an increase in size and the number of desmosomes and tonofibrils. Other epithelial cells show degenerative changes with loss of tonofibrils, detachment of desmosomes, nuclear wrinkling, and cytoplasmic vacuolization; in the upper layers of the epithelium, these changes are more pronounced. Cells in the granular layer show nuclear degeneration, margination, and condensation of chromatin. Virions are evident in nuclei of degenerated cells in the keratin layer by electron microscopy and are frequently in crystalline array.

Host immune responses to papillomavirus infection are not well understood, but infection usually occurs in the young followed by persistence of the wart for a variable period of time.

After regression the host is left immune to reinfection by the same virus. In man, antibody response to HPV infection is characterized by the appearance of IgM prior to the onset of regression; just after regression, both IgM and IgG antibodies are present, and long after regression only IgG is detectable (reviewed by von Krough, 1979). The conversion from IgM to IgG has also been observed in cattle experimentally infected with BPV (Lee and Olson, 1969b).

Rejection of papillomas appears to be closely associated with cell-mediated immunity. In cattle experimentally infected with papillomavirus, regression is preceded by infiltration of mononuclear leukocytes, mainly lymphocytes; this occurs generally in perivascular areas, but also as a diffuse scattering throughout the papilloma (Lee and Olson, 1969a). In man, regressing flat warts have a similar histological appearance with perivascular infiltration of mononuclear leukocytes in the upper dermis with epidermal invasion sharply confined to the papilloma (Tagami et al., 1974). The simultaneous regression of multiple warts at distant sites suggest that cell-mediated immunity plays a major role in papilloma rejection. Regression of flat warts has no effect, however, on plantar or palmar warts in the same individual, indicating that regression is HPV type-specific (Berman and Berman, 1978). A similar differential regression of warts has also been observed in cattle infected with multiple BPV types (Barthold et al., 1974).

3. Evidence for the Association of HPV with Anogenital Neoplasia

Infection of the human anogenital tract by HPV was first indicated by transmission experiments of cell-free extracts of anogenital warts (condylomata acuminata) to the skin of human volunteers (reviewed by Rowson and Mahy, 1967). These observations were later substantiated by direct observation of intranuclear virus particles in genital warts by electron microscopy (Dunn and Ogilvie, 1968), and later proven by detection of papillomavirus structural antigens in 50% of cases and DNA sequences of HPV-6 in about 65% of lesions (Woodruff et al., 1980; Kurman et al., 1981; Gissmann et al., 1983). In the majority of cases, typical exophytic condylomata are spread by sexual contact (Barrett et al., 1954; Teokharov, 1969; Oriel, 1971) and HPV structural antigens have been detected in condylomas occurring in the oral cavity (Jenson et al., 1982a), male urethra (Dean et al., 1983; Murphy et al., 1983), and urinary bladder (authors' unpublished results). The prevalence of genital condylomata is high, with an incidence of 50.34/100,000 population recorded in 1978 in England (Department of Health and Social Security, 1979). In the United States, the Centers for Disease Control (1983) estimated that the number of consultations for condylomata with private physicians increased from 169,000 in 1966 to 946,000 in 1981. Numerous clinical observations suggest that these lesions have malignant potential. Approximately 5% of squamous carcinomas of the vulva and 15% of penile squamous cancers develop in association with condylomata (Boxer and Skinner, 1977).

HPV infection of the female genital tract was thought to be associated with exophytic, papillary lesions based on experience with genital warts and cervical condylomata. zur Hausen (1976) proposed that HPV may be associated with genital cancers based on the proven oncogenicity of papillomaviruses in animals and humans and on the epidemiologic similarities of condylomata and genital cancer. The identification of koilocytotic cells (Koss and Durfee, 1956), commonly observed in condylomas, in flat cervical lesions traditionally classified as dysplasia suggested that HPV might play a role in cervical neoplasia (Meisels and Fortin, 1977). The observation by Hills and Laverty (1979) of papillomavirus-like particles in nuclei of koilocytes in a routine cervical smear provided inferential evidence for HPV infection of the cervix. Direct evidence, however, was provided by immunocytochemical and DNA hybridization studies (Kurman et al., 1982). The significance of the role of HPV in cervical neoplasia may be underscored by the fact that cytological studies have revealed that cellular alterations thought to be caused by HPV infection (koilocytosis) are present in the cervix of 1–2% of all women and 5–10% of young women screened (Ludwig et al., 1981).

Whereas 2–10% of squamous lesions of the cervix are exophytic condylomas, 70% of lesions previously classified as mild dysplasia (cervical intraepithelial neoplasia, CIN I) were reclassified by some (Meisels et al., 1982) as "flat condylomas." In addition, 25–35% or more of cervical lesions regarded as moderate to severe dysplasia/carcinoma *in situ* (CIS) (CIN II to CIN III, respectively), are associated with changes interpreted as condylomatous, and therefore have been reclassified by some as "atypical condyloma" (Meisels et al., 1982). Lesions with few if any atypical changes in the proliferating cells (basal and parabasal), but with atypical degenerative changes in the maturing cells, have been traditionally classified as a mild dysplasia (CIN I) and recently by some as a "flat condyloma." Lesions exhibiting nuclear pleomorphism, primarily in the proliferating cells, hyperchromatism, presence of atypical mitotic figures, and disturbance in the level of maturation have been referred to as moderate (CIN II) or severe dysplasia/CIS (CIN III). If there is evidence of papillomavirus atypia (koilocytosis) (Kurman et al., 1983), the lesion may be classified as dysplasia (mild, moderate, or severe) or CIN (I, II, or III) with evidence of HPV infection.

There is controversy over the appropriate terminology to be used to describe the various types of intraepithelial cervical lesions. In the past, all of these lesions were included within the category of dysplasia or CIN and were regarded as precursors to cervical squamous cell carcinoma. Detection of HPV antigens and DNA sequences in many of these lesions has led some investigators to attempt to distinguish HPV infection from lesions tht are truly neoplastic. Because there is considerable overlap in the morphology of these lesions and it is not clear at present whether all lesions that are viral are benign or whether a subset of these may progress to cancer, it is appropriate to retain the traditional classification of dysplasia or CIN until the behavior of these lesions has been established.

3.1. Immunological Studies

Intranuclear HPV antigens have been detected by immuno-cytochemical methods specific for papillomavirus structural antigens in association with mild dysplasia in 43% of cases, moderate dysplasia in 15% of cases, severe dysplasia in 17% of cases, and CIS in 10% of cases (Kurman et al., 1983). The lesions were generally present within metaplastic squamous epithelium in the transformation zone. Involvement of endocervical glands was frequently observed.

Mild dysplasias are characterized by a thickened epithelium composed of cells with varying degrees of atypical, degenerative nuclear changes overlying a hyperplastic zone of typical basal and parabasal cells. Cells displaying viral-induced nuclear degeneration are confined to the superficial and intermediate layers in which antigen distribution is either focal (Fig. 1) or diffuse (Fig. 2). Nuclei within the hyperplastic zone do not stain, although parabasal cells near the surface are occasionally positive. Moderate dysplasias show a greater degree of nuclear atypia and proliferation. The hyperplastic zone usually occupies one-half to two-thirds of the epithelium. Mitotic activity is prominent and abnormal mitotic figures are occasionally observed. Antigen localization is confined

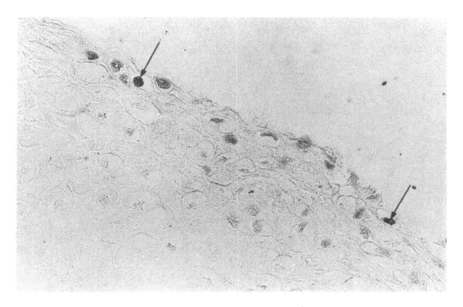

Fig. 1. Immunoperoxidase localization of HPV structural antigens in a cervical dysplasia. Focal distribution of the antigens is seen in superficial epithelial cells employing a papillomavirus genus-specific antiserum. Virus antigens (black precipitate, arrows) are localized in nuclei of cells showing HPV-induced atypia (no counterstain, PAP, ×395).

to the superficial layers of the epithelium, which is similar to the mild dysplasias. In severe dysplasia and CIS, virus structural antigens are usually present in areas of mild and moderate dysplasia immediately adjacent to the high-grade lesions. Rarely are antigens present directly within severe dysplasia. When present, however, the antigens are confined to the most superficial layers. When virus antigen-containing nuclei are present in moderate dysplasia, the positive cells merge imperceptibly with the high-grade lesions. The proliferating basal and parabasal cells in the high-grade lesions are generally indistinguishable from those of moderate dysplasia, making it difficult to distinguish cytologic changes attributable to viral infection from those associated with neoplastic transformation; however, a sharp demarcation is occasionally seen between low- and high-grade lesions (Fig. 3). Fewer positive nuclei are found in areas of moderate and mild dysplasia adjacent to the high-grade lesions than in mild and moderate dysplasias unassociated with high-grade lesions.

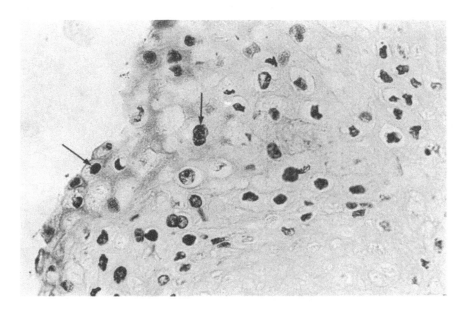

Fig. 2. Immunoperoxidase localization of HPV structural antigens in a diffuse distribution in a cervical dysplasia by employing a papillomavirus genus-specific antiserum. Virus antigens (black precipitate, arrows) are localized in degenerative nuclei of varying sizes and shapes and many nuclei do not stain (no counterstain, PAP, ×395).

Dysplasias with no demonstrable antigen have similar histologic alterations (koilocytosis, nuclear wrinkling, bi- and multinucleation, and dyskaryosis) as positive lesions. This discrepancy in antigen positivity (roughly 50% of lesions) has been noted in plantar and common warts (Jenson et al., 1982b), laryngeal papillomas (Lack et al., 1980; Costa et al., 1981), and condylomata of the vulva and vagina (Woodruff et al., 1980; Kurman et al., 1981), lesions all known to contain HPV. The reasons for lack of antigen are unknown, but could be related to low sensitivity of the immunocytochemical test or periodic cycling of viral genome expression of genes encoding structural polypeptides, perhaps modulated by the host immune system. Periodic antigen expression was observed by Lack et al. (1980), who showed that detection of HPV antigens in laryngeal papilloma increased from 48% when only one biopsy was performed to 100% when four or more sequential biopsies were taken.

The failure to detect viral antigens in the majority of more advanced cervical lesions could be the result of a disturbance in virus gene expression associated with neoplastic transformation.

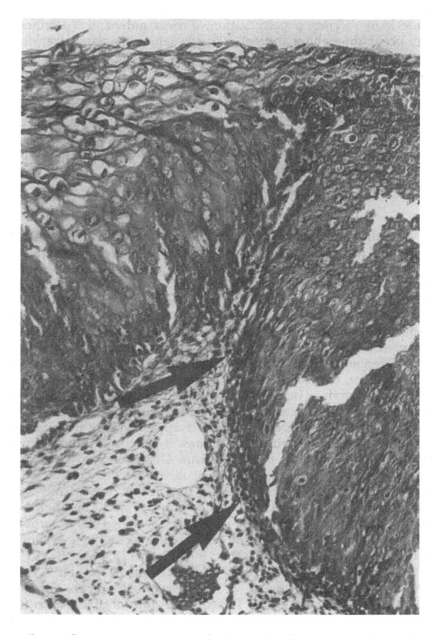

Fig. 3. Carcinoma *in situ* on right (arrows) adjacent to moderate dysplasia on left demonstrating a sharp demarcation between a high- and low-grade lesion. This lesion was positive for HPV structural antigens (hematoxylin and eosin, ×270).

This could also account for the decrease in the number of positive nuclei within mild and moderate dysplasias associated with high-grade lesions. Thus, a perturbation of virus polypeptide synthesis may occur throughout the entire lesion when neoplastic transformation occurs in part of it. Similar to this situation are lesions of EV in which benign wart-like skin lesions contain large number of virus particles; however, virus particles are scarce at the time of *in situ* carcinoma development and have never been detected after invasion occurs (Ruiter and Van Mullem, 1970). Similarly, infectious virus can be obtained in high quantities from benign cottontail rabbit papillomas, but have not been recovered after the lesion becomes malignant (Kidd and Rous, 1940).

3.2. DNA Hybridization

Recent studies have demonstrated the presence of HPV DNA sequences in a high percentage of cervical dysplasias. In a series of 13 biopsies, HPV DNA sequences were detected in four of seven mild dysplasias, three of three moderate dysplasias, and in a single case of severe dysplasia (Lancaster et al., 1983). This study was unable to distinguish the HPV type because the conditions of hybridization (nonstringent) were designed to detect papillomavirus common DNA sequences. Based on restriction enzyme digestions, four different DNA banding patterns emerged, indicating that, at the very least, four different HPV subtypes are capable of infecting the uterine cervix. The inability to detect viral sequences in three of seven mild dysplasias may have been because of the sensitivity of the hybridization reaction, which is approximately fivefold less sensitive than that of stringent reactions. It has the advantage, however, of detecting any papillomavirus DNA, circumventing the need for specific probes. Okagaki et al. (1983) demonstrated the presence of HPV sequences in 19/19 samples of cervical and vaginal intraepithelial neoplasms employing various conditions of hybridization stringency with molecularly cloned HPV probes. Gissmann et al. (1983), using HPV type-specific probes under stringent hybridization conditions, identified HPV types 6 and 11 DNA sequences in 86% of condylomata acuminata and HPV-11 in five of five "flat condylomas" or dysplasias of the cervix. In addition, they detected HPV type 11 sequences (but not HPV-6) in five of 27 cervical cancers (three invasive and two CIS). Although unable to detect HPV 11 in a series of dysplasias, Lancaster et al. (1983) were able to show that one of six invasive squamous cell carcinomas of the cervix harbored HPV-11 sequences. Another virus, HPV-10, isolated from flat warts of a patient with EV, hybridized extensively to HPV sequences in two of 37 invasive cervical cancers, as well as two condylomas (Green et al., 1982).

Employing nonstringent hybridization detection, Dürst et al. (1983) were able to identify and clone a new HPV DNA (type 16) from a biopsy of cervical cancer. DNA from this new virus type hybridized under stringent conditions to a high proportion of cervical cancers from German patients (11/18) and to a lower proportion of cervical cancers from Kenya and Brazil (8/23). Sequences representing this new virus were detected in only two of 33 condylomas and two of 20 cervical dysplasias. These results suggest that there may be regional differences in the HPV type infecting the cervix and that HPV-16 (at least in the German population) may be a virus that possesses a high degree of oncogenic potential because of the disparity in detection between dysplasia and carcinoma. In a study of 23 cervical and vaginal cases of dysplasia, Crum et al. (1984) correlated the presence of HPV-16 DNA sequences in seven of 10 cases with abnormal mitotic figures and aneuploidy; only one of the remaining 13 cases contained HPV-16 sequences. Thus, the presence of a specific HPV type(s) may be associated with lesions that present high risk to the individual.

Recently, DNA from an additional virus, HPV-18, has been molecularly cloned from a cervical cancer (Boshart et al., 1984). DNA sequences from this HPV have been detected in about 22% of invasive cervical cancers, but not in 25 cases of CIS and dysplasia that were tested. Interestingly, HPV-18 DNA sequences have been detected in HeLa cells. This cell line was established in 1951 from tumor tissue originally diagnosed as epidermoid carcinoma of the cervix (Gey et al., 1952), but was reclassified as an adenocarcinoma upon review of the original slides (Jones et al., 1971). As opposed to other papillomaviruses, HPV-18 DNA has been found only in the integrated state in cervical cancers and HeLa cells.

4. Detection of HPV Structural Antigens

4.1. Method of Analysis

The various antisera used to detect papillomavirus structural antigens have been derived either from virus obtained from pools of human plantar warts or bovine fibropapillomas. BPV-1 has been employed as an immunogen because of the availability of fibropapillomas, thereby ensuring a standardized source of virus. In addition, there is less of a chance of false positive reactions with endogenous proteins that may be present in preparations of HPV. BPV-1 virions purified by banding in CsCl and sedimentation through sucrose gradients are disrupted with 1% SDS and the virus suspension made 0.24M with 2-mercaptoethanol and heated to 68°C for 15 min. Antigen is diluted in saline and mixed with an equal amount of Freund's complete adjuvant and rabbits inoculated subcutaneously three times with decreasing doses of antigen over a period of 6 wk (Jenson et al., 1980). This hyperimmune serum [anti-BPV-1(SDS)] is reactive at 1:30 dilution with virus-positive (by electron microscopy) cutaneous and mucosal papillomas from a variety of species, including human, dog, cow, rabbit, deer, and horse; it does not react with virus-negative papillomas (Jenson et al., 1980). An antiserum derived from BPV-1 similar to BPV-1(SDS) is available from Dako Corp., Santa Barbara, CA.

Papillomavirus structural antigens are detectable by indirect immunofluorescence using anti-BPV-1(SDS) on acetone-fixed frozen sections and by the peroxidase–antiperoxidase (PAP) or biotin–avidin procedure on formalin-fixed, paraffin-embedded tissues. The latter are advantageous because of ease of sectioning, increased sensitivity, improved cytologic morphology, and the ability to perform retrospective studies (Kurman et al., 1984).

Four micron sections are cut from the paraffin-embedded tissue blocks, deparaffinized, cleared, and washed in phosphate buffered saline. After quenching of endogenous peroxidase activity with 0.3% hydrogen peroxide and methanol, the sections are incubated for 30 min with 10% egg albumin to reduce nonspecific staining. The primary antibody (diluted 1:400) is then added to the sections and allowed to react overnight. The secondary antibody [swine anti-rabbit immunoglobulin (Dakopatts Accurate Chemical and Scientific Corp., Westbury, NY)] is diluted 1:40 and left on the sections for 30 min. This is followed by a 30-min incubation with a rabbit peroxidase–antiperoxidase complex diluted 1:80 (Sternberger-Meyer Immunocytochemicals Inc., Jarretsville, MD). The reaction is developed by the addition of 0.03% 3,3'-diaminobenzidine and 0.3% hydrogen peroxide in Tris-HCl (pH 7.6) for 13 min. Sections are then rehydrated, cleared, and mounted. Sections can be counterstained with hexatoxylin. The reactions and all washings performed between incubations are with phosphate buffered saline (pH 7.4). For the biotin–avidin method (Hsu et al., 1981), the primary antibody can be used at a dilution of 1:1000–1:1600. After a 30-min incubation with the secondary antibody (biotinylated anti-rabbit IgG), an avidin–biotinylated horseradish peroxidase complex is added (Vector Laboratories, Burlingame, CA), and the reaction developed as with the PAP method.

The procedures that have been performed to ascertain the specificity of the antiserum on mucosal tissues have been detailed elsewhere (Kurman et al., 1981). The positive control is a section of a virus-positive (by electron microscopy) human plantar wart run in parallel with the lesion to be tested. The negative control is a serial section of the lesion being tested incubated with normal rabbit serum at the appropriate dilution.

4.2. Interpretation of Results

Localization of HPV structural antigens is invariably intranuclear and confined to the upper third of the epithelium, often directly on the surface. Positive staining occurs in a wide variety of cell types, ranging from those with enlarged rounded nuclei having a diffuse finely granular chromatin pattern, to those with ovoid and flattened nuclei displaying all degrees of pyknosis and nuclear wrinkling. The cytoplasm may exhibit perinuclear vacuolation or may contain a large vacuole that compresses the nucleus against the cell membrane. Positive cells near the surface may have scant cytoplasm and show no evidence of vacuolation. Cells with double nuclei are sometimes positive. Localization of virus antigens is therefore not confined to cells showing the classic features of koilocytosis.

Cells in which virus antigens have not been identified include those showing marked pleomorphism, multinucleation, and individual cell keratinization. Cells containing virus antigens cannot be distinguished morphologically from those that do not. The number of positive cells depends on the lesion. In general, cutaneous lesions have more positive nuclei than lesions obtained from mucosal surfaces. Mucosal lesions tend to have focal areas of positive nuclei; therefore careful scrutiny of the microscopic sections stained for HPV is necessary. In focal staining patterns positive cells are located in the most superficial layer. In about 85% of cases with demonstrable virus antigen, positive cells overlie a zone of proliferating basal and parabasal cells showing varying degrees of nuclear atypia. There may be a marked degree of mitotic activity in these cells and abnormal mitotic figures may also be present; these proliferating cells are never positive for virus structural antigens.

5.   Detection of HPV DNA Sequences

5.1.   Methods of Analysis

A number of techniques of molecular hybridization are used for the detection of viral sequences in tissues; each has certain advantages and disadvantages. When large amounts of tissue are available, analysis of hybridization kinetics provides the opportunity to accurately quantitate the amount of viral DNA present, as well as distinguish sequences that are closely related, but not identical, to the probe and determine the percent homology. Reactions are run under conditions of hybridization (T_m, 25°C), in which the rate of reassociation of the probe is optimal (Wetmur and Davidson, 1968). The kinetics of the reaction are second-order when the sequences in the tissue are identical to those of the probe; however, the reaction exhibits complex kinetics when probe sequences have partial homology to those in the tissue (Sharp et al., 1974).

DNA can be isolated from tissue by sectioning on a cryostat and lysing the sections with 0.6% SDS, 0.01M EDTA, followed by overnight digestion with proteinase K (50 µg/mL). Protein is removed by phenol and chloroform extractions and nucleic acids precipitated with ethanol. RNA is removed by treatment with heat-treated RNase A and the DNA reextracted with phenol and chloroform. for kinetic studies, DNA solutions are sheared to a uniform single-stranded piece size (about 500 nucleotides) by sonication. Probe DNAs are labeled to high-specific activity using either ³H-thymidine triphosphate or alpha ³²P-deoxynucleotide triphosphates by nick translation (Rigby et al., 1977). The concentration of probe to cell DNA is determined by the sensitivity desired. To detect one papillomavirus genome per cell would require 1.3 pg of probe per µg of cell DNA (Gelb et al., 1971). DNAs are mixed, denatured, brought to the appropriate salt concentration and temperature, and allowed to hybridize for various periods of time. The rate of reassociation can be determined by quantitating the amount of probe hybridized either by hydroxyapatite chromatography (Britten and Kohne, 1968) or S1 nuclease digestion (Sutton, 1971).

A more flexible method of hybridization is the Southern blotting technique (Southern, 1975). This technique offers variability in the stringency of the hybridization reaction, as well as determination of the state of the viral sequences in the specimen under analysis. Cell DNA (5–20 µg) can either be digested with restriction endonucleases or left undigested and electrophoresed through agarose gels. The DNA is denatured in situ with alkali, then neutralized and transferred to a nitrocellulose membrane. To facilitate transfer of DNA in gels containing undigested or Fo 1 sequences, DNA is depurinated by treatment of the gel with dilute HCl prior to denaturation (Wahl et al., 1979). After washing, the membrane is baked under vacuum for 2 h at 80°C and prehybridized in 10x Denhardt's (1966) solution (0.2% each of Ficoll, bovine serum albumin, polyvinylpyrrolidone) in 4x SSC (SSC = 0.15M NaCl, 0.015M sodium citrate), containing 50 μg/mL sonicated and denatured salmon sperm DNA for 4 h at 60°C. Stringent hybridizations (T_m, 25°C) are carried out in solution containing 1–5 $\times$ 10^6 counts/min ^{32}P-labeled nick-translated DNA (specific activity of 1–2 $\times$ 10^8 counts/min/μg DNA), 1M NaCl, 1x Denhardt's, 0.15M TES [tris(hydroxymethyl)methyl-2-aminoethanesulfonic acid], pH 7.5, with 50 μg/mL sonicated and denatured salmon sperm DNA in 50% formamide for 16–24 h at 37°C. The membranes are washed extensively in 0.1x SSC at 52°C, air dried, and exposed to X-ray film.

For nonstringent hybridizations (T_m, 43°C), total cellular DNA results in background hybridization that interferes with the detection of HPV sequences. For these reactions, Hirt (1967) supernatant fractions are isolated by lysing tissue sections as described above, but prior to deproteinization the viscous solutions are brought to 1M NaCl and kept at 4°C overnight to precipitate high molecular weight sequences. The high and low molecular weight fractions are separated by centrifugation at 12,000g for 20 min in the cold. The supernatant is deproteinized, and the DNA precipitated and used for Southern analysis. Reactions are carried out as described above, except human lymphocyte DNA is used in place of salmon sperm DNA and hybridizations contain 30% formamide. Membranes are washed extensively in 4x SSC at 52°C, air dried, and exposed to X-ray film. Since the papillomaviruses have conserved DNA sequences that can be detected under nonstringent hybridization conditions, any papillomavirus DNA can be employed as the probe.

5.2. Interpretation of Results

A major consideration associated with hybridization analysis of papillomaviruses is the degree of relatedness the probe has with the sequences present in the specimen under study. This is important with the Southern blotting technique because a moderate degree of sequence homology under stringent conditions of hybridization can yield a strong signal even though the probe and sequences in the sample represent different virus types. HPV-6 and HPV-11 share about 25% sequence homology under stringent conditions (Gissmann et al., 1982), and unless restriction enzyme analyses are performed, it is difficult to determine whether a signal is caused by HPV-6 or HPV-11 sequences. To distinguish these two virus types and their subtypes, PstI digestion has proven useful (Gissmann et al., 1983). An example of this cross hybridization is shown in Fig. 4. DNA from a laryngeal papilloma was digested with PstI and probed with either HPV-6 or HPV-11. Although both probes hybridized to the sample, the signal produced by the HPV-11 probe was strong and the PstI fragments consistent with the pattern for HPV-11a were detectable. However, the HPV-6 probe hybridized to a significant extent but failed to hybridize to two of the five fragments, and the molecular weight of these fragments was much lower than the 8 kb expected for a papillomavirus genome.

Hybridization of multiple samples with a mixture of HPV probes has proven useful for rapid analysis of DNA preparations that contain different HPV types. DNA from two cervical squamous cell cancers were digested with PstI, blotted, and hybridized under stringent conditions to a probe containing a mixture of HPV-11 and HPV-16 (Fig. 5). The PstI cleavage pattern for one of the cervical cancers is consistent with HPV-16 (Dürst et al., 1983), whereas the other cervical cancer has a PstI cleavage pattern representative of HPV-11a DNA (Gissmann et al., 1983).

To determine whether HPV sequences are present in a sample that represents an uncharacterized virus type, nonstringent hybridization is the only method of choice. Shown in Fig. 6 is a Southern blot analysis hybridized under nonstringent conditions (T_m, 43°C) using a BPV-1 probe on a series of low molecular weight DNA fractions derived from colposcopically directed biopsies of cervical dysplasias. The samples were previously digested with BamHI or HindIII (restriction enzymes that cleave papillomavirus DNA at a limited number of sites). Depending on the restriction enzyme used, different patterns emerge. For example, the pattern exhibited by viral sequences in biopsy #23 indicate that they are not cleaved with BamHI, but do appear to contain a single HindIII site. The reverse is true for biopsy #27. Biopsy #15 has a very strong background signal that is problematic with nonstringent hybridizations and could not be analyzed. Biopsy #19 has a complex restriction pattern. Both BamHI and HindIII digestion yield unit length (Fo III) 8 kb molecules, as well as smaller fragments. this suggests that the biopsy may contain more than one HPV type or subtype. Similar

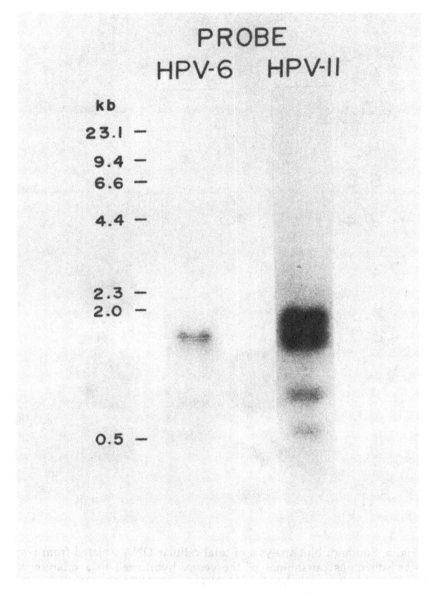

Fig. 4. Southern blot analysis of total cellular DNA isolated from a laryngeal papilloma probed with either molecularly cloned radiolabeled HPV-6 or HPV-11 DNA under stringent hybridization conditions. Prior to electrophoresis, the tumor DNA was digested with PstI. Size markers represent HindIII-digested lambda DNA run in parallel. The probes have been previously described (Gissmann et al., 1983).

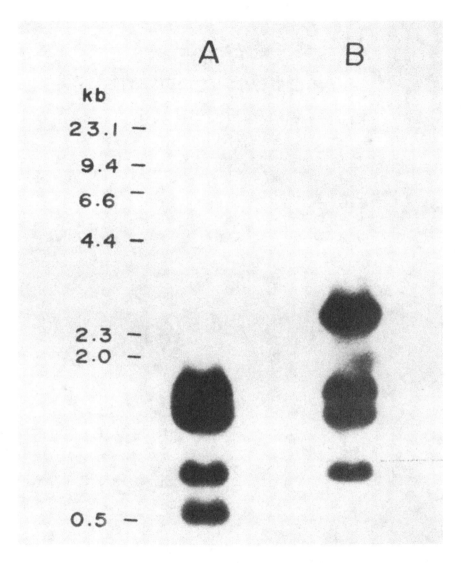

Fig. 5. Southern blot analysis of total cellular DNA isolated from two invasive squamous carcinomas of the cervix hybridized to a mixture of molecularly cloned radiolabeled HPV-11 and HPV-16 DNAs under stringent conditions. Prior to electrophoresis, the tumor DNAs were digested with PstI. The restriction pattern shown in panel A is consistent with HPV-11a DNA and the pattern in panel B represents HPV-16 DNA. Size markers represent HindIII-digested lambda DNA run in parallel. The probes have been previously described (Gissmann et al., 1983; Dürst et al., 1983).

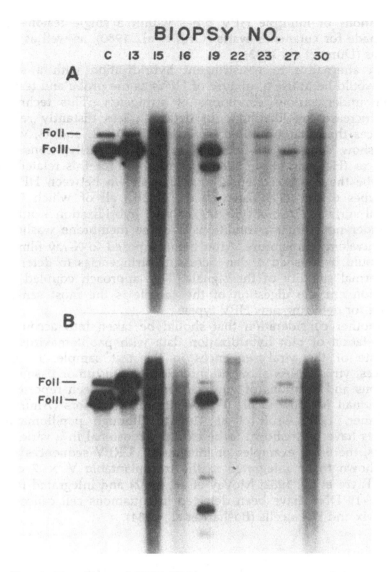

Fig. 6. Detection of HPV DNA sequences in cervical biopsies by Southern blot analysis employing a BPV-1 DNA probe under non-stringent conditions. Hirt supernatant fractions of the biopsies were digested with either BamHI (A) or HindIII (B) prior to electrophoresis. Lane C represents 10 ng of BamHI-digested HPV-1 DNA isolated from a pool of plantar warts. Biopsies #13, 15, 23, and 30 were diagnosed as mild dysplasia, #19 and 27 as moderate dysplasia, #16 as severe dysplasia, and #22 as squamous metaplasia. Fo II is nicked circular HPV-1 DNA and Fo III is unit length linear HPV-1 DNA.

observations of multiple HPV types within a single lesion have been made for cutaneous warts (Orth et al., 1980), as well as condylomas (Dürst et al., 1983).

An alternative to nonstringent hybridization with a single probe would be to use a mixture of HPVs as the probe and test the sample under various conditions of stringency. This technique could increase the likelihood of detecting less distantly related sequences than that exhibited between HPV-1, -2, and -4, which only show homology because of evolutionarily conserved sequences (Heilman et al., 1980). An example for this relatedness would be the 3–4% sequence homology shown between HPV-13 with types 6 and 11 (Pfister et al., 1983b), all of which infect mucosal surfaces. In this type of analysis, hybridization would be run under nonstringent conditions and the membrane washed at the equivalent temperature. After being exposed to X-ray film, the blot would be washed under increasing stringencies to determine the thermal stability of the signals. This approach coupled with restriction enzyme digestion of the sample is the most sensitive method for detecting new HPV types.

Another consideration that should be taken into account in interpretation of blot hybridization data with papillomaviruses is the state of the viral sequences in the test sample. In most instances, virus DNAs show no modifications in tumor tissue, but insertions and deletions of viral sequences have been reported in both human (Ostrow et al., 1982) and animal tumors (Amtmann and Sauer, 1980; Groff et al., 1983). Although papillomavirus genomes have been shown to be extrachromosomal in a variety of systems, there are examples of integration. CRPV sequences have been shown to be integrated in the transplantable V × 7 carcinoma (Favre et al., 1982; McVay et al., 1982) and integrated forms of HPV-18 DNA have been detected in squamous cell cancers of the cervix and HeLa cells (Boshart et al., 1984).

6. Papillomaviruses and Cancer

It is not clear what role, if any, HPV has in the genesis of anogenital cancer. The studies to date indicate an extremely high association of HPV with anogenital neoplasia, most notably premalignant and malignant lesions of the uterine cervix. Two parallels can be drawn to HPV and cervical cancer: the papilloma-to-carcinoma sequence in rabbits induced by CRPV and the evolution of pityriasis-like skin lesions in patients with EV to squamous carcinoma by HPV types 5 and 8. In both situations, secondary effectors (genetic background and other intrinsic factors, such as sunlight) appear to be involved with the transformation of the benign viral-induced lesion to cancer. The role of predisposing factors in cervical cancer, such as herpes simplex virus type-2 infection (zur Hausen, 1982) or cigaret smoking (Lyon et al., 1983; Trevathan et al., 1983), both of which are risk factors, and their interaction with HPV is unknown.

There is a close similarity of the clinical behavior of these papillomavirus-induced carcinomas to the natural history of cervical cancer and its precursors. Indirect evidence for HPV association in cervical neoplasia has been provided by morphologic, immunocytochemical, and molecular virologic studies. For the first time a venereally transmited agent can be linked through a series of morphologic transitions to a neoplasm. In addition, HPV structural antigens and HPV DNA sequences have been detected within all phases of the intraepithelial process leading to CIS and in a high proportion of invasive cancer. However, this does not establish HPV as the etiological agent of the disease.

Aside from the experimental data demonstrating the relationship of HPV and cervical cancer and the parallel to the papilloma-to-carcinoma sequence in rabbits and EV patients, no direct evidence exists that implicated HPV as a causal agent of the disease. The most definitive approach to answering this question would be the development of a vaccine administered to young women at high risk for the development of cervical cancer at the time that they become sexually active. A reduction in the incidence of dysplasia and carcinoma of the cervix would provide cogent evidence implicating certain HPV types as cofactors in the development of malignancy and would confirm the hypothesis that dysplasia is a precursor of cervical cancer.

References

Amtmann, E., H. Müller, and G. Sauer (1980), Equine connective tissue tumors contain unintegrated bovine papilloma virus DNA. *J. Virol.* **35**, 962–964.

Amtmann, E., and G. Sauer (1982), Bovine papilloma virus transcription: Polyadenylated RNA species and assessment of the direction of transcription. *J. Virol.* **43**, 59–66.

Barrett, T. J., S. J. Silbar, and J. P. McGinley (1954), Genital warts—a venereal disease. *J. Am. Med. Assoc.* **154**, 333–334.

Barthold, S. W., L. D. Koller, C. Olson, E. Studer, and A. Holtan (1974), Atypical warts in cattle. *J. Am. Vet. Med. Assoc.* **165**, 276–280.

Barthold, S. W., and C. Olson (1978), Common membrane neoantigen on bovine papilloma virus-induced fibroma cells from cattle and horses. *Am. J. Vet. Res.* **39**, 1643–1645.

Berman, A., and J. E. Berman (1978), Efflorescence of new warts: A sign of onset of involution in flat warts. *Br. J. Dermatol.* **99**, 179–182.

Boshart, M., L. Gissmann, H. Ikenberg, A. Kleinheinz, W. Scheurien, and H. zur Hausen (1984), A new type of papillomavirus DNA, its presence in genital cancer biopsies and in cell lines derived from cervical cancer. *EMBO J.* **3**, 1151–1157.

Boxer, R. J., and D. G. Skinner (1977), Condyloma acuminata and squamous carcinoma. *Urology* **9**, 72–78.

Britten, R. J., and D. E. Kohne (1968), Repeated sequences in DNA. *Science* **161**, 529–540.

Centers for Disease Control (1983), Condyloma acuminatum—United States, 1966–1981. *Morbid. Mortal. Weekly Report* **32**, 306–308.

Chen, E. Y., P. M. Howley, A. D. Levinson, and P. H. Seeburg (1982), The primary structure and genetic organization of the bovine papillomarivus type 1 genome. *Nature* **299**, 529–534.

Coggin, J. R., Jr., and H. zur Hausen (1979), Workshop on papillomaviruses and cancer. *Cancer Res.* **39**, 545–546.

Costa, J., P. M. Howley, M. C. Bowling, R. Howard, and W. C. Bauer (1981), Presence of human papilloma viral antigens in juvenile multiple laryngeal papilloma. *Am. J. Clin. Pathol.* **75**, 194–197.

Crum, C. P., H. Ikenberg, R. M. Richart, and L. Gissmann (1984), Human papillomavirus type 16 and early cervical neoplasia. *N. Eng. J. Med.* **10**, 880–883.

Danos, O., M. Katinka, and M. Yaniv (1982), Human papillomavirus 1a complete DNA sequence: A novel type of genome organization among papovaviridae. *EMBO J.* **1**, 231–236.

Dean, P., W. D. Lancaster, B. K. Chun, and A. B. Jenson (1983), Human papillomavirus structural antigens in squamous papillomas of the male urethra. *J. Urol.* **129**, 873–875.

Denhardt, D. T. (1966), A membrane filter technique for the detection of complementary DNA. *Biochem. Biophys. Res. Commun.* **23**, 641–646.

Department of Health and Social Security (1979), Sexually Transmitted Diseases, in *On the State of the Public Health: The Annual Report of the Chief Medical Officer of the Department of Health and Social Security for the Year 1978.* HMSO, London.

Dunn, A. E. G., and M. M. Ogilvie (1968), Intranuclear virus particles in human genital wart tissue: Observations on the ultrastructure of the epidermal layer. *J. Ultrastruct. Res.* **22**, 282–295.

Dürst, M., L. Gissmann, H. Ikenberg, and H. zur Hausen (1983), A new type of papillomavirus DNA from a cervical carcinoma and its prevalence in cancer biopsies from different geographic regions. *Proc. Natl. Acad. Sci. USA* **80**, 3812–3815.

Engel, L., C. A. Heilman, and P. M. Howley (1983), Transcriptional organization of bovine papillomavirus type 1. *J. Virol.* **47**, 516–528.

Favre, M., G. Orth, O. Croissant, and M. Yaniv (1975), Human papillomavirus DNA: Physical map. *Proc. Natl. Acad. Sci. USA* **72**, 4810–4814.

Favre, M., N. Jibard, and G. Orth (1982), Restriction mapping and physical characterization of the cottontail rabbit papillomavirus genome in transplantable VX2 and VX7 domestic rabbit carcinomas. *Virology* **119**, 298–309.

Gelb, L. D., D. E. Kohne, and M. A. Martin (1971), Quantitation of simian virus 40 sequences in African green monkey, mouse, and virus-transformed cell genomes. *J. Mol. Biol.* **57**, 129–145.

Gey, G. O., W. D. Coffman, and M. T. Kubicek (1952), Tissue culture studies of the proliferative capacity of cervical carcinoma and normal epithelium. *Cancer Res.* **12**, 264–265.

Gissmann, L., H. Pfister, and H. zur Hausen (1977), Human papilloma viruses (HPV): Characterization of four different isolates. *Virology* **76**, 569–580.

Gissmann, L., and H. zur Hausen (1980), Partial characterization of viral DNA from human genital warts (condylomata acuminata). *Int. J. Cancer* **25**, 605–609.

Gissmann, L., V. Diehl, H. -J. Schultz-Coulon, and H. zur Hausen (1982), Molecular cloning and characterization of human papilloma virus DNA derived from a laryngeal papilloma. *J. Virol.* **44**, 393–400.

Gissmann, L., L. Wolnick, H. Ikenberg, U. Koldovsky, H. G. Schnürch, and H. zur Hausen (1983), Human papillomavirus type 6 and type 11 DNA sequences in genital and laryngeal papillomas and some cervical cancers. *Proc. Natl. Acad. Sci.* **80**, 560–563.

Green, M., K. H. Brackmann, P. R. Sanders, P. M. Loewenstein, J. H. Freel, M. Eisinger, and S. A. Switlyk (1982), Isolation of a human papillomavirus from a patient with epidermodysplasisa verruciformis: Presence of related viral DNA genomes in human urogenital tumors. *Proc. Natl. Acad. Sci. USA* **79**, 4437–4441.

Groff, D. E., J. P. Sundberg, and W. D. Lancaster (1983), Extrachromosomal deer fibromavirus DNA in deer fibromas and virus-transformed mouse cells. *Virology* **131**, 546–550.

Heilman, C. A., M. -F Law, M. A. Israel, and P. M. Howley (1980), Cloning of human papilloma virus genomic DNAs and analysis of homologous polynucleotide sequences. *J. Virol.* **36**, 395–407.

Heilman, C. A., L. Engel, D. R. Lowy, and P. M. Howley (1982), Virus-specific transcription in bovine papillomavirus transformed mouse cells. *Virology* **119**, 22–34.

Hills, E., and C. R. Laverty (1979), Electron microscopic detection of papillomavirus particles in selected koilocytotic cells in a routine cervical smear. *Acta. Cytol.* **23**, 53–56.

Hirt, B. (1967), Selective extraction of polyoma DNA from infected mouse cell cultures. *J. Mol. Biol.* **26**, 365–369.

Hsu, S. -M., L. Raine, and H. Fanger (1981), The use of antiavidin antibody and avidin–biotin–peroxidase complex in immunoperoxidase techniques. *Am. J. Clin. Pathol.* **75**, 816–821.

Jablonska, S., J. Dabrowski, and K. Jakubowicz (1972), Epidermodysplasia verruciformis as a model in studies on the role of papovaviruses in oncogenesis. *Cancer Res.* **32**, 583–589.

Jenson, A. B., J. R. Rosenthal, C. Olson, F. Pass, W. D. Lancaster, and K. Shah (1980), Immunological relatedness of papillomaviruses from different species. *J. Natl. Cancer Inst.* **64**, 495–500.

Jenson, A. B., W. D. Lancaster, D. P. Hartmann, and E. L. Shaffer, Jr. (1982a), Frequency and distribution of papillomavirus structural antigens in verrucae, multiple papillomas, and condylomata of the oral cavity. *Am. J. Path.* **107**, 212–218.

Jenson, A. B., S. Sommers, C. Payling-Wright, F. Pass, C. C. Link, and W. D. Lancaster (1982b), Human papillomavirus: Frequency and distribution in plantar and common warts. *Lab. Invest.* **47**, 491–497.

Jenson, A. B., R. J. Kurman, and W. D. Lancaster (1984), Human Papillomaviruses, in *Textbook of Human Virology* (R. Belsche, ed.) Littleton, MA. Wright-PGS, pp. 951–968.

Jones, H. W., Jr., V. A. McKusick, P. S. Harper, K. -D. Wuu (1971), George Otto Gey (1899–1970). The HeLa cell and a reappraisal of its origin. *Obstet. Gynecol.* **38**, 945–949.

Kidd, J. G., and P. Rous (1940), A transplantable rabbit carcinoma originating in a virus-induced papilloma and containing the virus in a masked or altered state. *J. Exp. Med.* **71**, 813–838.

Koss, L. G., and G. R. Durfee (1956), Unusual patterns of squamous epithelium of the uterine cervix: Cytologic and pathologic study of koilocytotic atypia. *Ann. N.Y. Acad. Sci.* **63**, 1235–1261.

Kremsdorf, D., M. Favre, S. Jablonska, S. Obalek, L. A. Rueda, M. A. Lutzner, C. Blanchet-Bardon, P. C. van Voorst Vader, and G. Orth (1984), Molecular cloning and characterization of the genomes of nine newly recognized human papillomavirus types associated with epidermodysplasia verruciformis. *J. Virol.* **52**, 1013–1018.

Kremsdorf, D., S. Jablonska, M. Favre, and G. Orth (1983), Human papillomaviruses associated with epidermodysplasia verruciformis. II. Molecular cloning and biochemical characterization of human papillomavirus 3a, 8, 10, and 12 genomes. *J. Virol.* **48**, 340–351.

Krzyzek, R. A., S. L. Watts, D. L. Anderson, A. J. Faras, and F. Pass (1980), Anogenital warts contain several distinct species of human papillomavirus. *J. Virol.* **36**, 236–244.

Kurman, R. J., K. H. Shah, W. D. Lancaster, A. B. Jenson (1981), Immunoperoxidase localization of papillomavirus antigens in cervical dysplasia and vulvar condylomas. *Am. J. Obstet. Gynecol.* **140**, 931–935.

Kurman, R. J., L. E. Sanz, A. B. Jenson, S. Perry, and W. D. Lancaster (1982), Papillomavirus infection of the cervix. I. Correlation of histology with viral structural antigens and DNA sequences. *Int. J. Gynecol. Pathol.* **1**, 17–28.

Kurman, R. J., A. B. Jenson, and W. D. Lancaster (1983), Papillomavirus infection of the cervix. II. Relationship to intraepithelial neoplasia based on the presence of specific viral structural proteins. *Am. J. Surg. Pathol.* **7**, 39–52.

Kurman, R. J., A. B. Jenson, C. F. Sinclair, and W. D. Lancaster (1984), Detection of Human Papillomaviruses by Immunocytochemistry, in *Advances in Immunohistochemistry* (R. A. DeLillis, ed.) Masson, New York, pp. 201–221.

Lack, E. E., A. B. Jenson, H. G. Smith, G. B. Healy, F. Pass, and G. F. Vawter (1980), Immunoperoxidase localization of human papillomavirus in laryngeal papillomas. *Intervirol.* **14**, 148–154.

Laird, C. D., B. L. McConaughy, and B. J. McCarthy (1969), Rate of fixation of nucleotide substitutions in evolution. *Nature* **224**, 149–154.

Lancaster, W. D., and C. Olson (1980), State of bovine papilloma virus DNA in connective tissue tumors. *Cold Spring Harbor Conf. Cell. Prolif.* **7**, 223–232.

Lancaster, W. D. (1981), Apparent lack of integration of bovine papillomavirus DNA in virus-induced equine and bovine tumors and virus-transformed mouse cells. *Virology* **108**, 251–255.

Lancaster, W. D., and A. B. Jenson (1981), Evidence for papillomavirus antigens and DNA sequences in laryngeal papilloma. *Intervirol.* **15**, 204–212.

Lancaster, W. D., and C. Olson (1982), Animal papillomaviruses. *Microbiol. Rev.* **46**, 191–207.

Lancaster, W. D., R. J. Kurman, L. E. Sanz, S. Perry, and A. B. Jenson (1983), Human papillomavirus: Detection of viral DNA sequences and evidence for molecular heretogeneity in metaplasias and dysplasias of the uterine cervix. *Intervirol.* **20**, 202–212.

Law, M. -F. W. D. Lancaster, and P. M. Howley (1979), Conserved sequences among the genomes of papillomaviruses. *J. Virol.* **32**, 199–207.

Law, M. -F., D. R. Lowy, I. Dvoretzky, and P. M. Howley (1981), Mouse cells transformed by bovine papillomavirus contain only extrachromosomal viral DNA sequences. *Proc. Natl. Acad. Sci. USA* **78**, 2727–2731.

Lee, K. P., and C. Olson (1969a), Histochemical study of experimentally produced bovine fibropapillomas. *J. Invest. Dermatol.* **52**, 454–464.

Lee, K. P., and C. Olson (1969b), Precipitin response of cattle to bovine papilloma virus. *Cancer Res.* **29**, 1393–1397.

Lowy, D. R., I. Dvoretzky, R. Shober, M. -F. Law, L. Engel, and P. M. Howley (1980), In vitro tumorigenic transformation by a defined subgenomic fragment of bovine papilloma virus DNA. *Nature* **287**, 72–74.

Ludwig, M. E., D. M. Lowell, and V. A. LiVolsi (1981), Cervical condylomatous atypia and its relationship to cervical neoplasia. *Am. J. Clin. Pathol.* **76**, 255–262.

Lutzner, M., O. Croissant, M. -F. Ducasse, H. Kreis, J. Croisner, and G. Orth (1980), A potentially oncogenic human papillomavirus (HPV-5) found in two renal allograft recipients. *J. Invest. Dermatol.* **75**, 353–356.

Lutzner, M. A., G. Orth, V. Dutronquay, M. -F. Ducasse, H. Kreis, and J. Croisner (1983), Detection of human papillomavirus type 5 DNA in skin cancers of an immunosuppressed renal allograft recipient. *Lancet,* ii, 422–424.

Lyon, J. L., J. W. Gardner, D. W. West, W. M. Stanish, and R. M. Hebertson (1983), Smoking and carcinoma *in situ* of the uterine cervix. *Am. J. Public Health* **73**, 558–562.

McVay, P., M. Fretz, F. O. Wettstein, J. Stevens, and Y. Ito (1982), Integrated Shope virus DNA is present and transcribed in the transplantable rabbit tumour Vx-7. *J. Gen. Virol.* **60**, 271–278.

Meisels, A., and R. Fortin (1977), Condylomatous lesions of the cervix and vagina. I. Cytologic patterns. *Acta Cytol.* **20**, 505–509.

Meisels, A., C. Morin, and M. Casas-Cordero (1982), Human papillomavirus infection of the uterine cervix. *Int. J. Gynecol. Pathol.* **1**, 75–94.

Mellors, R. C. (1960), Tumor cell localization of the antigens of the Shope papilloma virus and Rous sarcoma virus. *Cancer Res.* **10**, 744– 46.

Murphy. W. M., Y. S. Fu, W. D. Lancaster, and A. B. Jenson (1983), Papillomavirus structural antigens in condyloma acuminata of the male urethra. *J. Urol.* **130**, 84–85.

Okagaki, T., L. B. Twiggs, K. R. Zachow, B. A. Clark, R. S. Ostrow, and A. J. Faras (1983), Identification of human papillomavirus DNA in cervical and vaginal intraepithelial neoplasia with molecularly cloned virus-specific DNA probes. *Int. J. Gynecol. Pathol.* **2**, 153–159.

Olson, D., D. E. Gordon, M. G. Robl, and K. P. Lee (1969), Oncogenicity of bovine papilloma virus. *Arch. Environ. Health* **19**, 827–837.

Oriel, J. D. (1971), Natural history of genital warts. *Br. J. Vener. Dis.* **47**, 1–13.

Orth, G., M. Favre, and O. Croissant (1977), Characterization of a new type of human papillomavirus that causes skin warts. *J. Virol.* **24**, 108–120.

Orth, G., F. Breitburd, and M. Favre (1978a), Evidence for antigenic determinants shared by the structural polypeptides of (Shope) rabbit papillomavirus and human papillomavirus type 1. *Virology* **91**, 243–255.

Orth, G., S. Jablonska, M. Favre, O. Croissant, M. Jarzabek-Chorzelska, and G. Rzesa (1978b), Characterization of two new types of human papilloma viruses in lesions of epidermodysplasia verruciformis. *Proc. Natl. Acad. Sci. USA* **75**, 1537–1541.

Orth, G., M.Favre, F. Breitburd, O. Croissant, S. Jablonska, S. Obalek, M. Jarzabek-Chorzelska, and G. Rzesa (1980), Epidermodysplasia verruciformis: A model for the role of papilloma viruses in human cancer. *Cold Spring Harbor Conf. Cell. Prolif.* **7**, 259–282.

Orth, G., S. Jablonska, M. Favre, O. Croissant, S. Obalek, M. Jarzabek-Chorzelska, and N. Jibard (1981), Identification of papillomaviruses in butcher's warts. *J. Invest. Dermatol.* **76**, 97–102.

Osato, T., and Y. Ito (1967), In vitro cultivation and immunofluorescence studies of transplantable carcinomas Vx2 and Vx7. Persistence of a Shope virus-related antigenic substance in the cell of both tumor. *J. Exp. Med.* **126**, 881–886.

Ostrow, R. S., R. Krzyzek, F. Pass, and A. J. Faras (1981), Identification of a novel human papilloma virus in cutaneous warts of meathandlers. *Virology* **108**, 1–27.

Ostrow, R. A., M. Bender, M. Niimura, T. Seki, M. Kawashima, F. Pass and A. J. Faras (1982), Human papillomavirus DNA in cutaneous primary and metastasized squamous cell carcinomas from patients with epidermodysplasia verruciformis. *Proc. Natl. Acad. Sci. USA* **79**, 1634–1638.

Pfister, H. (1984), Biology and biochemistry of papillomaviruss. *Rev. Physiol. Biochem. Pharmacol.* **99**, 111–181.

Pfister, H., A. Gassenmaier, F. Nürnberger, and G. Stüttgen (1983a), HPV-5 DNA in a carcinoma of an epidermodysplasia verruciformis patient infected with various human papillomavirus types. *Cancer Res.* **43**, 1436–1441.

Pfister, H., I. Hettich, U. Runne, L. Gissmann, and G. N. Chilf (1983b), Characterization of human papillomavirus type 13 from focal epithelial hyperplasia Heck lesions. *J. Virol.* **47**, 363–366.

Rigby, P. D. Rhodes, M. Dieckmann, and P. Berg (1977), Labeling deoxyribonucleic acid to high specific activity in vitro by nick translation with DNA polymerase I. *J. Mol. Biol.* **113**, 237–251.

Rous, P., and J. W. Beard (1935), The progression to carcinoma of virus-induced rabbit papillomas (Shope). *J. Exp. Med.* **65**, 523–548.

Rowson, K. E. K., and B. W. J. Mahy (1967), Human papova (wart) virus. *Bacteriol. Rev.* **31**, 110–131.

Ruiter, M., and P. J. van Mullem (1970), Behavior of virus in malignant degeneration of skin lesions in epidermodysplasia verruciformis. *J. Invest. Dermatol.* **54**, 324–331.

Schwarz, E., M. Dürst, C. Demankowski, O. Lattermann, R. Zech, E. Solfsperger, S. Suhai, and H. zur Hausen (1983), DNA sequence and genome organization of genital human papillomavirus type 6b. *EMBO J.* **2**, 2341–2348.

Sharp, P. A., U. Pettersson, and J. Sambrook (1974), Viral DNA in transformed cells. I. A study of the sequences of adenovirus 2 DNA in a line of transformed rat cells using specific fragments of the viral genome. *J. Mol. Biol.* **86**, 709–726.

Southern, E. M. (1975), Detection of specific sequences among DNA fragments separated by gel electrophoresis. *J. Mol. Biol.* **93**, 503–517.

Sutton, W. D. (1971), A crude nuclease preparation suitable for use in DNA reassociation experiments. *Biochim. Biophys. Acta* **240**, 522–531.

Tagami, H., A. Ogino, M. Takigawa, S. Imamura, and S. Ofuji (1974), Regression of plane warts following spontaneous inflammation. A histopathological study. *Br. J. Dermatol.* **90**, 147–154.

Teokharov, B. A. (1969), Non-gonococcal infections of the female genitalia. *Br. J. Vener. Dis.* **45**, 150–160.

Trevathan, E., P. Layde, L. A. Webster, J. B. Adams, B. B. Benigno, and H. Ory (1983), Cigarette smoking and dysplasia and carcinoma *in situ* of the uterine cervix. *J. Am. Med. Assoc.* **250**, 499–502.

von Krough, G. (1979), Warts: Immunologic factors of prognostic significance. *Int. J. Dermatol.* **18**, 195–204.

Wahl, G. M., M. Stern, and G. R. Stark (1979), Efficient transfer of large DNA fragments from agarose gels to diazobenzyloxymethyl-paper and rapid hybridization using dextran sulfate. *Proc. Natl. Acad. Sci. USA* **76**, 3683–3687.

Wetmur, J. G., and N. Davidson (1968), Kinetics of renaturation of DNA. *J. Mol. Biol.* **31**, 349–370.

Wettstein, F. O., and J. G. Stevens (1984), Variable-sized free episomes of Shope papilloma virus DNA are present in all non-virus-producing noeplasms and integrated episomes are detected in some. *Proc. Natl. Acad. Sci. USA* **79**, 790–794.

Woodruff, J. D., L. Braun, R. Cavallieri, P. Gupta, F. Pass, and K. V. Shah (1980), Immunological identification of papillomavirus antigen in paraffin-processed condyloma tissues from the female genital tract. *Obstet. Gynecol.* **56**, 727–732.

zur Hausen, H. (1976), Condylomata acuminata and human genital cancer. *Cancer Res.* **36**, 530.

zur Hausen, H. (1982), Human genital cancer: Synergism between two virus infections or synergism between a virus infection and initiating events? *Lancet* ii, 1370–1372.

Human Epstein-Barr Virus and Cancer

Toyoro Osato, Fumio Mizuno,

Shigeyoshi Fujiwara, and

Shigeki Koizumi

Department of Virology, Cancer Institute, Hokkaido University School of Medicine, Sapporo, Japan

1. Introduction

Herpesviruses are ubiquitous in various species, including humans, and some are causally associated with naturally occurring tumors. The Epstein-Barr virus (EBV), which was first discovered in a culture of African Burkitt's lymphoma in 1964 by Epstein and coworkers Achong and Barr as a previously unknown viral agent, is now considered to be one such oncogenic herpesvirus. EBV can readily convert normal human B lymphocytes in vitro into blast cells with infinite replicative capabilities and is capable of inducing lymphomas in cotton-top marmosets. EBV widely infects humans in early childhood without any serious diseases, followed by life-long persistence of the virus. EBV is therefore a human ubiquitous viral agent with oncogenic potential. Knowledge of these characteristic features of EBV is essential to understand the functions of this virus in humans.

2. EBV Virion, Antigens, and Genome

2.1. EBV Virion

EBV (Epstein et al, 1964; Epstein and Achong, 1979a) is an approximately 150-nm diameter enveloped particle with an icosahedral capsid consisting of 162 capsomeres. The virus contains a double-stranded linear DNA molecule with a molecular mass of 10^8 daltons. The EBV virion includes a number of polypeptides; the molecular weight of the main component of the capsid is 160,000 and the viral envelope has mainly 350,000, 220,000, and 85,000 polypeptides. EBV is a member of the γ-herpesvirus subfamily of the herpesvirus family.

2.2. EBV-Related Antigens

Several different antigens are linked to EBV infection and oncogenesis, as has been determined by immunofluorescence and immunoprecipitation with SDS-polyacrylamide gel electrophoresis.

2.2.1. Viral Capsid Antigen (VCA)

VCA (Henle and Henle, 1966; Ernberg and Klein, 1979) is usually stained in acetone-fixed, EBV-producer Burkitt's lymphoma P3HR-1 cells by the virus-infected, healthy donor serum. This antigen consists of several polypeptides (Thorley-Lawson et al., 1982), mainly 160,000, which are sensitive to cytosine arabinoside (ara-C) and phosphonoacetic acid (PAA) and represent late, structural viral components.

2.2.2. Early Antigen Complex (EA)

EA (Ernberg and Klein, 1979; Henle et al., 1970) is an antigen complex appearing early in replicative, cytocidal EBV infection. The antigen complex can be visualized in EBV genome-positive, nonproducer Burkitt's Raji cells superinfected with nontransforming P3HR-1 strain EBV. This staining is evident when using serum from patients with Burkitt's lymphoma, nasopharyngeal carcinoma, or infectious mononucleosis. Two immunofluorescence patterns are known: one is a diffuse staining in both the nucleus and the cytoplasm (EA-D); and the other is restricted to the perinuclear cytoplasm (EA-R). EA consists of more than 10 polypeptides, mainly 145,000, 95,000, and 35,000 (Thorley-Lawson et al., 1982). All the polypeptides are resistant to ara-C and PAA, indicating that the EA complex consists of early, nonstructural viral proteins. EA seems to carry the virus-specific DNA polymerase activity (Miller et al., 1977; Ooka et al., 1979).

2.2.3. Membrane Antigen Complex (MA)

MA (Ernberg and Klein, 1979; Klein et al., 1966) is divided into two categories—early and late MA—both of which are observed as membrane immunofluorescence on viable cell surfaces. Early MA is a nonstructural viral protein that was first demonstrated in a biopsy of Burkitt's lymphoma cells and can also be seen on the newly EBV-transformed lymphocytes. The early MA is also detected in the early stage of superinfection of nonproducer cells, such as Daudi, in the presence of ara-C or PAA. The late MA is sensitive to ara-C and PAA and is identical in antigenicity with the EBV virion envelope. This type of MA is observed on the surface of producer cells such as P3HR-1. MA consists of several polypeptides, mainly 350,000, 220,000, and 85,000 (Thorley-Lawson et al., 1982), and generates specific neutralizing antibody to EBV. MA is also a target antigen for antibody-dependent cellular cytotoxicity (ADCC) against EBV infection and transformation (Pearson and Orr, 1976; Jondal, 1976; Aya et al., 1980a).

2.2.4. Lymphocyte-Detected Membrane Antigen (LYDMA)

LYDMA (Ernberg and Klein, 1979; Svedmyr and Jondal, 1975) is believed to be a nonvirion, EBV-specific cell surface antigen exclusively detected by cellular cytotoxicity of virus-sensitized T cells. This particular antigen probably plays an important role in the protection against EBV-induced oncogenesis.

2.2.5. Nuclear Antigen (EBNA)

EBNA (Ernberg and Klein, 1979; Reedman and Klein, 1973) is detected in the nucleus as the earliest EBV expression in cases of nonpermissive, transformable EBV infection. This antigen readily brings to mind the T antigen in SV40 and polyoma virus transformation. EBNA is an EBV-determined, DNA-binding protein, is consistently expressed in EBV-transformed cells, and is the most probable EBV-transforming protein. The molecular weight of native EBNA is 200,000, in which 48,000 and 53,000 components are involved (Luka et al., 1980). The 48,000 protein is probably EBV-specific and the 53,000 component seems to be of cellular origin; the latter is widely linked with carcinogenesis. EBNA is also composed of more components (Matsuo et al., 1978; Spelsberg et al., 1982). According to the recent development of EBV molecular biology, there are at least two kinds of EBNA, EBNA1 (Summers et al., 1982) and EBNA2 (Hennessy and Kieff, 1983), the molecular weights of which are 76,000 and 82,000, respectively. EBNA1 is closely associated with chromosomal DNA, but EBNA2 may not be.

2.3. EBV Genome

Analyses of the EBV genome has been long hampered by the lack of a proper in vitro permissive system for viral replication and also because of the large size of the viral genome. However, knowledge has rapidly accumulated through the use of molecular cloning techniques. The structure of the EBV genome outlined in Fig. 1 shows a linear double-stranded DNA molecule with a molecular mass of 1.15×10^8 daltons, composed of 1.7×10^5 base pairs. There is a direct tandem repeat sequence (TR) at each end of the viral DNA. Inside the genome, there are four direct tandem repeats (IR1–IR4) and five regions of unique nucleotide sequences (U1–U5) (Kieff et al., 1982). As for induction of EBV-related antigens, the EcoRI-E region is considered to be responsible for VCA synthesis, BamHI-L for MA, BamHI-H for EA-R, and BamHI-d through B for EA-D (Hummel and Kieff, 1982; Hummel et al., 1984; Glaser et al., 1983). On the other hand, EBNA seems to be related to BamHI-K as EBNA1 and BamHI-V·X·H as EBNA2 (Summers et al., 1982; Dambaugh et al., 1984). There is a report that BamHI-M is also responsible for the nuclear antigen (Grogan et al., 1983). For immortalization and transformation, BamHI-D through T and BamHI-X·H·F regions are reportedly necessary (Stoerker et al., 1983; Griffin and Karran, 1984). As for LYDMA, Dhet region may be responsible (Hennessy et al., 1984). The complete nucleotide sequence of EBV has been recently established (Baer et al., 1984).

3. Oncogenicity of EBV

3.1. Oncogenic Properties of EBV

It is rather difficult to prove that EBV is the causative agent of human malignancies such as Burkitt's lymphoma (Burkitt, 1958); however, this particular virus is currently considered to be oncogenic for the following reasons: (1) EBV can convert normal

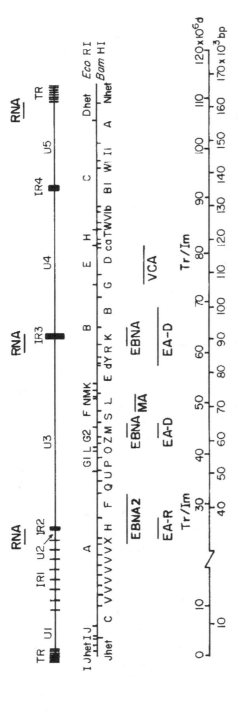

Fig. 1. Structure and function of EBV genome. EA, VCA, MA, EBNA, and transformation/immortalization activity (Tr/Im) are considered to be closely associated with the underlined EBV DNA regions, respectively. Three different DNA regions are transcribed (underlined RNAs) in nonproducer transformed cells.

human and new world monkey (cotton-top marmosets) B lymphocytes in vitro into lymphoblasts with infinite replicative capabilities. In such transformed cells, EBV DNA and EBNA are both detectable, as demonstrated by nucleic acid hybridization and immunofluorescence, respectively (Pope, 1979). (2) EBV can induce B cell lymphomas in marmosets. In such animal tumors, both EBV DNA and EBNA are also detected (Miller, 1979). These findings strongly suggest that EBV should be considered to be in the same category of known animal tumor viruses such as SV40 and polyoma virus.

3.2. In Vitro Transformation of Human Lymphocytes by EBV

When B cell-rich fractions are collected from human umbilical cord blood or adult human peripheral blood and inoculated with B95-8 strain EBV, several steps are involved sequentially in the transformation process. First, EBNA appears as early as 10 h after EBV exposure, followed by blastogenesis within 18 h. Cellular DNA synthesis is evident by 36 h and, finally, EBNA-positive, cellular DNA-synthesizing lymphoblasts began to divide and proliferate rapidly with high frequency establishment of B cell lines (Takada and Osato, 1979; Robinson and Smith, 1981).

Host ranges of EBV infection and transformation are narrow. The target cells are limited to B cells of humans and some new world monkeys (Pope, 1979). However, human B lymphocytes are highly susceptible to EBV, and under ordinary experimental conditions the frequencies of EBV-infectable cell fractions are 5–10% of unfractionated lymphocytes and 20–40% of a T cell-depleted, B cell-rich population, in terms of EBNA synthesis (Takada and Osato, 1982). All B cell subpopulations are susceptible to EBV (Koizumi et al., 1984). Although normal lymphocytes in ordinary culture conditions have a limited number of divisions, the presence of EBV gives the cells continuous, infinite proliferating capabilities. With exposure to EBV, B cells grow rapidly in suspension, form clumps, and readily established B lymphoblast cell lines within 1 mo. In these cell lines, EBV DNA and EBNA can be found in all of the cells. Since EBV-infected, transformed B cells are polyclonal in origin, as judged from the diversity of their surface and cytoplasmic immunoglobulin expressions, the virus can be categorized as a polyclonal B cell activator (Nilsson, 1979).

EBV-transformed cells have multiple virus genomes, approximately 10 copies per cell. The resident EBV genomes are mostly present in the form of closed circular episomes (Nonoyama and

Pagano, 1972; Lindahl et al., 1976). A small number, however, are probably integrated into the cellular DNA (Kieff et al., 1982; Kaschka-Dierich et al., 1976). Three different EBV DNA regions are transcribed in nonproducer transformed cells; the right end of U5 (EcoRI-Dhet), IR3 and its neighboring areas (BamHI-R·K), and a right portion of IR1 together with U2 (BamHI-V·X·H), thereby suggesting that the three regions in the viral genome are closely associated with the transformation by EBV. Further, the BamHI-X·H fragments are lacking in nontransforming P3HR-1 EBV DNA (Kieff et al., 1982), and more recently marker rescue and transfection experiments also suggest that BamHI-X·H·F and BamHI-D through T regions are responsible for EBV-induced immortalization and transformation (Stoerker et al., 1983; Griffin and Karran, 1984). As for EBNA synthesis, cells transfected by BamHI-K and M fragments reportedly become antigen-positive (Summers et al., 1982; Grogan et al., 1983).

When normal human B lymphocytes are exposed to transforming B95-8 strain EBV and immediately seeded into semisolid agar, discrete colonies can be grossly seen after 3~4 wk (Mizuno et al., 1976; Katsuki and Hinuma, 1976). Although blast cells composing these colonies do not usually have chromosome abnormalities or grow subcutaneously in adult nude mice (Nilsson, 1979; Giovanella et al., 1979), there are a very few colonies that become visible within 1 wk after seeding the EBV-exposed normal B cells in agar. These rapidly growing transformed cells have a high plating efficiency in agar, reveal chromosome translocations several months after culture initiation, and form subcutaneous tumors in adult nude mice (Aya et al., 1981).

3.3. Experimental Tumorigenesis In Vivo by EBV

EBV can induce polyclonal lymphoproliferation when inoculated into cotton-top marmosets. Furthermore, Burkitt's lymphoma-like B cell malignancy developed in some of these animals and the tumors were considered to be monoclonal, as judged from cell surface markers and chromosome investigations (Miller, 1979). The marmoset lymphoma cells were positive for EBV DNA copies and also EBNA immunofluorescence, as are Burkitt's lymphoma cells in humans. In addition, marmoset lymphocytes transformed in vitro by EBV can produce lymphomas when transplanted to autologous host animals. Old world monkeys, such as rhesus and cynomolgus, commonly used in virological studies, are not susceptible to EBV oncogenesis.

4. Ubiquity of EBV in Humans

As EBV efficiently infects human B lymphocytes in vitro and readily converts the target into blast cells with infinite replicative capabilities, it is important to assess how this potentially oncogenic EBV is distributed among human populations.

4.1. Natural History of EBV Infection in Humans

Seroepidemiological studies reveal that EBV is a widespread viral agent with a latent, inapparent infection in man. The presence of EBV is not limited to patients with certain diseases such as Burkitt's lymphoma, or to the population in certain geographical areas such as tropical Africa; rather the virus is present worldwide, as detected by antibody tests (Henle and Henle, 1979b). In addition, EBV is often shed orally in seropositive healthy persons (Gerber et al., 1972; Chang et al., 1973). The ubiquity of EBV is also known from the finding that a large number of lymphoid cell lines established from seropositive humans living all over the world all harbor EBV genomes (Nilsson, 1979).

Primary infection of humans with EBV is generally seen in young children with an inapparent infection and without any serious disorder; however, the percentages of healthy carriers probably differ in age in some countries (Henle and Henle, 1979b). The vast majority of young children are seropositive in Africa and Asia. This may be attributed to the low economic levels, questionable hygienic states, and overcrowding. Nearly all of the newborn babies are positive for EBV antibodies, in reflection of the high seropositivity of their mothers. After the level of the mother-derived antibodies reaches a minimum within several months, the number of seropositive children increases rapidly, with more than 80% positive at 2–3 yr, and nearly 100% positive by the time adolescence is reached. In contrast, the age of primary EBV infection is generally higher in western countries, particularly among high socioeconomic groups. Approximately 50% are still EBV-seronegative, even at adolescence. Most, however, are seropositive when tested at various ages during adulthood.

EBV infects humans through the respiratory tract and is considered to replicate in salivary glands and the respiratory mucosa (Niederman et al., 1973; Morgan et al., 1979; Sixbey et al., 1984; Wolf et al., 1984). The virus will then reach the lymph nodes where B cells are the targets for latent infection and transformation. Most EBV-infected, transformed cells, however, will be suppressed or eliminated in normal individuals by specific and nonspecific defense mechanisms, including cytotoxic T cells, NK cells, K cells, EBV antibodies, and interferon. A small number of the latently infected cells may enter the viral productive cycle or divide, under normal circumstances, but the events are well controlled in healthy individuals. Thus, no massive viral production or infinite replication of the infected, transformed cells are observed, and there are no life-threatening situations. The basic features of EBV infection in vivo, therefore, are latency and persistence. Once infected with EBV, the virus persists in a small fraction of B cells and infected individuals remain seropositive all their lives (Henle, 1979).

4.2. Abnormality in Natural History of EBV Infection

EBV infection is usually symptomless throughout the life of an individual, as is generally the case with herpesvirus infections. However, EBV is potentially oncogenic and infected cells can proliferate without restraint. The abnormality in the natural history of EBV infection often shows a close association with disturbances in the immunological system. Since the EBV targets are B cells, the infection itself tends to primarily affect the immune system.

5. Epstein-Barr Virus and Human Cancer

Human malignancies with which EBV has long been linked are Burkitt's lymphoma and nasopharyngeal carcinoma. In addition, the significance of EBV in opportunistic tumorigenesis seems to be closely associated in patients with immunosuppression and immunodeficiency.

5.1. Burkitt's Lymphoma and EBV

EBV was first suggested as a possible human tumor viral agent when discovered in cultures of Burkitt's lymphoma cells in 1964 (Epstein et al., 1964; Epstein and Achong, 1979a). Burkitt's lymphoma (Burkitt, 1958) is highly endemic in tropical Africa, the so-called Burkitt's belt, which has high temperatures and humidity. The tumor most frequently occurs in the lower jaw and has a peak incidence in 6~8-yr-old children. This particular lymphoma is the most common malignancy in African children, occurring annually in 10~20 per 100,000 children living in the endemic areas. The histopathology is also characteristic as "starry sky" appearance, in which histiocytes are seen scattered throughout the tumor cell population. Clinically, the tumor is highly sensitive to chemotherapy, although it grows and develops rapidly and metastasizes. Burkitt's lymphoma is also endemic in New Guinea, which also has high temperatures and humidity, and is sporadic in other areas in the world (Epstein and Achong, 1979b).

Such endemic development of Burkitt's lymphoma strongly suggested the possible presence of causative, infectious agent(s), and a number of attempts were made at detection and isolation. EBV has been singled out as the most important candidate for the following reasons (Epstein and Achong, 1979b). First, EBV genomic DNA persists in the Burkitt's tumor cells with the expression of EBNA in the nucleus, the antigen which is a possible EBV-transforming protein. Second, Burkitt's lymphoma patients have high EBV-related antibody titers, some of which are rather negative in healthy subjects. Change in antibody titers during the disease is often a good parameter to predict patients' prognosis. Third, Burkitt's tumors are B cell lymphomas and normal B cells are the targets for transformation by EBV. Fourth, EBV can induce B cell lymphomas in cotton-top marmosets. The relation between EBV and Burkitt's lymphoma supports the concept of viral oncogenesis.

It is important to perform longitudinal EBV seroepidemiology studies on Burkitt's lymphoma in tropical Africa, to further elucidate the relationship between the virus and this particular tumor. A large-scale seroepidemiological survey was made on over 40,000 African children from 1972–1977 in the endemic West Nile district of Uganda, by the International Agency for Research on Cancer (de-Thé, 1979). A large number of serum samples were obtained from healthy children from 1972–1974. Lymphoma later developed in some of the donors. In 14 patients, detailed studies on EBV antibodies, before and after the occurrence of Burkitt's lymphoma, revealed that all of these children were already EBV-seropositive with high antibody titers before the onset of the disease. These African children with high EBV antibody titers had 30 times the risk of Burkitt's lymphoma occurring than did children with average EBV antibody titers. These seroepidemiological investigations clearly indicate that Burkitt's lymphoma is not directly associated with a primary EBV infection, but rather possibly caused by prolonged, unusual EBV events in predisposed children in endemic areas of tropical Africa.

The mechanism of the occurrence and development of Burkitt's lymphoma has not been fully clarified. EBV exists worldwide, yet Burkitt's lymphomas are seen in certain limited areas, mostly in tropical Africa. EBV can readily convert normal B cells in vitro to lymphoblasts with infinite growth capabilities. The lymphoma incidence, however, is very low. Although this particular lymphoma is cytogenetically characterized by a specific translocation between chromosomes no. 8 and 14 (Manolov and Manolova, 1972; Zech et al., 1976; Manolova et al., 1979), EBV-transformed lymphocytes in vitro are generally free of chromosome changes. In addition, all Burkitt's tumors are not necessarily positive for the EBV genome. Thus, cofactors other than EBV, immunologic, physiologic, genetic, and environmental factors are probably required for the manifestation of this particular malignancy.

Tropical Africa, where Burkitt's lymphoma is endemic, also has high rates of malaria, and the malaria infection may be an important cofactor linked to Burkitt's tumor (Epstein and Achong, 1979b; Burkitt, 1969; Klein, 1979b). It is plausible that chronic malaria infection may not only stimulate EBV-infected cells, leading to their active proliferation, but might also alter the sensitivity and responsiveness of target normal B lymphocytes to EBV. Therefore, EBV-infected cells in patients with chronic malaria may be less stable and have a greater potential for chromosome abnormalities. Above all, when the no. 8 and 14 chromosome translocation occurs, such EBV-infected lymphocytes may present as a malignant Burkitt's cell proliferating indefinitely, having escaped from immune surveillance mechanisms. Malaria infection itself generally affects host immune systems in such a manner as to make them favorable for tumor growth. There is a report that the T-cell control of EBV-infected B cells is lost during malaria (Whittle et al., 1984). The administration of antimalaria drugs in "Burkitt's belt" reportedly reduced the incidence of this particular lymphoma (de-Thé, 1982). There is also a report in which the development of EBV-induced lymphoma was significantly increased in marmosets experimentally infected with a malaria agent (Leibold et al., 1976).

The vast majority of patients with Burkitt's lymphoma live in tropical Africa and most of the tumors have both EBV DNA and 8;14 reciprocal translocation [t(8q24; 14q32)] (Manolov and Manolova, 1972; Zech et al., 1976; Manolova et al., 1979). In contrast, the majority of sporadic Burkitt's lymphomas outside of Africa are free of EBV DNA, but have the characteristic translocation (Kaiser-McCaw, et al., 1977). In both the endemic and sporadic Burkitt's lymphomas, another two specific chromosome abnormalities consisting of 8;2 and 8;22 reciprocal translocations are known (Miyoshi et al., 1979; van den Berghe et al., 1979).

Based on the observation of the specific chromosome translocations, the following mechanism has been proposed concerning the occurrence of Burkitt's lymphoma (Klein, 1981; Klein, 1983). In human B lymphocytes, a gene responsible for cell proliferation is located in a region of the long arm of the no. 8 chromosome (8q24). When this particular gene is transposed to the immunoglobulin heavy-chain gene locus on chromosome no. 14, the κ-chain gene locus on chromosome no. 2, or the λ-chain gene locus on chromosome no. 22 through the translocation of 8q24, the gene responsible for B cell proliferation will be abnormally activated and may lead to the development of Burkitt's lymphoma cells. This particular gene is now understood to be one of the cellular oncogenes (c-*onc*) that are normally present in human cells and represent homologs of animal retroviral oncogenes. Recent reports demonstrate that the c-*myc* gene (a c-*onc*), which is located at 8q24 and is homologous to the avian myeloblastosis viral (v) myc gene, is transposed to the end of the long arm of the no. 14 chromosome, and also to nos. 2 and 22, in Burkitt's tumor cells. This transposed c-*myc* gene is highly transcribed in this particular lymphoma. It has also been claimed that another c-*onc Blym*-1, was activated in Burkitt's lymphoma (Diamond et al., 1983).

On the other hand, a single resident EBV genome in virus-transformed, EBNA-positive lymphoblasts can be seen in the no. 14 chromosome (Yamamoto et al., 1978). When the EBV genome-containing chromosome no. 14 segregated out of mouse–human hybrid cells, the tumorigenicity of such cells became decreased in nude mice (Yamamoto et al., 1980). It is therefore considered possible that the presence of EBV genome in highly active sites of B lymphocytes, such as chromosomes no. 14, 22, and 2, may be of primary importance in the oncogenesis of EBV-associated lymphomas, including Burkitt's tumors. The EBV genome is also seen in the no. 1 chromosome (Henderson et al., 1983), in which *Blym*-1 gene may be present (Morton et al., 1983).

Taken together, interactions between several different causes and factors, including the presence of the EBV genome, the participation of cellular oncogenes, and the presence of malaria infection, may be necessary for the high risk and high frequency occurrence of this particular Burkitt's lymphoma.

As for the cellular origin of EBV-associated lymphomas, the following experiment is relevant (Aya et al., 1981). When human lymphocytes are seeded onto semisolid agar immediately after EBV exposure, transformed colonies usually become grossly visible after 3~4 wk. However, there are a small number of colonies that grow rapidly and can be isolated within 1 wk of incubation. The transformed cells composing such colonies showed high recloning efficiencies comparable to Burkitt's lymphoma cells, and chromosome translocations were evident as early as 6 mo. These colonies could generate subcutaneous tumor growth when injected into adult nude mice. These results suggest that the cells possessing a potentially highly oncogenic nature, although very small in number, may occur at the initiation of EBV infection.

The following data are of interest in connection with the high incidence of Burkitt's lymphoma in tropical Africa. Fusobacterium, a common oral flora in humans, produces n-butyric acid as the terminal metabolite. The extracts of Euphorbia plants widely used as herbal drugs in tropical Africa contain tumor promoters such as 12-O-tetradecanoyl phorbol-13-acetate (TPA). A remarkable induction of the latent EBV was evident when nonproducer Burkitt's lymphoma cell lines were exposed to both n-butyric acid and the plant extracts (Ito et al., 1981). It became further evident that a very small amount of these plant extracts remarkably enhanced transformation of human lymphocytes by EBV in a semisolid agar condition (Mizuno et al., 1983).

5.2. EBV and Nasopharyngeal Carcinoma

Another clinical malignancy that has long been suspected to have a causal relation to EBV infection is nasopharyngeal carcinoma, particularly the anaplastic type. It was first reported in 1966 that some patients had remarkably high serum antibody titers to this particular virus (Old et al., 1966). Nasopharyngeal carcinoma is frequently encountered among the Chinese in southern mainland China, Hong Kong, Taiwan, Singapore, and Malaysia. The peak incidence is seen at ages 45–55, and over 50 patients of a 100,000 population are diagnosed annually in the highly endemic areas of southern China. Nasopharyngeal carcinoma is the most common tumor seen in the middle-aged male Chinese, and ranks as the second most common tumor in females in the endemic areas of China. This particular malignancy is also frequently seen among the Eskimos in Alaska and the East African people. The incidence is generally low in other parts of the world (de-Thé, 1979; Klein, 1979a).

Like Burkitt's lymphoma, the causal relationship between EBV infection and nasopharyngeal carcinoma may be as follows (Klein, 1979a). First, the EBV genome is found in tumor cells with the expression of EBNA in the nucleus. Second, EBV-related antibodies in patients are not only high in titer, but also qualitatively distinct from those seen in healthy individuals. Furthermore, a change in antibody patterns in the course of the disease is often closely associated with the prognosis. As compared with Burkitt's lymphoma, however, the relation between EBV and this malignancy is less well understood because of the lack of both in vitro and in vivo models. The mode and mechanism of EBV infection in normal nasopharyngeal epithelial cells is not clear. Since the local tissues are rich in lymphocytes, some of which may latently involve EBV, nasopharyngeal epithelial cells may be infected with the virus through cell fusion with the virus-containing lymphocytes (Yamamoto et al., 1975/76). Although the nasopharyngeal epithelial cells are not susceptible to the ordinary EBV inoculation, they seem to allow EBNA synthesis by the implantation of EBV receptors onto the surface of the epithelial cells (Shapiro and Volsky, 1983). There is also a report that wild-type EBV from fresh oropharyngeal washings can infect to epithelial cells, but not laboratory EBV strains (Sexbey et al., 1983).

A large-scale study of EBV seroepidemiology in nasopharyngeal carcinoma was recently carried out in endemic southern China and yielded etiological information of EBV in this particular tumor, as well as providing insight into preventive medicine (Zeng et al., 1983). In the survey from 1978–1980, VCA-IgA antibodies, which are considered to be a good indication for the detection of the tumor, were assayed in 150,000 individuals aged 30 and older. Three thousand five hundred residents were VCA-IgA-positive and 55 had nasopharyngeal carcinoma at the time. The remaining positive healthy individuals were then checked periodically for the occurrence of the tumor, and 32 additional nasopharyngeal carcinoma patients were diagnosed during the next 3 yr. Thus, the EBV-specific IgA antibody test is important for the early detection of nasopharyngeal carcinoma in endemic areas.

In southern China, nearly all persons are seroconverted in their early life and individual patients with nasopharyngeal carcinoma had previously been infected with EBV before the occurrence of the tumor. Therefore, the development of this particular tumor does not seem to be simply associated with EBV infection. Since the malignancy is most frequently seen in the Chinese, a racial genetic factor has to be considered. In this respect, the association of certain HLA types with the patients has been noted and discussed (Simons et al., 1975; Levine, 1983). On the other hand, environmental factors may also be important, such as carcinogenic and tumor promoter substances in smoked fish and salt fish, a daily food among these people (Henle et al., 1979; Ho, 1972). Euphorbia plants native to southern China activate the latent EBV (Ito et al., 1981) and markedly enhance the lymphocyte transformation (Mizuno et al., 1983). The extracts of such Euphorbia plants with tumor promoter substances are used as herbal drugs. More than 500 plant species commonly used in medicine were tested and 16 had the capacity to activate the latent EBV. No significant promoter activity was found in 100 representative Chinese food ingredients (Zeng, 1982).

5.3. EBV and Opportunistic Lymphoma

EBV, which is ubiquitous and potentially oncogenic to humans, infects B cells of the immune system in young children and persists throughout life. Therefore, both primary and past EBV infections tend to become serious in patients with immunosuppression and immunodeficiency. In this sense, the opportunistic development of lymphoma occasionally seen in primary and secondary immunologic abnormalities has attracted interest as a causal association with EBV.

5.3.1. Fatal Infectious Mononucleosis

Rare, fatal cases of infectious mononucleosis probably fall into the category of EBV-associated opportunistic lymphomas. Infectious mononucleosis was first identified in 1968 as an EBV infectious disease (Henle et al., 1968; Henle and Henle, 1979a). This particular illness is a self-limiting, benign hematologic disease manifested as a result of primary EBV infection among adolescents and young adults, with a 50% incidence after a 3~4 wk incubation period. Oral excretion of EBV is frequently evident in the acute phase, with an appearance of EBNA-positive lymphoblastoid cells in peripheral blood. Atypical lymphocytes characteristic of the disease are mainly T cells generated in response to B cell proliferation induced by EBV infection. Therefore, the pathogenesis of infectious mononucleosis is considered to be represented by the immunopathological reaction of EBV-infected, transformed B cells with specific killer T cells, and nonspecific suppressor T cells. In addition to T cells, other specific and nonspecific mechanisms, including K cells (antibody-dependent cellular cytotoxicity), NK cells, and interferon, are also important to effectively eliminate the infected, transformed cells.

Thus, infectious mononucleosis is basically considered to be a disease reflecting the oncogenicity of EBV, although its manifestation is benign and temporary. This particular illness may therefore have a potential risk of unlimited growth of EBV-infected, transformed lymphocytes if a patient is in an immunologically suppressed or deficient state. There are reports, albeit rare, of life-threatening and fatal cases of infectious mononucleosis caused by massive proliferation and invasion of EBNA-positive blast cells (Bar et al., 1974; Britton et al., 1978; Robinson et al., 1980; Thestrup-Pedersen et al., 1980; Crawford et al., 1979). Among the cases, X-linked lymphoproliferative syndrome, Duncan's disease, occurs on a definite genetic background possibly linked to EBV-specific immunodeficiency (Purtilo, 1981). Since the family members with Duncan's disease have a recessive gene on the X chromosome, male family members are at high risk for infinite, fatal proliferation of EBV-infected B cells, although they look healthy before the EBV infection. More than 100 patients with severe, life-threatening infectious mononucleosis have been reported in several such families in North America (Purtilo et al., 1982).

B cells are polyclonally activated in vitro in EBV infection and transformation, and EBNA-positive lymphoblastoid cells appearing in infectious mononucleosis are also polyclonal. Furthermore, the above-described life-threatening illnesses seem to be expressed as a polyclonal immunoblastoma or a polyclonal immunoblastic sarcoma (Robinson et al., 1980; Thestrup-Pedersen et al., 1980; Crawford et al., 1979; Purtilo, 1981). In contrast, Burkitt's lymphoma is a monoclonal malignancy (Epstein and Achong, 1979b). It has therefore been speculated that there is a sequential malignant progression from polyclonal, benign infectious mononucleosis to polyclonal continuous lymphoproliferation, including immunoblastoma and immunoblastic sarcoma, and eventually to a monoclonal tumor such as Burkitt's lymphoma. Our recent experience lends support to this idea (Abo et al., 1982). A 1-yr-old Japanese boy with severe infectious mononucleosis was treated with a large dose of corticosteroid. He had been repeatedly ill with signs and symptoms of infectious mono for 1.5 yr, then Burkitt's lymphoma followed. The tumor was positive for EBV DNA and EBNA with a typical starry sky appearance and a specific translocation between chromsomes 10 and 17. This particular case is considered important in terms of not only the view of opportunistic lymphoma by EBV, but also in view of progressive development of a monoclonal malignant tumor from a polyclonal benign EBV infection of B cells.

5.3.2. Organ Transplantation and EBV-Carrying Lymphoma

The use of immunosuppressive drugs in organ transplantation appears to be closely associated with the development of opportunistic lymphomas by EBV. It has been noted that lymphomas occurred in some of the recipients of transplanted kidneys, the majority of which were positive for EBV DNA (Hanto et al., 1981). Such EBV-carrying lymphomas were also seen in cases of heart implantation (Saemundsen et al., 1982; Weintraub and Warnke, 1982). In organ transplant recipients, latent EBV is generally activated. The virus is shed orally in high frequency (Strauch et al., 1974; Chang et al., 1978), and EBV-related antibody titers are also highly elevated. In addition, the recipients often have a decreased EBV-specific killer T cell activity, which results in lowering the capacity to eliminate EBV-infected cells in the body (Crawford et al., 1981; Gaston et al., 1982). It is therefore understood that in organ transplantation, the latent EBV tends to be highly activated to reveal its potential oncogenicity because of secondary immunodeficiency caused by the long-term administration of immunosuppressive drugs. The EBV-carrying lymphomas occurring in these occasions are mostly polyclonal, although conversion of a polyclonal lymphoproliferation to a monoclonal malignancy has been reported (Hanto et al., 1982).

5.3.3. Primary Immunodeficiency and Lymphoma Development

Ataxia telangiectasia, known as a representative primary immunodeficiency disorder, has a high frequency of lymphoma development. In this particular disease, EBV antibody response is unusual, with a high prevalence of EA antibodies and high VCA antibody titers, but with very low EBNA antibody levels (Joncas et al., 1977; Berkel et al., 1979). Basically, patients' helper T cell functions are much decreased and the EBV-specific killer T cell activity may also be lowered. EBNA-positive cells are sometimes detected in the peripheral blood. These features probably indicate that in these patients the EBV infection status is elevated, although the infected B lymphocytes are poorly eliminated because of reduced immunologic capacities. As a result, it is plausible that EBV-infected, EBNA-positive cells tend to proliferate and increase in these patients. An EBV genome-carrying lymphoma occurred in a patient with ataxia telangiectasia (Saemundsen et al., 1981). Similar unusual immune response to EBV is evident in Wiskott-Aldrich syndrome (Vilmer et al., 1984; Okano et al., 1984) and massive proliferation of EBV-infected, transformed cells occurred in a patient (Okano et al., 1984).

6. Protection Against EBV-Induced Oncogenesis

EBV widely infects humans in early life and there is a lifetime viral persistence, without serious disease. In the ordinary symbiotic relationship between EBV and man, not only antibodies to EBV capsid antigen VCA, but also antibodies to the virus-transforming protein EBNA are detectable in sera from infected healthy individuals. This suggests that EBNA-positive cells apparently occur even by reexposure to EBV or reactivation of the virus, but can be effectively eliminated by normal immunlogic defense mechanisms. The EBNA antibodies will thus be frequently generated by the exposed nuclear antigen.

6.1. Possible Defense Mechanisms

The healing mechanism of infectious mononucleosis described in section 5.3.1 represents the strength of the immunological protection against EBV invasion. Although the virus-specific killer T cells appearing in mononucleosis are not detectable in healthy infected individuals, EBV-specific memory T cells are regularly present for the surveillance of the infected, transformed cells to promptly induce killer T cells (Rickinson et al., 1981). Such specific killer T cells are also seen in Burkitt's lymphoma and nasopharyngeal carcinoma tissues (Klein et al., 1976). While in general the function of the EBV killer T cells induced in vitro are HLA restricted, such HLA restriction may not be the case in infectious mononucleosis (Seeley et al., 1981).

On the other hand, NK cells were shown to be activated early in response to EBV-transformed cells before the appearance of specific killer T cells (Tanaka et al., 1980). Therefore, the nonspecific NK cells may initially play an important role in the protection against EBV invasion. The activities of such NK cells and T cells are considered to be enhanced by interferon, which is induced at the beginning of EBV infection (Thorley-Lawson, 1981; Kikuta et al., 1984).

EBV-infected, transformed cells can also be eliminated promptly by the mechanism of the virus-specific, antibody-dependent, cell-mediated cytotoxicity in seropositive healthy persons, before the induction of killer T cells (Pearson and Orr, 1976; Jondal, 1976; Aya et al., 1980a). Such antibody-dependent cytotoxicity is also highly enhanced in the presence of a small amount of interferon (Aya et al., 1980b).

6.2. EBV Vaccine

A vaccine directed against EBV infection and oncogenesis has been proposed (Epstein, 1976) and is actively discussed relative to the recent progress in antigen purification methods and genetic engineering techniques. It is anticipated that the EBV vaccine will prevent infectious mononucleosis in western countries by the administration to seronegative adolescents and young adults, as well as protect people in tropical Africa and southeast Asia from Burkitt's lymphoma and nasopharyngeal carcinoma.

An experimental EBV vaccine, containing purified EBV-specific membrane antigen MA obtained from human lymphoid cells (MA is known to generate neutralization activity and also antibody-dependent cellular cytotoxicity activity),was recently proven to be effective in animals (Epstein et al., 1982; Pearson et al., 1982). Another MA vaccine is being developed on the basis of gene engineering, based on the recent identification of the EBV DNA region encoding the MA antigen (Kieff, 1982).

Although the successful application of vaccine for the protection of chickens against lymphoma induced by the ubiquitous Marek's disease virus is a beautiful model for the EBV vaccine, there are certain difficulties (Klein, 1982). One is that of timing for the administration of vaccine because of the widespread nature of EBV in early life, especially in endemic areas of nasopharyngeal carcinoma and Burkitt's lymphoma. Another problem is whether or not EBV vaccine will alter the natural symbiotic relation between the virus and man. EBV vaccine, however, is expected to lower the risk of nasopharyngeal carcinoma, a tumor that is one of the most common malignancies in one-fourth of the world population: the Chinese people.

7. Summary

Important aspects of the human Epstein-Barr virus and cancer are summarized as follows.

(1) EBV infects resting normal human B lymphocytes, as target cells, resulting in their activation and conversion to polyclonal lymphoblasts. The transformed B cells have infinite replicative capabilities under the continued functional expression of the resident EBV genome. (2) EBV, on the other hand, is a widespread, ubiquitous virus present in human beings early in life. However, immunological surveillance mechanisms are sufficiently potent in healthy indi-

viduals to protect them against the infinite growth of the infected lymphocytes. (3) Both primary and secondary immunodeficiency states will extend EBV events so that massive polyclonal B cell proliferation of EBV genome-carrying B cells will occur. (4) There may be conversion of such polyclonal lymphoproliferation into monoclonal malignant lymphoma. This is possibly the case of selective clonal growth of polyclonal EBV-induced transformed cells caused by a genetic error. Burkitt's lymphoma is possibly one of such examples. (5) The oncogenic potential of EBV appears dependent upon cofactors. Among them, immunodeficiency, genetic predisposition, and environmental circumstances are experimentally and clinically suggested to be the key cofactors in EBV oncogenesis. (6) The activation and unusual expression of cellular oncogenes may be closely associated with the mechanism of carcinogenesis. In this respect, events occurring in Burkitt's lymphoma in connection with chromosome translocation suggest a possible association of cellular oncogenes with EBV-induced oncogenesis. (7) It has long been suggested that EBV plays an important role in the occurrence of nasopharyngeal carcinoma. However, knowledge is yet limited, both in vitro and in vivo, as compared with B cell malignancy induced by the virus, including the mechanism of EBV infection to nasopharyngeal epithelial cells.

Acknowledgment

We thank M. Ohara of Kyushu University for generous help with this manuscript and Mrs. J. Kusajima-Matsumoto for secretarial assistance.

References

Abo, W., K. Takada, M. Kamada, M. Imamura, T. Motoya, M. Iwanaga, T.Aya, S. Yano, T. Nakao, and T. Osato (1982), Evolution of infectious mononucleosis into Epstein-Barr virus carrying monoclonal malignant lymphoma. *Lancet* i, 1272–1276.

Aya, T., F. Mizuno, and T. Osato (1980a), Immunologic cytotoxicity against autologous human lymphocytes transformed or infected by Epstein-Barr virus: Role of antibody-dependent cellular cytotoxicity in healthy individuals. *J. Natl. Cancer Inst.* **65**, 265–271.

Aya, T., T. Osato, and T. Kishida (1980b), Protection against Epstein-Barr virus oncogenesis. Cooperative effect of lymphocytes, antibodies and interferon. *Proc. Japan. Acad.* **56**, 523–527.

Aya, T., T. Osato, T. Tomiyasu, and O. Shiratori (1981), Malignancy of Epstein-Barr virus (EBV)-transformed human lymphocytes. *Int. Workshop on Herpesviruses*, p. 267, Bologna, Italy.

Baer, R., A. T. Bankier, M. D. Biggin, P. L. Deininger, P. J. Farrell, T. J. Gibson, G. Hatfull, G. S. Hudson, S. C. Satchwell, C. Séguin, P. S. Tuffnell, and B. G. Barrell (1984), DNA sequence and expression of the B95-8 Epstein-Barr virus genome. *Nature* **310**, 207–211.

Bar, R. S., C. J. DeLor, K. P. Clausen, P. Hurtubise, W. Henle, and J. F. Hewetson (1974), Fatal infectious mononucleosis in a family. *N.Engl. J. Med.* **290**, 363–367.

Berkel, A. I., W. Henle, G. Henle, G. Klein, F. Ersoy, and Ö. Sanal (1979), Epstein-Barr virus-related antibody patterns in ataxia telangiectasia. *Clin. Exp. Immunol.* **35**, 196–201.

Britton, S., M. Andersson-Anvret, P. Gergely, W. Henle, M. Jondal, G. Klein, B. Sandstedt, and E. Svedmyr (1978), Epstein-Barr virus immunity and tissue distribution in a fatal case of infectious mononucleosis. *N. Engl. J. Med.* **298**, 89–92.

Burkitt, D. (1958). A sarcoma involving the jaws in African children. *Brit. J. Surg.* **46**, 218–223.

Burkitt, D. P. (1969), Etiology of Burkitt's lymphoma—An alternative hypothesis to a vectored virus. *J. Natl. Cancer Inst.* **42**, 19–28.

Chang, R. S., J. P. Lewis, and C. F. Abildgaard (1973), Prevalence of oropharyngeal excreters of leukocyte-transforming agents among a human population. *N. Engl. J. Med.* **289**, 1325–1329.

Chang, R. S., J. P. Lewis, R. D. Reynolds, M. J. Sullivan, and J. Neuman (1978), Oropharyngeal excretion of Epstein-Barr virus by patients with lymphoproliferative disorders and by recipients of renal homografts. *Ann. Intern. Med.* **88**, 34–40.

Crawford, D. H., M. A. Epstein, B. G. Achong, S. Finerty, J. Newman, S. Liversedge, R. S. Tedder, and J. W. Stewart (1979), Virological and immunological studies on a fatal case of infectious mononucleosis. *J. Infect.* **1**, 37–48.

Crawford, D. H., J. M. B. Edwards, P. Sweny, A. V. Hoffbrand, and G. Janossy (1981), Studies on long-term T-cell-mediated immunity to Epstein-Barr virus in immunosuppressed renal allograft recipients. *Int. J. Cancer* **28**, 705–709.

Dambaugh, T., K. Hennessy, L. Chamnankit, and E. Kieff (1984), U2 region of Epstein-Barr virus DNA may encode Epstein-Barr nuclear antigen 2. *Proc. Natl. Acad. Sci. USA* **82**, 7632–7636.

de-Thé, G. (1979), Demographic Studies Implicating the Virus in the Causation of Burkitt's Lymphoma; Prospects for Nasopharyngeal Carcinoma, in *The Epstein-Barr Virus* (Epstein, M. A. and B. G. Achong, eds.) Springer-Verlag, Berlin.

de-Thé, G. (1982), Discussion, IVth Int. Symp. Nasopharyngeal Carcinoma, Kuala Lumpur, Malaysia.

Diamond, A., G. M. Cooper, J. Ritz, and M. -A. Lane (1983), Identification and molecular cloning of the human B*lym* transforming gene activated in Burkitt's lymphomas. *Nature* **305**, 112–116.

Epstein, M. A. (1976), Epstein-Barr virus—Is it time to develop a vaccine program? *J. Natl. Cancer Inst.* **56**, 697–700.

Epstein, M. A. and B. G. Achong, eds. (1979a), *The Epstein-Barr Virus*, Springer-Verlag, Berlin.

Epstein, M. A. and B. G. Achong (1979b), The relationship of the virus to Burkitt's lymphoma, in *The Epstein-Barr Virus* (Epstein, M. A. and B. G. Achong, eds.) Springer-Verlag, Berlin.

Epstein, M. A., B. G. Achong, and Y. M. Barr (1964), Virus particles in cultured lymphoblasts from Burkitt's lymphoma. *Lancet* **1**, 702–703.

Epstein, M. A., J. R. North, A. J. Morgan, and J. L. Thompson (1982), Abstracts, IVth Int. Symp. on Nasopharyngeal Carcinoma, Kuala Lumpur, Malaysia.

Ernberg, I. and G. Klein (1979), EB virus-induced antigens, in *The Epstein-Barr Virus* (Epstein, M. A. and B. G. Achong, eds.) Springer-Verlag, Berlin.

Gaston, J. S. H., A. B. Rickinson, and M. A. Epstein (1982), Epstein-Barr-virus-specific T-cell memory in renal-allograft recipients under long-term immunosuppression. *Lancet* **1**, 923–925.

Gerber, P., M. Nonoyama, S. Lucas, E. Perlin, and L. I. Goldstein (1972), Oral excretion of Epstein-Barr virus by healthy subjects and patients with infectious mononucleosis. *Lancet* **ii**, 988–989.

Giovanella, B., K. Nilsson, L. Zech, O. Yim, G. Klein, and J. S. Stehlin (1979), Growth of diploid, Epstein-Barr virus-carrying human lymphoblastoid cell lines heterotransplanted into nude mice under immunologically privileged conditions. *Int. J. Cancer* **24**, 103–113.

Glaser, R., A. Boyd, J. Stoerker, and J. Holliday (1983), Functional mapping of the Epstein-Barr virus genome: Identification of sites coding for the restricted early antigen, the diffuse early antigen, and the nuclear antigen. *Virology* **129**, 188–198.

Griffin, B. E. and L. Karran (1984), Immortalization of monkey epithelial cells by specific fragments of Epstein-Barr virus DNA. *Nature* **309**, 78–82.

Grogan, E. A., W. P. Summers, S. Dowling, D. Shedd, L. Gradoville, and G. Miller (1983), Two Epstein-Barr viral nuclear neoantigens distinguished by gene transfer, serology, and chromosome binding. *Proc. Natl. Acad. Sci. USA* **80**, 7650–7653.

Hanto, D. W., K. Sakamoto, D. T. Purtilo, R. L. Simmons, and J. S. Najarian (1981), The Epstein-Barr virus in the pathogenesis of posttransplant lymphoproliferative disorders. *Surgery* **90**, 204–213.

Hanto, D. W., G. Frizzera, K. J. Gajl-Peczalska, K. Sakamoto, D. T. Purtilo, H. H. Balfour, R. L. Simmons, and J. S. Najarian (1982), Epstein-Barr virus-induced B-cell lymphoma after renal transplantation. *N. Engl. J. Med.* **306**, 913–918.

Henderson, A., S. Ripley, M. Heller, and E. Kieff (1983), Chromosome site for Epstein-Barr virus DNA in a Burkitt tumor cell line and in lymphocytes growth-transformed in vitro. *Proc. Natl. Acad. Sci. USA* **80**, 1987–1991.

Henle, G. (1979), Infectious Mononucleosis, in *Epstein-Barr Virus Oncogenesis* (Osato, T., ed.) Hokkaido University School of Medicine, Sapporo.

Henle, G. and W. Henle (1966), Immunofluorescence in cells derived from Burkitt's lymphoma. *J. Bacteriol.* **91**, 1248–1256.

Henle, G. and W. Henle (1979a), The Virus as the Etiologic Agent of Infectious Mononucleosis, in *The Epstein-Barr Virus* (Epstein, M. A. and B. G. Achong, eds.) Springer-Verlag, Berlin.

Henle, W. and G. Henle (1979b), Seroepidemiology of the Virus, in *The Epstein-Barr Virus* (Epstein, M. A. and B. G. Achong, eds.) Springer-Verlag, Berlin.

Henle, G., W. Henle, and V. Diehl (1968), Relation of Burkitt's tumor-associated herpes-type virus to infectious mononucleosis. *Proc. Natl. Acad. Sci. USA* **59**, 94–101.

Henle, W., G. Henle, B. A. Zajac, G. Pearson, R. Waubke, and M. Scriba (1970), Differential reactivity of human serums with early antigens induced by Epstein-Barr virus. *Science* **169**, 188–190.

Henle, W., G. Henle, and E. T. Lennette (1979), The Epstein-Barr virus. *Sci. Am.* **241**, 48–59.

Hennessy, K. and E. Kieff (1983), One of two Epstein-Barr virus nuclear antigens contains a glycine-alanine copolymer domain. *Proc. Natl. Acad. Sci. USA* **80**, 5665–5669.

Hennessy, K., S. Fennewald, M. Hummel, T. Cole, and E. Kieff (1984), A membrane protein encoded by Epstein-Barr virus in latent growth-transforming infection. *Proc. Natl. Acad. Sci. USA* **81**, 7207–7211.

Ho, H. C. (1972), Current knowledge of the Epidemiology of Nasopharyngeal Carcinoma—A Review, in *Oncogenesis and Herpesviruses* (Biggs, P. M., G. de Thé, and L. N. Payne, eds.) Int. Agency Res. Cancer, Lyon.

Hummel, M. and E. Kieff (1982), Mapping of polypeptides encoded by the Epstein-Barr virus genome in productive infection. *Proc. Natl. Acad. Sci. USA* **79**, 5698–5702.

Hummel, M., D. Thorley-Lawson, and E. Kieff (1984), An Epstein-Barr virus DNA fragment encodes messages for the two major envelope glycoproteins (gp350/300 and gp220/200). *J. Virol.* **49**, 413–417.

Ito, Y., M. Kishishita, T. Morigaki, S. Yanase, and T. Hirayama (1981), Induction and Intervention of Epstein-Barr Virus Expression in Human Lymphoblastoid Cell Lines: A Simulation Model for Study of Cause and Prevention of Nasopharyngeal Carcinoma and Burkitt's Lymphoma, in *Cancer Campaign* (Grundmann, E., G. R. F. Krueger, and D. V. Ablashi, eds.) Gustav Fischer Verlag, Stuttgart.

Joncas, J., N. Lapointe, F. Gervais, and M. Leyritz (1977), Unusual prevalence of Epstein-Barr virus early antigens (EBV-EA) antibodies in Ataxia telagiectasia, *J. Immunol.* **119**, 1857–1859.

Jondal, M. (1976), Antibody-dependent cellular cytotoxicity (ADCC) against Epstein-Barr virus-determined membrane antigens. I. Reactivitiy in sera from normal persons and from patients with acute infetious mononucleosis. *Clin. exp. Immunol.* **25**, 1–5.

Kaiser-McCaw, B., A. L. Epstein, H. S. Kaplan, and F. Hecht (1977), Chromosome 14 translocation in African and North American Burkitt's lymphoma. *Int. J. Cancer* **19**, 482–486.

Kaschka-Dierich, C., A. Adams, T. Lindahl, G. W. Bornkamm, G. Bjursell, G. Klein, B. C. Giovanella, and S. Singh (1976), Intracellular forms of Epstein-Barr virus DNA in human tumor cells in vivo. *Nature* **260**, 302–306.

Katsuki, T. and Y. Hinuma (1976), A quantitative analysis of the susceptibility of human leukocytes to transformation by Epstein-Barr virus. *Int. J. Cancer* **18**, 7–13.

Kieff, E. (1982), Discussion, IVth Int. Symp. Nasopharyngeal Carcinoma, Kuala Lumpur, Malaysia.

Kieff, E., T. Dambaugh, M. Heller, W. King, A. Cheung, V. van Santen, M. Hummel, C. Beisel, S. Fennewald, K. Hennessy, and T. Heineman (1982), The biology and chemistry of Epstein-Barr virus. *J. Infect. Dis.* **146**, 506–517.

Kikuta, H., F. Mizuno, S. Yano, and T. Osato (1984), Interferon production by Epstein-Barr virus in human mononuclear leukocytes. *J. Gen. Virol.* **65**, 837–841.

Klein, G. (1979a), The Relationship of the Virus to Nasopharyngeal Carcinoma, in *The Epstein-Barr Virus* (Epstein, M. A. and B. G. Achong, eds.) Springer-Verlag, Berlin.

Klein, G. (1979b), Lymphoma development in mice and humans: Diversity of initiation is followed by convergent cytogenetic evolution. *Proc. Natl. Acad. Sci. USA* **76**, 2442–2446.

Klein, G. (1981), The role of gene dosage and genetic transpositions in carcinogenesis. *Nature* **294**, 313–318.

Klein, G. (1982), Discussion, IVth Int. Symp. Nasopharyngeal Carcinoma, Kuala Lumpur, Malaysia.

Klein, G. (1983), Specific chromosomal translocation and the genesis of B-cell-derived tumors in mice and men. *Cell* **32**, 311–315.

Klein, E., S. Becker, E. Svedmyr, M. Jondal, and F. Vánky (1976), Tumor infiltrating lymphocytes. *Ann. NY Acad. Sci.* **276**, 207–216.

Klein, G., P. Clifford, E. Klein, and J. Stjernswärd (1966), Search for tumor-specific immune reactions in Burkitt lymphoma patients by the membrane immunofluorescence reaction. *Proc. Natl. Acad. Sci. USA* **55**, 1628–1635.

Koizumi, S., W. Abo, F. Mizuno, and T. Osato (1984), Analysis of Epstein-Barr virus infection and transformation of human lymphocytes by two-color immunofluorescence for viral nuclear antigen and immunoglobulin synthesis. 6th Intl. Congress of Virology, Sendai, Japan.

Leibold, W., G. Huldt, T. D. Flanagan, M. Andersson, M. Dalens, D. H. Wright, A. Voller, and G. Klein (1976), Tumorigenicity of Epstein-Barr virus (EBV)-transformed lymphoid line cells in autologous squirrel monkeys. *Int. J. Cancer* **17**, 533–541.

Levine, P. H. (1983), Cellular Immunity and Genetics in Nasopharyngeal Carcinoma: An Overview, in *Nasopharyngeal Carcinoma: Current Concepts* (Prasad, U., D. V. Ablashi, P. H. Levine, and G. R. Pearson, eds.) University of Malaya, Kuala Lumpur.

Lindahl, T., A. Adams, G. Bjursell, G. W. Bornkamm, C. Kaschka-Dierich, and U. Jehn (1976), Covalently closed circular duplex DNA of Epstein-Barr virus in a human lymphoid cell line. *J. Mol. Biol.* **102**, 511–530.

Luka, J., H. Jörnvall, and G. Klein (1980), Purification and biochemical characterization of the Epstein-Barr virus-determined nuclear antigen and an associated protein with a 53,000-dalton subunit. *J. Virol.* **35**, 592–602.

Manolov, G. and Y. Manolova (1972), Marker band in one chromosome 14 from Burkitt lymphomas. *Nature* **237**, 33–34.

Manolova, Y., G. Manolov, J. Kieler, A. Levan, and G. Klein (1979), Genesis of the 14q+ marker in Burkitt's lymphoma. *Hereditas* **90**, 5–10.

Matsuo, T., N. Hibi, S. Nishi, H. Hirai, and T. Osato (1978), Studies on Epstein-Barr virus-related antigens. III. Purification of the virus-determined nuclear antigen (EBNA) from non-producer Raji cells. *Int. J. Cancer* **22**, 747–752.

Miller, G. (1979), Experimental Carcinogenicity by the Virus In Vivo, in *The Epstein-Barr Virus* (Epstein, M. A. and B. G. Achong, eds.) Springer-Verlag, Berlin.

Miller, R. L., R. Glaser, and F. Rapp (1977), Studies of an Epstein-Barr virus-induced DNA polymerase. *Virology* **76**, 494–502.

Miyoshi, I., S. Hiraki, I. Kimura, K. Miyamoto, and J. Sato (1979), 2/8 translocation in a Japanese Burkitt's lymphoma. *Experientia* **35**, 742–743.

Mizuno, F., T. Aya, and T. Osato (1976), Growth in semisolid agar medium of human cord leukocytes freshly transformed by Epstein-Barr virus. *J. Natl. Cancer Inst.* **56**, 171–173.

Mizuno, F., S. Koizumi, T. Osato, J. O. Kokwaro, and Y. Ito (1983), Chinese and African Euphorbiaceae plant extracts: Markedly enhancing effect on Epstein-Barr virus-induced transformation. *Cancer Lett.* **19**, 199–205.

Morgan, D. G., J. C. Niederman, G. Miller, H. W. Smith, and J. M. Dowaliby (1979), Site of Epstein-Barr virus replication in the oropharynx. *Lancet* ii, 1154–1157.

Morton, C. C., R. Taub, A. Diamond, M. A. Lane, G. M. Cooper, and P. Leder (1984), Mapping of the human B*lym*-1 transforming gene activated in Burkitt lymphomas to chromosome 1. *Science* **223**, 173–175.

Niederman, J. C., G. Miller, H. A. Pearson, J. S. Pagano, and J. M. Dowaliby (1976), Infectious mononucleosis Epstein-Barr-virus shedding in saliva and the oropharynx. *N. Engl. J. Med.* **294**, 1355–1359.

Nilsson, K. (1979), The Nature of Lymphoid Cell Lines and Their Relationship to the Virus, in *The Epstein-Barr Virus* (Epstein, M. A. and B. G. Achong, eds.) Springer-Verlag, Berlin.

Nonoyama, M. and J. S. Pagano (1972), Separation of Epstein-Barr virus DNA from large chromosomal DNA in non-virus-producing cells. *Nature N. Biol.* **238**, 169–171.

Okano, M., F. Mizuno, T. Osato, Y. Takahashi, Y. Sakiyama, and S. Matsumoto (1984), Wiskott-Aldrich syndrome and Epstein-Barr virus-induced lymphoproliferation. *Lancet* ii, 933–934.

Old, L. J., E. A. Boyse, H. F. Oettgen, E. de Harven, G. Geering, B. Williamson, and P. Clifford (1966), Precipitating antibody in human serum to an antigen present in cultured Burkitt's lymphoma cells. *Proc. Natl. Acad. Sci. USA* **56**, 1699–1704.

Ooka, T., G. Lenoir, and J. Daillie (1979), Characterization of an Epstein-Barr virus-induced DNA polymerase. *J. Virol.* **29**, 1–10.

Pearson, G. R., R. Chase, and L. F. Qualtiere (1982), IVth Int. Symp. on Nasopharyngeal Carcinoma, Kuala Lumpur, Malaysia.

Pearson, G. R. and T. W. Orr (1976), Antibody-dependent lymphocyte cytotoxicity against cells expressing Epstein-Barr virus antigens. *J. Natl. Cancer Inst.* **56**, 485–488.

Pope, J. H. (1979), Transformation by the Virus In Vitro, in *The Epstein-Barr Virus* (Epstein, M. A. and B. G. Achong, eds.) Springer-Verlag, Berlin.

Purtilo, D. T. (1981), Immune deficiency predisposing to Epstein-Barr virus-induced lymphoproliferative diseases: The X-linked lymphoproliferative syndrome as a model. *Adv. Cancer Res.* **34**, 279–312.

Purtilo, D. T., K. Sakamoto, V. Barnabei, J. Seeley, T. Bechtold, G. Rogers, J. Yetz, and S. Harada (1982), Epstein-Barr virus-induced diseases in boys with the X-linked lymphoproliferative syndrome (XLP). Update studies of the registry. *Am. J. Med.* **73**, 49–56.

Reedman, B. M. and G. Klein (1973), Cellular localization of an Epstein-Barr virus (EBV)-associated complement-fixing antigen in producer and non-producer lymphoblastoid cell lines. *Int. J. Cancer* **11**, 499–520.

Rickinson, A. B., D. J. Moss, L. E. Wallace, M. Rowe, I. S. Misko, M. A. Epstein, and J. H. Pope (1981), Long-term T-cell-mediated immunity to Epstein-Barr virus. *Cancer Res.* **41**, 4216–4221.

Robinson, J. and D. Smith (1981), Infection of human B lymphocytes with high multiplicities of Epstein-Barr virus: Kinetics of EBNA expression, cellular DNA synthesis, and mitosis. *Virology* **109**, 336–343.

Robinson, J. E., N. Brown, W. Andiman, K. Halliday, U. Francke, M. F. Robert, M. Andersson-Anvret, D. Horstmann, and G. Miller (1980), Diffuse polyclonal

B-cell lymphoma during primary infection with Epstein-Barr virus. *N. Engl. J. Med.* **302**, 1293–1297.

Saemundsen, A. K., A. I. Berkel, W. Henle, G. Henle, M. Anvret. Ö. Sanal, F. Ersoy, M. Çaglär and G. Klein (1981), Epstein-Barr-virus-carrying lymphoma in a patient with ataxia-telangiectasia. *Brit. Med. J.* **282**, 425–427.

Saemundsen, A. K., G. Klein, M. Cleary, and R. Warnke (1982), Epstein-Barr-virus-carrying lymphoma in cardiac transplant recipient. *Lancet* **ii**, 158.

Seeley, J., E. Svedmyr, O. Weiland, G. Klein, E. Moller, E. Ericksson, K. Andersson, and L. Van der Waal (1981), Epstein-Barr virus-selective T cells in infectious mononucleosis are not restricted to HLA-A and B antigens. *J. Immunol.* **127**, 293–300.

Shapiro, I. M. and D. J. Volsky (1983), Infection of normal human epithelial cells by Epstein-Barr virus. *Science* **219**, 1225–1228.

Simons, M. J., G. B. Wee, S. H. Chan, K. Shanmugaratnam, N. E. Day and G. B. de-Thé (1975), Probable identification of an HL-A second-locus antigen associated with a high risk of nasopharyngeal carcinoma. *Lancet* **i**, 142–143.

Sixbey, J. W., J. G. Nedrud, N. Raab-Traub, R. A. Hanes, and J. S. Pagano (1984), Epstein-Barr virus replication in oropharyngeal epithelial cells. *New Engl. J. Med.* **310**, 1225–1230.

Sixbey, J. W., E. H. Vesterinen, J. G. Nedrud, N. Raab-Traub, L. A. Walton, and J. S. Pagano (1983), Replication of Epstein-Barr virus in human epithelial cells infected in vitro. *Nature* **306**, 480–483.

Spelsberg, T. C., T. B. Sculley, G. M. Pikler, J. A. Gilbert, and G. R. Pearson (1982), Evidence for two classes of chromatin-associated Epstein-Barr virus-determined nuclear antigen. *J. Virol.* **43**, 555–565.

Stoerker, J., J. E. Holliday, and R. Glaser (1983), Identification of a region of the Epstein-Barr virus (B95-8) genome required for transformation. *Virology* **129**, 199–206.

Strauch, B., N. Siegel, L. -L. Andrews, and G. Miller (1974), Oropharyngeal excretion of Epstein-Barr virus by renal transplant recipients and other patients treated with immunosuppressive drugs. *Lancet* **1**, 234–237.

Summers, W. P., E. A. Grogan, D. Shedd, M. Robert, C. -R. Liu, and G. Miller (1982), Stable expression in mouse cells of nuclear neoantigen after transfer of a 3,4-megadalton cloned fragment of Epstein-Barr virus DNA. *Proc. Natl. Acad. Sci. USA* **79**, 5688–5692.

Svedmyr, E. and M. Jondal (1975), Cytotoxic effector cells specific for B cell lines transformed by Epstein-Barr virus are present in patients with infectious mononucleosis. *Proc. Natl. Acad. Sci. USA* **72**, 1622–1626.

Takada, K. and T. Osato (1979), Analysis of the transformation of human lymphocytes by Epstein-Barr virus. I. Sequential occurrence from the virus-determined nuclear antigen synthesis, to blastogenesis, to DNA synthesis. *Intervirology* **11**, 30–39.

Takada, K. and T. Osato (1982), Simple assay method for susceptibility of human lymphocytes to Epstein-Barr virus infection. *Intervirology* **18**, 87–91.

Tanaka, Y., K. Sugamura, Y. Hinuma, H. Sato, and K. Okochi (1980), Memory of Epstein-Barr virus-specific cytotoxic T cells in normal seropositive adults as revealed by an in vitro restimulation method. *J. Immunol.* **125**, 1426–1431.

Thestrup-Pederson, K., V. Esmann, S. Bisballe, J. R. Jensen, G. Pallesen, J. Hastrup, M. Madsen, K. Thorling, M. Grazia-Masucci, A. K. Saemundsen, and I. Ernberg (1980), Epstein-Barr-virus-induced lymphoproliferative disorder converting to fatal Burkitt-like lymphoma in a boy with interferon-inducible chromosomal defect. *Lancet* **ii**, 997–1002.

Thorley-Lawson, D. A. (1981), The transformation of adult but not newborn human lymphocytes by Epstein-Barr virus and phytohemagglutinin is inhibited by interferon: The early suppression by T cells of Epstein Barr infection is mediated by interferon. *J. Immunol.* **126**, 829–833.

Thorley-Lawson, D. A., C. M. Edson, and K. Geilinger (1982), Epstein-Barr virus antigens—A challenge to modern biochemistry. *Adv. Cancer Res.* **36**, 295–348.

van Den Berghe, H., C. Parloir, S. Gosseye, V. Englebienne, G. Cornu, and G. Sokal (1979), Variant translocation in Burkitt lymphoma. *Cancer Genet. Cytogenet.* **1**, 9–14.

Weintraub, J. and R. A. Warnke (1982), Lymphoma in cardiac allo-transplant recipients. *Transplantation* **33**, 347–351.

Whittle, H. C., J. Brown, K. Marsh, B. M. Greenwood, P. Seidelin, H. Tighe, and L. Wedderburn (1984), T-cell control of Epstein-Barr virus-infected B cells is lost during *P. falciparum* malaria. *Nature* **312**, 449–450.

Wolf, H., M. Haus, and E. Wilmes (1984), Persistence of Epstein-Barr virus in the parotid gland. *J. Virol.* **51**, 795–798.

Yamamoto, K., T. Matsuo, and T. Osato (1975/76), Appearance of Epstein-Barr virus-determined nuclear antigen in human epithelial cells following fusion with lymphoid cells. *Intervirology* **6**, 115–121.

Yamamoto, K., F. Mizuno, T. Matsuo, A. Tanaka, M. Nonoyama, and T. Osato (1978), Epstein-Barr virus and human chromosomes: Close association of the resident viral genome and the expression of the virus-determined nuclear antigen (EBNA) with the presence of chromosome 14 in human–mouse hybrid cells. *Proc. Natl. Acad. Sci. USA* **75**, 5155–5159.

Yamamoto, K., T. Osato, O. Shiratori, S. Makino, and K. Katagiri (1980), Epstein-Barr virus and human chromosomes. Growth characteristics in culture and nude mice of the virus-positive, chromosome 14-containing human–mouse hybrid cells. *Pproc. Japan. Acad.* **56**, 519–522.

Zech, L., U. Haglund, K. Nilsson, and G. Klein (1976), Characteristic chromosomal abnormalities in biopsies and lymphoid-cell lines from patients with Burkitt and non-Burkitt lymphomas. *Int. J. Cancer* **17**, 47–56.

Zeng, Y. (1982), Discussion, IVth Int. Symp. Nasopharyngeal Carcinoma, Kuala Lumpur, Malaysia.

Zeng, Y., J. M. Zhong, L. Y. Li, P. Z. Wang, H. Tang, Y. R. Ma, J. S. Zhu, W. J. Pan, Y. X. Liu, Z. N. Wei, J. Y. Chen, Y. K. Mo, E. J. Li, and B. F. Tan (1983), Follow-up studies on Epstein-Barr virus IgA/VCA antibody-positive persons in Zangwu county, China. *Intervirology* **20**, 190–194.

Hepatitis B Virus and Hepatocellular Carcinoma

Hubert E. Blum, Myron J. Tong, and Girish N. Vyas

1. Introduction

Malignant tumors of the liver are of either epithelial origin (heaptocellular carcinoma, cholangiocarcinoma, biliary cystadenocarcinoma, squamous carcinoma, mucoepidermoid carcinoma), mesenchymal origin (hemangiosarcoma, undifferentiated embryonal sarcoma, fibrosarcoma, leiomyosarcoma, leiomyoblastoma, malignant mesenchymoma), or mixed origin (hepatoblastoma, mixed hepatic tumor, carcinosarcoma).

Heaptocellular carcinoma (HCC) is the major malignant primary liver tumor throughout the world, the most prevalent tumor in some of the most populous countries, and one of the world's most frequent malignancies. HCC is not only one of the most frequent carcinomas worldwide; it is clinically also one of the most malignant in terms of progression, outcome, and poor response to treatment. Thus, HCC is one of the leading worldwide causes of death from cancer (Kew, 1982; Okuda and Mackay, 1982).

Infection with hepatitis B virus (HBV) is endemic throughout much of the world, with an estimated 200 million persistently infected people, presenting a major public health problem (Robinson, 1977; McCollum and Zuckerman, 1981; Tiollais et al., 1981; Vyas and Blum, 1984). HBV infects only humans and certain nonhuman primates, and belongs to a group of hepatotropic DNA (hepadna) viruses that includes the woodchuck heaptitis virus (WHV), the ground squirrel hepatitis virus (GSHV), and the Pekin duck hepatitis B virus (DHBV). In humans, HBV infection is associated with a wide spectrum of clinical presentations, ranging from the inapparent carrier state, acute and fulminant hepatitis, to various forms of chronic liver disease and liver cirrhosis, and is involved in the development of hepatocellular carcinoma (Szmuness, 1978; Brechot et al., 1980; Beasley et al., 1981; Brechot et al., 1981b; Koshy et al., 1981; Shafritz and Kew, 1981; Shafritz et al., 1981; Brechot et al., 1982a; Popper et al., 1982; Szmuness et al., 1982; Dejean et al., 1983; Koshy et al., 1983; Kew, 1984; Shafritz and Lieberman, 1984; Vyas et al., 1984).

The role of a hepatitis virus in the etiology of HCC was first suggested by Payet et al. (1956) and by Steiner and Davis (1957), based on the observations that the incidence of HCC appeared to correlate with the incidence of viral hepatitis. With the availability of specific serologic markers for HBV infection in the early 1970s, a close association between HBV infection and the development of HCC was established (Denison et al., 1971; Velasco et al., 1971; Ohbayashi et al., 1972; Tepfer, 1972; Blumberg et al., 1975; Prince, 1975; Prince et al., 1975; Larouze et al., 1976; Tabor et al., 1977, Szmuness, 1978; Beasley et al., 1981; Beasley, 1982; Beasley et al., 1982; Beasley and Hwang, 1984). Apart from the geographic correlation between hepatitis B surface antigen (HBsAg) carrier prevalence and HCC incidence, the integration of HBV DNA into the genome of malignantly transformed hepatocytes and the development of HCC in the woodchuck model of hepadna viruses (Gerin, 1984; Wain-Hobson, 1984) provide additional support for the concept of a causal relationship between HBV and HCC in humans.

Important advances have been made during the past few years in the study of the biology of HBV and the virus/host cell interaction at the molecular level. The HBV genome has been cloned by recombinant DNA technologies and its detailed structure, including the complete nucleotide sequence, has been determined. The genetic organization of the genome has been established and viral genes have been expressed in vitro in various cell culture systems. Using cloned HBV DNA, viral nucleic acids have been identified and characterized in serum and liver of infected individuals by molecular hybridization techniques.

We will review here the structure, mode of replication, and genetic organization of the HBV genome, molecular analyses of HBV infection, epidemiologic, clinical, and molecular evidence for a relationship between HBV infection and the development of HCC, clinical presentation and management of patients with HCC, as well as current and future strategies for the prophylaxis against HBV and prevention of this malignancy.

2.   Structure and Biology of Hepatitis B Virus

2.1.   Structure of the Hepatitis B Virus

The hepatitis B virion (Dane particle) (Dane et al., 1970) has a diameter of approximately 42 nm. It consists of an electron-dense internal core structure (nucleocapsid) with a diameter of 28 nm and an envelope of about 7 nm thickness (Dane et al., 1970) (Fig. 1). the envelope of the virion contains the hepatitis B surface antigen (HBsAg), which shares antigenic determinants with the incomplete viral particles (22 nm spherical and filamentous forms) (Almeida et al., 1971). The nucleocapsid contains the hepatitis B core antigen (HBcAg) and its cryptic antigenic determinant hepatitis B e antigen (HBeAg) (Takahashi et al., 1979; MacKay et al., 1981), the viral DNA with a protein covalently attached to the 5' end of the minus-strand (Gerlich and Robinson, 1980), a DNA polymerase (Kaplan et al., 1973; Robinson and Greenman, 1974), and a protein kinase (Albin and Robinson, 1980).

2.2.   Structure of the Hepatitis B Virus Genome

The hepatitis B virus (HBV) genome is a small circular DNA molecule (Robinson et al., 1974) (Fig. 2) that is partially double-stranded. The single-stranded region varies between 15 and 60% in length in different molecules (Summers et al., 1975; Hruska et al., 1977; Landers et al., 1977), displaying a preferred minimum length of 650–700 nucleotides (Delius et al., 1983). The complete minus-

Hepatitis B virion

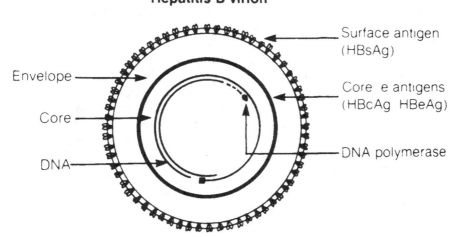

Fig. 1. Structure of HBV (Dane particle).

strand is a constant length of about 3200 nucleotides and has a
nick with a protein covalently attached to its 5' end (Gerlich and
Robinson, 1980), preventing phosphorylation of the DNA by
polynucleotide kinase. The 5' end of the incomplete plus-strand is
200–300 nucleotides downstream from the 5' end of the minus-
strand, creating a cohesive overlap that maintains the circular structure of virion DNA (Summers et al., 1975; Charnay et al., 1979;
Sattler and Robinson, 1979; Siddiqui et al., 1979). DNAs of this
size and structure, including the single-stranded region and a DNA
polymerase that functions to fill in the gap by elongation from the
3' end of the incomplete plus-strand (Kaplan et al., 1973; Robinson
and Greenman, 1974; Summers et al., 1975; Hruska et al., 1977;
Landers et al., 1977), have been found so far in only HBV, WHV
(Summers et al., 1978), GSHV (Marion et al., 1980a), and DHBV
(Mason et al., 1980).

The DNAs of all four hepadna viruses have been cloned in
bacteria (Wain-Hobson, 1984) and the complete nucleotide
sequences of HBV (Galibert et al., 1979; Pasek et al., 1979;
Valenzuela et al., 1980; Ono et al., 1983), WHV (Galibert et al.,
1982), and DHBV (Mandart et al., 1984) DNAs have been established.

2.3. Genetic Organization of the Hepatitis B Virus Genome

The minus-strand of virion DNA contains four open reading
frames based on the three reading phases of the nucleotide
sequence and the position of AUG start and TAA, TGA, or TAG
stop codons. A comparison of the nucleotide sequence of the reading frames with the available information on the gene products,
HBsAg and HBcAg (molecular weight, amino acid composition,
and sequence), allowed the identification and localization of these
viral genes in the genome (Fig. 3). These coding regions include the
region that codes for HBsAg (gene S) and a contiguous region
upstream termed presurface region (preS gene), the region that
codes for HBcAg (gene C), and two hypothetical regions coding for
the DNA polymerase (gene P) and the X protein (gene X), whose
existence have not yet been conclusively demonstrated. Through
extensive overlapping of gene P with genes preS/S, X, and C (Fig.
3), the small HBV genome can code for all four genes that account
for the known functions of the virus.

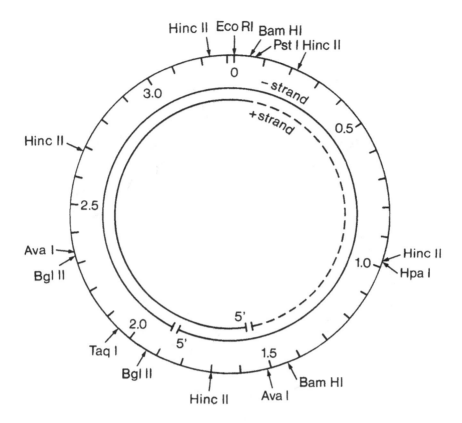

Fig. 2. Physical structure and restriction enzyme cleavage sites of HBV genome (HBsAg subtype adw₂), from Siddiqui et al. (1979).

2.4. Replication of the Hepatitis B Virus Genome

Based on work with the DHBV (Mason et al., 1982; Summers and Mason, 1982), replication of HBV is strikingly different from all other animal DNA viruses and involves the reverse transcription of an RNA intermediate by a virus-encoded reverse transcriptase. This life cycle is typical for the RNA-containing retroviruses, many of whom are tumor viruses (Varmus, 1982).

As illustrated in Fig. 4, upon internalization into host cells the infecting viral genome is made double-stranded and serves as a template for the transcription of its minus-strand into a full-length viral RNA molecule that either serves as messenger RNA or as template (pregenome) for the reverse transcription into minus-

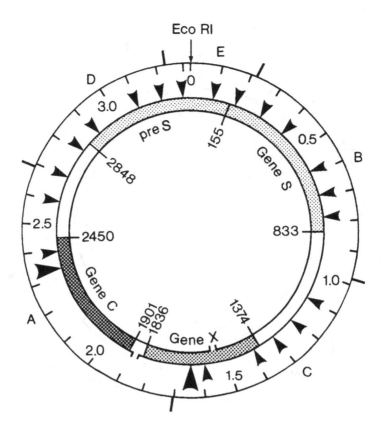

Fig. 3. Genetic organization of HBV genome and localization of HBsAg gene (gene S), HBcAg gene (gene C), DNA polymerase gene (arrows), and HBxAg gene (gene X).

strand DNA. These minus-strand DNA species are then made partially double-stranded to give mature virion DNA. Viral DNA replication is therefore asymmetric with separate pathways for plus- and minus-strand synthesis, and involves the reverse transcription of an RNA intermediate. In addition to the DHBV (Mason et al., 1982; Summers and Mason, 1982), this mechanism has also been demonstrated to be operative in GSHV (Weise et al., 1983) and human HBV (Blum et al., 1983a; Fowler et al., 1984), indicating that this mode of replication is central to the life cycle of all hepadna viruses.

PROPOSED RETROVIRAL MODE
OF REPLICATION OF HBV GENOME

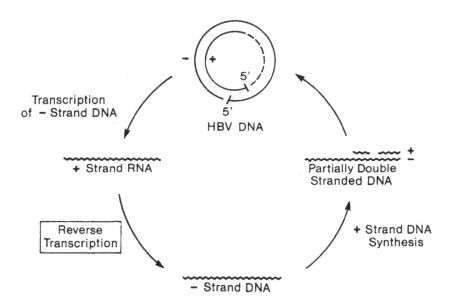

Fig. 4. Retroviral mode of replication of HBV DNA.

3. Molecular Analyses of Hepatitis B Virus Infection and Hepatocellular Carcinoma

3.1. Immunochemical Detection of Viral Antigens

HBV infection in humans is associated with the expression of the viral gene products, HBsAg, HBcAg/HBeAg, and DNA polymerase, and synthesis of the respective antibodies (anti-HBs, anti-HBc, anti-HBe), depending on the clinical presentation and course of the disease (Vyas and Blum, 1984). The laboratory diagnosis of HBV infection is therefore established by the specific and sensitive demonstration of these viral gene products or their corresponding antibodies in serum by radioimmunoassays and in tissues by immunohistochemical techniques.

The study of the expression of viral genes at the cellular level in conjunction with the localization and quantitation of viral DNA and RNA is of great interest in view of the biological interplay between gene expression, host immune response, and clinical course of the HBV infection (Vyas et al., 1984).

The viral gene products, namely HBsAg and HBcAg, can be detected using rabbit anti-HBs and anti-HBc as primary antibodies and peroxidase-labeled anti-rabbit IgG as the secondary antibody. As shown in Fig. 5A, in a patient with HBeAg-positive chronic active hepatitis B, HBsAg is localized in the cytoplasm of infected hepatocytes with a clearly focal tissue distribution of antigen-positive cells next to antigen-negative hepatocytes. A similar tissue distribution is found in this patient's liver for HBcAg (Fig. 5B), with the viral antigen localized predominantly in the nuclei. In contrast, no expression of HBsAg or HBcAg is detectable in this patient's HCC (Fig. 5C), indicating a significant biological difference between the infected normal and the malignantly transformed hepatocytes. Immunohistochemical detection of the viral antigens thus provides important information about the expression of viral genes at the tissue, cellular, and subcellular level.

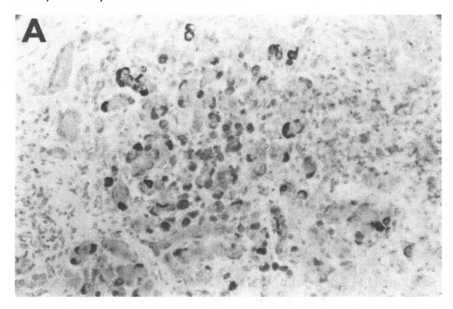

Fig. 5A. Immunohistochemical detection of HBV antigens in liver of a patient with HBeAg-positive chronic active hepatitis B. (A) HBsAg in nontumorous liver, (B) HBcAg in nontumorous liver, (C) HBsAg/HBcAg in hepatocellular carcinoma.

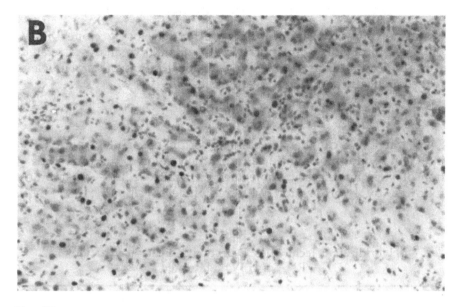

Fig. 5B.

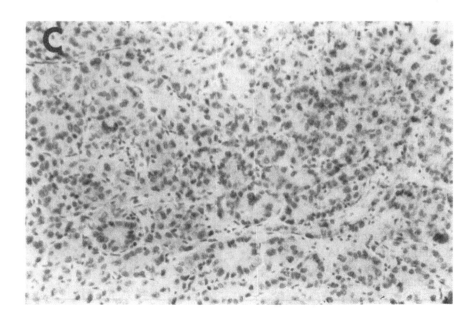

Fig. 5C.

3.2. Molecular Hybridization Analyses

Three molecular hybridization techniques using cloned HBV DNA as a probe allow quantitative and qualitative analyses related to the detection, characterization, and localization of viral nucleic acid sequence in serum and liver (Table 1).

3.2.1. Dot Blot Hybridization Analysis

Viral DNA can be detected in serum of patients with HBV infection by dot blot hybridization, which involves the immobilization of viral nucleic acid molecules on a nitrocellulose membrane followed by hybridization with radiolabeled cloned HBV DNA.

Table 1
Hybridization Techniques: Detection and Characterization of
DNA/RNA of HBV and Related Viruses

	Dot blot	Transfer blot (Southern/Northern)	In situ hybridization
DNA	+	+	+
RNA	+	+	+
Quantitation	+	+	+
Sensitivity (DNA)	0.1–0.5 pg	0.5–1 pg (per molecular species)	single copy (per cell)
Characterization			
RNA size classes	−	+	−
DNA size classes	−	+	−
DNA conformation	−	+	−
DNA integration	−	+	−
Restriction analysis	−	+	−
Replicative forms (ssDNA)	+	+	+
Single-cell analysis	−	−	+
Tissue pattern of viral DNA, RNA transcripts	−	−	+
Detection of rare/focal nucleic acid sequences	−	−	+
Combination of DNA/RNA hybridization with immunohistochemistry	−	−	+

Annealing of the radiolabeled probe to viral DNA results in hybrid molecules that can be detected by autoradiography and quantitated by densitometry or liquid scintillation counting, relative to standards of known amounts of cloned viral DNA.

The dot blot hybridization assay is specific for the detection of HBV DNA since an unrelated radiolabeled probe (e.g., pBR322) or DNA from an unrelated virus (e.g., Visna cDNA) does not result in a detectable hybrid formation, as illustrated in Fig. 6. This assay is easy to perform and readily identifies HBV DNA in the serum from a carrier serologically positive for HBsAg, HBeAg, and anti-HBc (D, Fig. 6). This result unequivocally indicates active viral replication in the liver and high infectivity of the serum from patient D. In contrast, three patients serologically positive for HBsAg, anti-HBc, and anti-HBe (A, B, and W, Fig. 6) are negative for serum HBV DNA. Patient C had HBsAg-negative chronic hepatitis. However, because of the relative insensitivity of the dot blot hybridization technique (limit of detection, about 0.1 pg HBV DNA, equivalent to approximately 30,000 viral copies), negative results do not exclude the presence of Dane particles in serum or active viral replication in the patient's liver. On the other hand, several studies have now established that dot blot analyses are more sensitive for the detection of HBV in the serum than radioimmunoassays for HBeAg and tests for DNA polymerase activity (Bonino et al., 1981; Berninger et al., 1982; Monjardino et al., 1982; Lieberman et al., 1983; Scotto et al., 1983). Additionally, HBV DNA has been detected by dot blot analyses in HBsAg-negative sera with and without antibodies to viral antigens (Shafritz et al., 1982; Wands et al., 1982; Scotto et al., 1983).

These findings provide evidence that both HBsAg-positive/ HBeAg-negative and HBsAg-negative patients with or without antibodies to HBV antigens (the so-called non-A, non-B hepatitis) may have active HBV replication in their livers and should be considered potentially infectious. Dot blot hybridization thus provides a sensitive and direct means for detecting HBV in the serum. The results redefine the serological patterns with epidemiological importance in identifying individuals with high levels of serum HBV, regardless of their HBsAg, HBeAg, or anti-HBe status.

Dot blot hybridization can also be applied for the detection of viral DNA or RNA in tissue extracts or subcellular fractions for the presence and average number of viral copies per cell as analyses preliminary to a more detailed characterization of viral nucleic acid sequences by transfer blots.

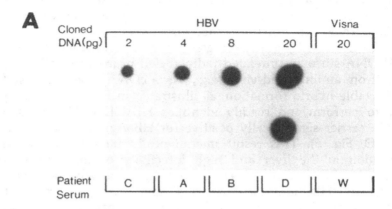

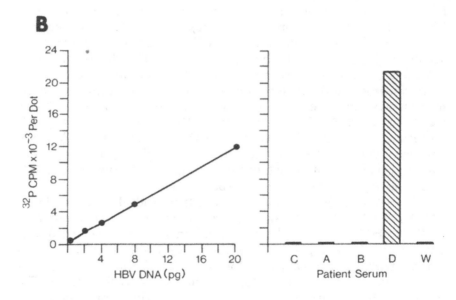

Fig. 6. Dot blot hybridization analyses of HBV DNA extracted from serum. (a) Autoradiogram of dot blot after hybridization of 2, 4, 8, and 20 pg of cloned HBV DNA (positive control) and 20 pg of cloned Visna cDNA (negative control) and sera from patients C, A, B, D, and W (*see* text) with ^{32}P-labeled cloned HBV DNA as a probe. (b) Quantitation of hybridization in (a) by liquid scintillation counting.

3.2.2. Transfer Blot Hybridization Analyses

The presence and state of viral DNA/RNA in liver tissues have been studied in detail by transfer blot hybridizations. The principle of this technique is the separtion of DNA or RNA molecules according to size by electrophoresis through agarose, followed by transfer to nitrocellulose under conditions preserving the relative positions of the nucleic acids in the gel. The immobilized DNA or RNA molecules are then hybridized with a ^{32}P-labeled HBV DNA probe and the presence and position of the nucleic acid species complementary to the probe are detected by autoradiography. This technique was first described by Southern (1975) for the analysis of DNA molecules and is popularly termed Southern blot analysis. In keeping with this terminology, the transfer blots for the characterization of RNA molecules were then termed Northern blots.

Southern blot analyses of DNA extracted from the liver tissue have been extensively used in characterization of the state of HBV DNA in various forms of liver disease. These studies have demonstrated that HBV DNA in hepatocytes can exist in a free, extrachromosomal form, as well as integrated into the cellular genome.

The hybridization pattern in a patient with active viral replication is characterized by the presence of large amounts of low molecular weight (<3.2 kb), nascent DNA molecules (Fig. 7). These species were shown to be predominantly single-stranded and of minus-strand polarity, demonstrating the asymmetric replication of the HBV genome (Blum et al., 1983a). By contrast, in a cell line derived from a human hepatocellular carcinoma (PLC/PRF/5; Alexander cells), the HBV DNA is predominantly integrated into the host genome and detectable as DNA species larger than 3.2 kb produced by restriction endonuclease digestion of cellular DNA (Fig. 8). As a result of flanking nucleotide sequences from the cellular genome, the viral DNA is generally of a molecular weight higher than that of free viral DNA of 3.2 kb.

Free viral DNA has been generally found in the liver of HBeAg-positive patients (Brechot et al., 1981a), whereas integrated forms are predominantly associated with HBeAg-negative chronic liver disease and hepatocellular carcinoma (Brechot et al., 1981b; Shafritz and Kew, 1981; Shafritz et al., 1981; Chen et al., 1982a; Brechot et al., 1982a,b). It is important, however, to recognize that analyses of hepatocellular DNA, without hydrolysis with restriction endonucleases, have shown free episomal or extrachromosomal replicative forms of a molecular weight higher than 3.2 kb in

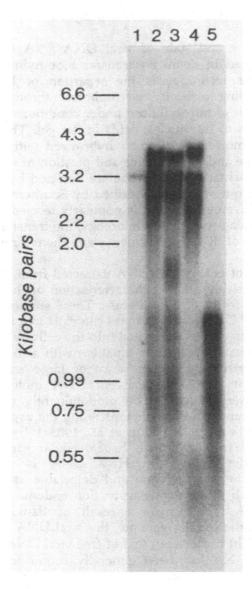

Fig. 7. Southern blot hybridization analysis of DNA (20 μg/lane) extracted from the liver of a patient with HBeAg-positive chronic active hepatitis B with ^{32}P-labeled cloned HBV DNA as a probe. Lane 1, 5 pg cloned HBV DNA as positive control and size marker; Lane 2, liver DNA undigested; Lane 3, liver DNA digested with EcoRI; Lane 4, liver DNA digested with single-stranded specific nuclease S 1; Lane 5, liver DNA heat-denatured.

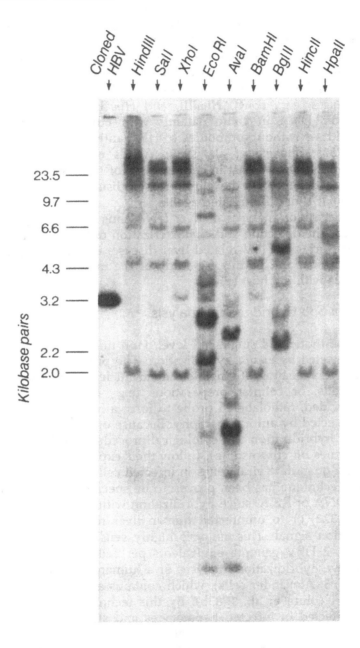

Fig. 8. Southern blot hybridization analysis of DNA (20 μg/lane) extracted from a human hepatoma cell line (PLC/PRF/5; Alexander cells) with ³²P-labeled cloned HBV DNA as a probe after digestion with restriction endonucleases indicated on top.

several HBsAg-negative patients with histologically proven chronic liver disease (Figus et al., 1984). Thus, free viral DNA with molecular weights higher than 3.2 kb may be misinterpreted as integrated forms, unless hepatocellular DNA is concurrently tested without hydrolysis, as well as after hydrolysis with different restriction endonucleases, e.g., EcoRI, HindIII, and HincII. Others have also shown HBV DNA in some patients with HBsAg-negative liver disease with or without antibodies to HBV antigens (Brechot et al., 1981b, 1982a; Shafritz et al., 1982; Wands et al., 1982). These findings imply that, at least in certain cases of serologically defined non-A, non-B hepatitis, the chronic liver disease may in fact be caused by HBV or HBV-related agents.

Southern blot analyses of liver DNA thus provide a powerful method for the detection and characterization of viral DNA species in various forms of HBV-related liver disease, including hepatocellular carcinoma, and permit the study of the molecular interaction of the virus with the host cell.

3.2.3. *In Situ* Hybridization Analysis

At the tissue and single cell level, viral nucleic acid sequences can be detected by *in situ* hybridization. The principle of this technique is the annealing of single-stranded nucleic acid molecules in tissues, cells, or cellular preparations (e.g., chromosomes) to a single-stranded, radiolabeled probe to form a hybrid molecule that can be detected by autoradiography. Because of the combination of molecular hybridization and cytological procedures, it is possible to localize genes on chromsomes, follow their expression in cells, and detect and quantitate viral genes in infected cells.

The technique has been proven to be specific for the detection of HBV DNA or RNA, since hybridization with an unrelated probe (e.g., pBR322) or to uninfected human liver results in a negative hybridization signal. This assay is highly sensitive and detects as little as 1–2 HBV genome equivalents per cell, as determined by comparative hybridization analyses of a human hepatoma cell line (PLC/PRF/5; Alexander cells), which contains about four copies of HBV DNA (Blum et al., 1983b). By this technique, HBV DNA is readily detected in infected hepatocytes and shows a highly focal tissue distribution with infected cells next to uninfected cells (Fig. 9), similar to the pattern obtained for viral antigens (Figs. 5a,b). The patients with active viral replication display a predominantly cytoplasmic hybridization pattern (Fig. 9). These cytoplasmic viral nucleic acid species are mostly single-stranded and of minus-strand

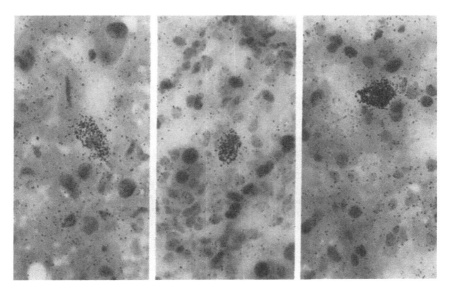

Fig. 9. *In situ* hybridization analyses of liver from a patient with HBeAg-positive chronic active hepatitis B with ^{3}H-labeled cloned HBV DNA as a probe.

polarity, demonstrating at the cellular level the asymmetric replication of HBV DNA (Blum et al., 1983a). In contrast to infected non-tumorous liver (NTL), no replicating HBV DNA species could be detected in the adjacent hepatocellular carcinoma (Fig. 10, HCC), indicating that malignantly transformed hepatocytes are nonpermissive for viral replication, possibly dependent on the degree of differentiation of the carcinoma cells.

Because of the high sensitivity of the *in situ* hybridization assay and visualization of the infected cells, HBV DNA could be demonstrated not only in the hepatocytes, but also in the bile duct epithelium, endothelial cells, and smooth muscle cells of blood vessel walls (Blum et al., 1983b).

The *in situ* hybridization assay thus provides a specific and sensitive tool for the localization and quantitation of viral nucleic acids at the single cell level and for the identification of individuals with active viral replication of HBV DNA not previously possible with other nucleic acid analyses. This assay is particularly useful since it requires only a fraction of the liver needle biopsy obtained routinely for diagnostic purposes and should permit investigators

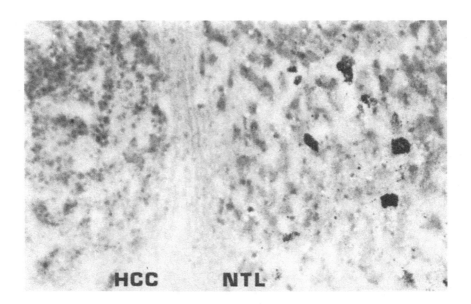

Fig. 10. *In situ* hybridization analysis of nontumorous liver (NTL) and hepatocellular carcinoma (HCC) from a patient with HBe-Ag-positive chronic active hepatitis B with ^{3}H-labeled cloned HBV DNA as a probe.

follow the natural course of HBV infection and select and monitor the patients undegoing antiviral regimens.

In applying the technique of *in situ* hybridization (see below) for the localization and quantitation of HBV DNA and gene-specific RNA (mRNA) in combination with immunoperoxidase staining for viral antigens, it is possible to determine the number of viral copies and their expression at the cellular level and to correlate these data with the histopathological findings in the same biopsy and with the available clinical-biochemical and serological findings of the patients (Blum et al., 1984b). Such studies should permit an insight into the molecular biology of HBV in infected human liver and an understanding of the pathogenetic mechanisms leading to viral persistence, chronicity of HBV infection, and development of HCC in man.

4.   Presence of Hepatitis B Virus DNA in Nonhepatocytes

A new and exciting aspect of the biology of HBV is the presence of viral DNA in nonhepatocytes. As summarized in Table 2,

Table 2
HBV DNA in Nonhepatocytes

Cells/tissues	Reference
Bile duct epithelium, endothelial cells, smooth muscle cells	Blum et al., 1983b
Kaposi's sarcoma	Siddiqui, 1983
Skin tissue, kidney, pancreas	Dejean et al., 1984
Lymphoblastoid cells from bone marrow	Romet-Lemonne et al., 1983; Elfassi et al., 1984
White blood cells	Lie-Injo et al., 1983
Peripheral mononuclear cells	Pontisso et al., 1984
Spleen	Blum, 1984

HBV DNA has been detected in bile duct epithelium, endothelial and smooth muscle cells of patients with HBV infection (Blum et al., 1983b), skin tissue from patients with Kaposi's sarcoma (Siddiqui, 1983), pancreas, kidney, and skin (Dejean et al., 1984), lymphoblastoid cells cultured from the bone marrow of a patient with recent HBV infection (Romet-Lemonne et al., 1983; Elfassi et al., 1984), leukocytes (Lie-Injo et al., 1983), peripheral mononuclear cells (Pontisso et al., 1984), and spleen (Fig. 11) (Blum et al., 1984a). All these findings indicate that the host cell range for HBV is more extensive than has been appreciated previously. The biological significance and pathological potential of the presence of HBV DNA in nonhepatocytes, however, remain to be defined.

5.   Presence, State, and Molecular Structure of Hepatitis B Viral DNA in Hepatocellular Carcinoma

The presence, state, and molecular structure of viral DNA in HCCs from humans and woodchucks, and in cell lines derived from human tumors, have been analyzed in great detail in an attempt to define the genetic contribution of HBV/WHV to the development of this malignancy.

5.1.   Presence of Viral DNA in Hepatocellular Carcinoma

The presence of viral DNA in human HCC tissue was first detected by Lutwick and Robinson (1977) and Summers et al. (1978). Subsequently, these findings were confirmed and extended

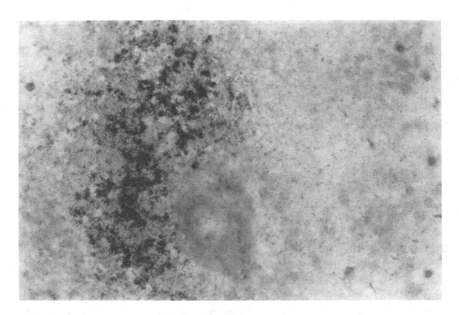

Fig. 11. *In situ* hybridization analysis of spleen from a patient with HBeAg-positive chronic active hepatitis B with ^{3}H-labeled cloned HBV DNA as a probe.

(Brechot et al., 1980; Shafritz and Kew, 1981; Shafritz et al., 1981; Brechot et al., 1981b; Koshy et al., 1981; Brechot et al., 1982a,b; Shafritz, 1982; Chen et al., 1982b; Dejean et al., 1983; Shafritz and Rogler, 1984; Brechot et al., 1984; Tiollais et al., 1984; Robinson et al., 1984), including cell lines derived from human HCCs (Marion et al., 1980b; Edman et al., 1980; Chakraborty et al., 1980; Zaslavsky et al., 1980; Twist et al., 1981; Koshy et al., 1981; Marquardt et al., 1982; Koike et al., 1983; Koshy et al., 1983; Dejean et al., 1983; Miller and Robinson, 1983; Monjardino et al., 1983; Koshy et al., 1984; Tiollais et al., 1984). Also in the woodchuck, viral DNA has been detected in HCC tissues of infected animals (Summers et al., 1978; Mitamura et al., 1982; Ogston et al., 1982; Gerin, 1984).

Although most HCCs from infected humans or woodchucks contain viral DNA, it should be emphasized that in some tumors there is no viral DNA detectable at a level of sensitivity of about 0.01 genome copies (equivalent to 50 bp) per cell (Summers et al., 1978; Shafritz and Kew, 1981; Koshy et al., 1981; Robinson et al., 1984; Gerin, 1984). Similarly, not all cell lines derived from human

HCC tissues contain detectable HBV DNA sequences (Koshy et al., 1981).

The absence of detectable viral DNA in some HCCs suggests that HBV/WHV DNA does not make a genetic contribution to the development of these malignancies or that the continuing presence of viral DNA is not required for the maintenance of the malignant phenotype (*see* section 7).

5.2. State of Viral DNA in Hepatocellular Carcinoma

Southern blot analyses of DNA isolated from HCC tissues and human hepatoma cell lines have revealed the presence of unintegrated/replicating forms of viral DNA in some human HCCs (Summers et al., 1978; Brechot et al., 1981b; Chen et al., 1982a; Tiollais et al., 1984; Robinson et al., 1984), in PLC/PRF/5 cells derived from a human HCC (Zaslavsky et al., 1980; Marquardt et al., 1982), as well as in woodchuck HCCs (Mitamura et al., 1982; Ogston et al., 1982). In most HCC tissues and human hepatoma cell lines positive for HBV DNA, however, HBV or WHV nucleotide sequences were found to be integrated into the host cellular genome. As demonstrated for PLC/PRF/5 cells (Fig. 8) derived from a human HCC (Alexander et al., 1976), there are at least eight HBV DNA-containing bands apparent after digestion of DNA with the restriction endonuclease *Hind*III, an enzyme that cleaves cellular DNA at specific sites, but not HBV DNA of all HBsAg subtypes reported so far. This HBV DNA hybridization pattern was shown to be identical for PLC/PRF/5 cells from an early passage (1978) and cells continuously passaged since then (Miller and Robinson, 1983), indicating that once established, the integration of HBV DNA into the host cellular genome is stable, at least at this level of analysis.

The number of cellular DNA fragments containing viral nucleic acid sequences (usually one to four), the site of integration into the cellular genome, and the average number of viral copies per cell (ranging from 0.05 to 4 in most cases studied) varies from HCC to HCC (Shafrtiz and Rogler, 1984; Tiollais et al., 1984; Tiollais and Wain-Hobson, 1984; Robinson et al., 1984; Varmus, 1984; Ogston et al., 1982; Gerin, 1984). It is therefore difficult to assess which of the viral insertions, if any, is of significance for the development of this neoplasia. Attempts to determine the importance of integrated viral DNA in hepatoma cells have been confounded further by the demonstration of a significantly different pattern of integration and viral copy numbers per cell in three hepatoma cell lines derived from the same tumor (Twist et al., 1981). The relationship between a specific viral insertion and the developmentof HCC is therefore unclear and not defined as yet.

5.3. Molecular Structure of Integrated Viral DNA Sequences and Relation to Host Cellular Genome

Studies on the molecular structure of viral DNA sequences integrated into host cellular DNA of HCC tissues and HCC-derived cell lines were aimed at an understanding of how the integration event or the integrated nucleic acid sequences might induce the development of this neoplasia.

The genetic organization of integrated viral DNA species and their flanking cellular sequences were investigated in human HCCs (Dejean et al., 1983; Fung et al., 1984; Shafritz and Rogler, 1984), in human hepatoma cell lines (Dejean et al., 1983; Koshy et al., 1983; Koike et al., 1983), and in woodchuck HCCs (Ogston et al., 1982; Shafritz and Rogler, 1984). Cloning and sequence analyses of viral DNA and their flanking cellular DNA have demonstrated unequivocally that viral nucleic acid sequences are integrated into the cellular genome of HCCs and HCC-derived cell lines. All integrated HBV/WHV DNA sequences characterized to date were found to be highly disordered, representing subgenomic viral DNA fragments as a result of deletions. In addition, most integrated viral sequences in HCCs display some degree of rearrangement with inversions and/or duplications, suggesting that these integrated viral sequences do not play a role in the normal life cycle of the virus as they do in retroviruses (Varmus, 1982). By comparison, integrated WHV DNA isolated from a chronically infected liver that never developed HCC did not contain internal rearrangements, but was colinear with the cloned viral genome except for a deletion of about 500 bp (Rogler and Summers, 1984). Further, Shafritz and Rogler (1984) presented evidence for modifications (deletions or rearrangements) of cellular sequences flanking the integrated viral DNA in human and woodchuck HCCs. Again, in chronically infected woodchuck liver no rearrangement of flanking cellular sequences could be detected (Rogler and Summers, 1984). At what stage of the development of HCCs these deletions/rearrangements in both viral and cellular DNA occur and whether they are of oncogenic significance remains uncertain.

Although HBV DNA seems to integrate randomly into the liver cell genome, the integration with respect to the viral genome appears to take place preferentially in the single-stranded region close to the 5' end of the plus-strand (Koshy et al., 1983). This mechanism involves the interaction of the DNA polymerase switching from the cellular template to the single-stranded region of the HBV genome during cellular replication. Cellular DNA then joins the strand of the viral genome through recombination, followed by completion of the single-stranded region and ligation of the plus-strand with cellular DNA. Based on the analyses of host–viral junctions of two clones from human HCC, Tiollais et al. (1984) suggest a mechanism of integration that involves a specific initial event mediated through a palindromic sequence. More analyses are needed, however, to establish the molecular mechanisms leading to the integration of viral genes into the host cellular genome.

To date there is no evidence that the hepadna virus genome carries one of the approximately 20 known cellular oncogenes. Also, none of the cloned flanking cellular sequences examined so far correspond to a known oncogene (Dejean et al., 1983). Furthermore, no rearrangement or amplification of known cellular oncogenes has been observed in human HCCs tested so far (Fung et al., 1984).

Although HBV DNA or DNA extracted from PLC/PRF/5 hepatoma cells appear to transform NIH/3T3 cells after transfection (Koshy et al., 1984; Robinson et al., 1984), the transformants did not contain viral DNA or RNA at a level of sensitivity of approximately 0.2 viral genomes (equivalent to 600 bp) per cell.

All these findings suggest that the presence and/or expression of any HBV/WHV gene is not essential for the initiation or maintenance of the malignant transformation of hapatocytes.

6. Expression of Viral Genes in Hepatocellular Carcinoma

HBV antigens in serum of patients with HCC are predominantly the product of nontumorous liver cells (see Figs. 5A and B). HCC cells, by comparison, rarely express HBsAg, and HBcAg seems to be absent (Fig. 5C) (Nayak et al., 1977; Thung et al., 1979). Indeed, there appears to exist an inverse relationship between the expression of HBsAg and the degree of differentiation of malignant hepatocytes (Goudeau et al., 1979; Goudeau et al., 1981). The lack of expression of viral antigens in HCC cells can be caused by (i) deletions and rearrangements of the integrated viral sequences, resulting in products antigenically distinct from the HBV antigens synthesized during the normal life cycle of the virus; or (ii) a lack of transcription and/or translation of viral genes in HCCs and HCC-derived cell lines in spite of functionally intact integrated HBV DNA sequences. This latter mechanism was shown to be operative in a HBsAg-negative HCC by transfecting mouse L cells with a HBV DNA-containing clone derived from the tumor, resulting in the synthesis and secretion of characteristic HBsAg particles into the culture medium (Dejean et al., 1982). Furthermore, HBcAg, whichis normally not expressed in PLC/PRF/5 cells in vitro, is expressed when the cells are grown in vivo after subcutaneous injection into nude mice (Marquardt et al., 1984) or when the cells are grown in vitro in the presence of 5-azacytidine (Yoakum et al., 1983; Yoakum, 1984). These findings indicate that the expression of viral genes integrated into HCC cells and possibly also into nonmalignant hepatocytes is regulated by mechanisms as yet not clearly defined. One potential mechanism could be related to the hypermethylation of specific genes, as shown for the core gene in in vitro cultures of PLC/PRF/5 cells (Miller and robinson, 1983) and its expression in the presence of 5-azacytidine (Yoakum et al., 1983; Yoakum, 1984). Further studies are required, however, in order to elucidate the molecular mechanisms regulating the expression of viral genes integrated into the host cellular genome and their significance, if any, for the malignant transformation of hepatocytes.

7. Molecular Mechanisms of Malignant Transformation of Hepatocytes

The basic observation that tumor cells inherit in some stable way the transformed phenotype suggests that the oncogenic transformation may be a result of genetic alterations. Indeed, cancer-causing genes (oncogenes) responsible for the maintenance of the transformed state were first clearly identified in certain retroviruses (v-*onc*) (Bishop, 1982,1983; Varmus, 1982). Nineteen v-*onc* genes have been identified and isolated, and DNA sequences homologous to the transforming genes of some retroviruses have also been found in nontransformed cells. DNA sequences homologous to most of the known v-*onc* genes have been detected in a variety of normal uninfected cells, including cells of human origin. The structural similarities between these cellular oncogenes (c-*onc* and their viral homologues suggest that the c-*onc* genes may also have oncogenic potential, a concept that is supported by several lines of evidence (Cooper, 1982; Slamon et al., 1984). These cellular oncogenes are active in normal cells and probably represent essential cellular constituents.

Following a discussion of the concept of expression or over-expression of a viral or cellular oncogene as the molecular basis for the malignant transformation of hepatocytes, four models of oncogenesis will be discussed.

1. Expression of v-*onc* induces transformed phenotype (Bishop, 1983).

   The mechanism of malignant transformation has been demonstrated for a number of acute retroviruses, including replication competent (e.g., Rous sarcoma virus) and replication defective viruses (e.g., murine and feline sarcoma viruses, Abelson leukemia virus, avian acute leukemia virus). These acute retroviruses carry an oncogene (v-*onc*) and their own promoter, integrate into the host genome at random, induce neoplastic disease in host animals rapidly (usually within 2–4 wk) and with high efficiency (approximately 100%), and transform target cells in tissue culture.

2. "Malignant" expression of c-*onc* through viral promoter insertion induces transformed phenotype (Bishop, 1983).

   This mechanism of malignant transformation has been shown for a number of chronic retroviruses, including avian leukosis virus and murine leukemia virus. These chronic retroviruses do not possess a transforming gene (v-*onc*), but carry a promoter and integrate at specific sites into the host genome. Through over-expression of a cellular oncogene (c-*onc*), these viruses induce neoplasia after a prolonged latent period (usually 4–12 mo) and with low efficiency (20–60%) and do not transform target cells in tissue culture.

3. "Malignant" expression of c-*onc* through translocation induces transformed phenotype (Rowley, 1983).

   Chromosomal aberrations/translocations, such as human c-myc *onc* gene in Burkitt's tumor cell line from chromosome 8 to 14, human c-mos *onc* gene in

    acute myeloblastic leukemia cells from chromosome
    8–21, human c-abl *onc* gene in chronic myelogeneous
    leukemia cells from chromosome 9 to 22/Philadelphia
    chromosome can be induced either by viruses (EBV/
    Burkitt) or by mutagens or other carcinogens and
    bring the c-*onc* under the influence of a different pro-
    moter, resulting in increased c-*onc* transcripts, leading
    in turn to malignant transformation of the cells.

4.   "Malignant" expression of c-*onc* through mutation
     induces transformed phenotype.
     The mutation of a cellular oncogene, induced by a
     virus, mutagen, or other carcinogen, leads to the
     conversion of a proto-oncogene into an active
     oncogene with the malignant transformation of cells
     without abnormal level of expression of the cellular
     oncogene (e.g., T 24 human bladder carcinoma)
     (Reddy et al., 1982).

Both the c-*onc* translocation and the c-*onc* mutation model of
carcinogenesis would not require the continuing presence of the
carcinogen (virus, mutagen, or other carcinogen) for the maintenance of the malignant state and would conform with the "hit-
and-run" mechanism postulated for the oncogenic potential or
herpes simplex viruses (Galloway and McDougall, 1983).

Although there is no evidence to date that HBV or WHV carry
their own oncogene, similar to acute retroviruses, or induce HCC
through a promoter insertion mechanism, similar to chronic retroviruses, the c-*onc* translocation and mutation model are possible
mechanisms, particularly since they accommodate HBV/WHV as
well as mutagens and other carcinogens implicated as etiologic
cofactors in the development of HCC (Okuda and Mackay, 1982).
Further studies are needed to establish whether HBV/WHV induce
HCC by any of the mechanisms described above or whether they
have some other direct transforming effect. In addition, the evidence available to date does not exclude the possibility that HBV/
WHV have no direct transforming effect on infected hepatocytes,
but rather trigger HCC formation in a more indirect way, such as
through chronic liver injury and liver regeneration. Such a concept
is indeed supported by the fact that liver injury leading to cirrhosis
over many years greatly increases the risk of developing HCC
(Szmuness, 1978; Beasley et al., 1981; Kew, 1982) and could conform with c-*onc* activation mechanism, since it was shown that the
expression of the cellular oncogene *ras* is increaased during liver
regeneration (Goyette et al., 1983).

The hepatotoxicity and mutagenicity of a carcinogenic metabolite produced by certain strains of fungus (*Aspergillus flavus*) contaminating food in areas of high HBV endemicity may be caused by the activated form of aflatoxin B1 (AFB1) causing covalent modification of guanine residues leading to alkali-labile sites in DNA (Meunch et al., 1983). The in vitro sequence specificity of alkali-labile sites induced by AFB1 also occur in vivo with the quantitative formation of AFB1-DNA adducts within the ribosomal RNA gene sequences of liver DNA from AFB1 treated rats (Irvinand Wogan, 1984). Refinement of this experimental approach, especially in the WHV-infected woodchucks, may be useful in defining the precise relationship between covalent AFB1-DNA interactions possibly underlying the oncogenic expression of WHV infection in the animal model.

8.   Epidemiology of Hepatocellular Carcinoma

8.1.   Geographic Distribution

Although less common in the United States, hepatocellular carcinoma is one of the most prevalent malignancies in some areas of the world. In certain Asian and African countries, HCC has been reported to be one of the most common causes of death. Many of these countries in which HCC is prevalent also have high carrier rates for the HBV. In Asia, reports from countries such as China, Hong Kong, and Taiwan indicate that the HBsAg carrier rate is up to 17% of the population, and these countries share the problem of a high incidence of HCC. In Africa, reports from South Africa, Uganda, Mozambique, and West Africa parallel those in Asia with respect to HCC and HBV carrier rates. Beasley et al. (1981) have found, in a prospective study in Taiwan, that the relative risk of HCC in chronic carriers of HBsAg is 223.

In the United States, HCC occurs less frequently, with a reported annual incidence of approximately 9000 cases/yr, which is similar to that reported for Hodgkin's disease (Chlebowski et al., 1984). However, recent analysis of HCC mortality by race showed that although the Chinese constituted only 0.7% of the population in New York, up to 10% of the HCC deaths occurred in this racial group (Szmuness et al., 1978). An autopsy study from Los Angeles showed that the percentage of cirrhotic patients who developed HCC was highest among the Asians (48%), followed by the blacks (8.3%), and lowest in the Caucasian race (<1%) (Peters et al., 1977).

Therefore, the racial distribution of HCC in the United States reflects the high incidence of this malignancy in the country of origin of the patients.

8.2. Role of HBV and Cirrhosis

As previously mentioned, the majority of cases of HCC in Asia and Africa are associated with chronic HBV infection. In certain countries in Africa and Asia, the HBsAg carrier rate in the general population is high, and the reported prevalence of HBsAg positivity in HCC is up to 80%. In addition, the presence of other HBV markers, such as anti-HBs and anti-HBc, are often positive in the HCC patients who are HBsAg-negative. HCC is, therefore, seldom detected in patients who are negative for HBV markers in these countries. In contrast, HCC is very uncommon in Greenland, Sardinia, and parts of South America, despite a high prevalence (5–10%) of HBsAg carriers in the population (Vyas and Blum, 1984; Lai, personal communication from Sardinia).

In areas of the world where the HBV carrier rate is low, the incidence of HCC is also much reduced. Although chronic infection by the HBV is closely associated with eventual development of HCC, the virus has not been shown to be directly oncogenic in experimental systems and its direct role as an oncogenic agent requires further investigation.

The majority of chronic carriers of the HBV remain asymptomatic carriers for life, and only a minority develops chronic liver disease and HCC. In autopsy studies, between 60 and 90% of HCC cases arise in a setting of cirrhosis. HCC occurs in other diseases associated with cirrhosis, such as alcoholic liver disease (Brechot et al., 1982a), hemochromatosis, primary biliary cirrhosis, and cryptogenic cirrhosis (Okuda and Mackay, 1982), but shows a lower incidence than in cirrhosis caused by chronic infection by the hepatitis B virus. Therefore, the factors associated with development of cirrhosis may also contribute to the eventual occurrence of HCC. In patients with HBsAg-positive HCC, the majority have underlying cirrhosis and only a small number of HBsAg-positive patients develop HCC in the absence of a cirrhotic liver. Thus, both the presence of a chronic HBV carrier state and a background of cirrhosis may contribute to the development of HCC.

8.3. Sex, Genetic, and Host Factors

HCC is a malignancy that occurs most often in males. Reported series have shown a male over female predominance from 5:1 to 7:1. The reasons for the male predominance have not been elucidated.

It has been previously noted that family clustering of HCC cases occurs. In the majority of these families, evidence for hepatitis B infection has been strong, as shown by the presence of either HBsAg or HBV antibodies (Tong et al., 1979). Our recent experience with HBsAg-positive HCC cases has yielded 10 such families with two or more cases of HCC in each family. Although a lack of evidence for autosomal recessive inheritence in chronic HBV infections has been reported (Vyas, 1974), familial clustering of HBV infections has been reported by many investigators. However, further studies are needed to determine if family susceptibility to develop HCC exists in those infected by the HBV. Family clustering of HCC has not been reported in HBsAg-negative cases.

Other factors that have been implicated in development of HCC include heavy cigaret smoking (Yu et al., 1983). The relative risk factor in cases of HBsAg-negative HCC was 2.6 compared to light and nonsmokers, and indicated that HBV infection and cigaret smoking are independent risk factors for HCC.

Exposure to environmental and chemical agents has been associated with HCC. Aflatoxin B1(AFB), produced by *Aspergillus flavus*, has been detected in food products in many areas where there is a high incidence of HCC. It was concluded that in these areas of heavy aflatoxin contamination, there was a direct correlation with the incidence of HCC. Moreover, aflatoxin has been shown to cause hepatocellular carcinoma in laboratory animals, especially if these animals are rendered cirrhotic prior to exposure to the aflatoxin. In certain areas of Africa and Asia, aflatoxin may play a contributory role in the development of HCC. However, it does not appear to play a significant role in the cases of HCC that arise in areas of low aflatoxin exposure, such as the United States.

The risk factors so far identified for development of HCC include the male sex, chronic hepatitis B infection, presence of cirrhosis, alcohol consumption, cigaret smoking, and possible exposure to carcinogens such as aflatoxin.

8.4. Aflatoxin B1 and HBV in Hepatocellular Carcinoma

Aflatoxin B1 and chronic HBV infection epidemiologically correlate with the geographic distribution of HCC. Integration of HBV DNA into the cellular genome of HCCs and the in vivo formation of adducts between AFB and nucleic acids lead us to suggest that hepatocytes with integrated HBV DNA preferentially acumulate AFB; the AFB adducts formed may then initiate cell transformation by modifying the expression of critical host genes. The altered molecular biology of liver cells in HCC is evidenced by the fact that HBV does not replicate in HCC tissues or cell lines. The effect of AFB on the expression of cellular genes such as endogenous retrovirus(es) and possibly cellular oncogene(s) can be analyzed in HCC cell lines with and without integrated HBV DNA. In addition, human HCC cell tissues can be probed for HBV sequences and AFB DNA adducts at the single-cell level. The presence of HBV and AFB can be correlated with the expression of putative transforming genes, providing a new insight into the interaction between liver cells, HBV, and AFB in the pathogenesis of HCC.

9.   Clinical Aspects of Hepatocellular Carcinoma

9.1.   Presenting Signs and Symptoms

HCC often arises in a setting of chronic liver disease. Thus, the signs and symptoms may be either caused by the liver cancer or secondary to the underlying cirrhosis. the most common presenting signs include an abdominal mass that may be painful on paplation and may involve the epigastrium and right upper quadrant. Ascites, peripheral edema, as well as a vascular bruit, may be evident over the tumor site. Jaundice is uncommon and when present, is usually mild. Again, it should be emphasized that the presenting signs and symptoms in these patients may be caused by HCC or the presence of chronic liver disease, and it may be difficult to clearly differentiate their symptoms. Patients who present with bone pain would have discernible lesions on radiologic examination, and those with respiratory insufficiency would have metastatic lesions on their chest X-rays.

In 121 patients from the Los Angeles area, the most common presenting symptoms included right upper-quadrant pain, abdominal fullness, weight loss, anorexia, and ascites, which occurred in 20–54% of patients (Chlebowski et al., 1984). Other symptoms included fever, bone pain from metastases, respiratory insufficiency secondary to pulmonary involvement, and gastrointestinal bleeding. Hemoperitoneum secondary to intraabdominal rupture of the tumor may also occur. A small number of patients were clinically asymptomatic and the primary liver cancer was discovered because of incidental laboratory abnormalities and was diagnosed on further investigation.

9.2. Paraneoplastic Manifestations

The paraneoplastic manifestation described in HCC include hypercalcemia, hypoglycemia, hyperlipidemia, and symptoms stemming from increased levels of human gonadotropin. Hypercalcemia is rare, and possible mechanisms that have been implicated include tumors producing a parathyroid hormone-like substance, osteoclast activating factor, and prostaglandin. The hypoglycemia may be related to a relative deficiency of glucose-6-phosphatase, which is required for breakdown of glycogen stores, and may be caused by an acquired enzyme defect from growth of the liver tumor, or to replacement of the liver by the HCC resulting in depletion of glycogen storage sites in the nontumor liver cells. The latter is seen more often during the terminal stages of HCC. Both hypercholesteremia and hyperlipidemia have been described in HCC patients. The mechanism involved is postulated to be caused by a malfunction of the negative feedback system resulting in increased production of the lipids. Increased human chorionic gonadotropin has been reported in young male patients with HCC, leading to early puberty and enlarged genitals.

9.3. Laboratory Tests

Routine laboratory tests of liver function reveal many abnormalities. In the 121 patients from our report, 18% had abnormal serum bilirubin levels, 93% had increases inserum aspartate aminotransferase values, 35% had elevated alanine aminotransferase values, and 93% had an increased alkaline phosphatase (Chlebowski et al., 1984). Taken together, 97% had at least one abnormal test of liver function. However, these tests were not diagnostic for HCC. Other laboratory tests may show a hematocrit of less than 36% in 55% of patients. Other abnormal tests may include hypercalcemia, hypoclycemia, and hyperlipidemia, which are considered paraneoplastic syndromes associated with HCC, as discussed in more detail above.

The serum alphafetoprotein (AFP) is a more specific test for HCC (Heyward et al., 1982). Significant elevation of AFP levels was noted 2–6 yr preceding clinical onset of the HCC. The AFP level is normally elevated in the pregnant female and is at its highest level during the latter stages of pregnancy. At birth, the levels return toward normal, i.e., 5–10 nanograms/mL. In 1963, AFP was found to be elevated in mouse hepatomas and this test was subsequently found to be useful for the diagnosis of HCC in man. Our previous study of 100 HCC patients from Taiwan showed that over 75% of patients had AFP levels greater than 20 ng/mL (Chien et al., 1981). In this study, approximately 25% of patients had normal AFP values, 25–35% had levels between 20 and 400 ng/mL, and 45% had AFP levels about 400 ng/mL. Some patients had AFP values as high as 2×10^5 ng/mL. However, patients with chronic active hepatitis may have values of AFP ranging from 20 to 400 ng/mL. Levels of AFP above 400 ng/mL are diagnostic for HCC and should be used in conjunction with other diagnostic modalities. In the early detection of human HCC, determination of AFP levels is not a reliable indicator (Chen et al., 1984). Carcinoembryonic antigen, serum ferritin, and alpha-1-antitrypsin levels have not been shown to be clinically useful at present. More recently, we reported the use of abnormal prothrombin as a marker for HCC (Liebman et al., 1984). Conversion of inactive prothrombin to an active biological form of prothrombin requires the carboxylation of glutamic acid residues on the precursor molecule. This modification is vitamin K-dependent and catalyzed by a carboxylase. In normal individuals, the precursoe molecule, or abnormal prothrombin, is absent in the circulation since it is fully converted to active prothrombin in the liver cell. Patients with HCC have unusually high circulatory levels of abnormal prothrombin that is unresponsive to vitamin K. In 75 HCC patients from the United States and Taiwan, 75% had high levels of abnormal prothrombin. When used in combination with AFB, the diagnostic accuracy of HCC was increased to 93% and demonstrated efficacy for the monitoring of patients undergoing therapy.

The HBsAg is positive in up to 80% of Asian patients (Chien et al., 1981). Our study from Los Angeles, which included all ethnic groups, showed that 52% were HBs-Ag-positive (Tong et al., 1981). The presence of a positive test for HBsAg and an elevated AFP level is strongly suggestive of HCC and requires immediate attention.

9.4. Diagnosis

The diagnosis of HCC rests on clinical, laboratory, and radiologic findings and histologic confirmation. Patients with underlying chronic liver disease (cirrhosis) who acutely decompensate should be further investigated for HCC. Others with abdominal masses associated with pain, weight loss, and anorexia should also arouse suspicion for HCC. Laboratory tests should initially include a serum AFP. Twenty-five percent of HCC patients have normal AFPs, but levels above 400 ng/mL in this clinical setting is strongly indicative of HCC. If levels above 20 ng/mL but below 400 ng/mL, are encountered, the AFP should be repeated at regular intervals; if a steady rise is noted, further investigation is warranted.

Radiologic modalities that have been used for diagnosis of HCC include technetium sulfur colloid (tech 99) liver scan, gallium scan, abdominal ultrasound, computerized axial tomography, and hepatic angiography. Up to 95% of HCC will show up as filling defects in the liver scan. Gallium scans were positive in the majority of these cases and show up as a "hot spot." Ultrasound delineates "small tumors" of 3-cm size and also aids in differentiating between solid and cystic lesions in the liver (Chen et al., 1982b). Abdominal CT scan is a very useful diagnostic modality and is positive in the majority of patients. Hepatic angiography is helpful in delineating the vascular composition of the tumors, as well as in locating lesions. Our recent studies have shown that the diagnostic accuracy of the above tests are: 95% for liver scans, 82% for abdominal ultrasound, 79% for abdominal CT scans, and 93% for hepatic angiography. Proper radiologic procedures should be chosen on the basis of the information that is desired.

9.5. Treatment

In our report of 121 patients in Los Angeles, only 12% were suitable candidates for surgical resection (Chlebowski et al., 1984). The majority of patients who presented with signs and symptoms of this malignancy had large tumors in the setting of cirrhosis, both of which are contraindications for surgical intervention. Recently, mass screening for HCC using AFP in China has been successful in detecting subclinical cases in which the tumor sizes were less than 3.5 cm in diameter (Tang et al., 1982). Detection of these early lesions increased the resectability rate to over 60% and significantly increased the survival rate. However, in the United States where the overall incidence of HCC is much lower, screening with AFP has not been initiated. Thus, in a selected population of patients with HCC who have subclinical lesions, surgery remains the only curative treatment.

Hepatic artery ligation alone or in combination with selective catheter placement for infusion chemotherapy has been attempted in patients with HCC. Also, arterial embolization of tumor-supplying vessels has been reported to have limited success.

Studies utilizing chemotherapeutic agents, such as 5-fluorouracil, adriamycin, and 5-methyl CCNU, have not shown increased survival rates in patients with HCC. The initial limited success with adriamycin in earlier studies was not reproducible and at present there are no chemotherapeutic regimens with proven efficacy. Since regression of aflatoxin B1-induced HCC in rats has been reported with reduced glutathione, this harmless antioxidant merits investigation as a potential antitumor agent in humans (Novi, 1981).

Immunotherapy using interferon is currently under investigation. Also, isotope immunotherapy utilizing antiferritin antibodies in patients with HCC is being studied in the United States.

In summary, therapeutic trials in patients with HCC have been uniformly disappointing and treatment for this malignancy remains a challenge for the years to come.

9.6. Natural History and Prognosis

The prognosis of HCC is poor. In a series of 211 patients from Hong Kong, the median survival of untreated patients was only 3.5 wk (Lai et al., 1981). In our series from Los Angeles, which included treated patients, the median survival was 18 wk (Chlebowski et al., 1984). An elevated serum bilirubin level above 2 mg/dL, presence of pulmonary metastasis, and patient's age of more than 45 yr significantly decreased survival. The reason for the short survival is that the majority of patients presents with large tumors and chronic liver disease. The hepatic reserve is such that a large amount of liver tissue must be replaced by tumor before signs and symptoms of HCC appear. Thus, in the majority of cases of HCC, the disease is advanced and liver function has already been compromised at the time of diagnosis. The extent of the cancer, as well as the presence of cirrhosis, significantly decreases survival.

9.7. Strategies of Prophylaxis Against HBV and Prevention of Hepatocellular Carcinoma

Considering the poor response to treatment, the efforts to deal with HCC as a worldwide public health problem will have to be directed toward the development of strategies of prophylaxis and prevention of this neoplasia.

The pathogenesis of HCC, being most likely multifactorial and dependent on the geographic area, dictates an approach that takes these various etiologic factors into account. Undoubtedly, the most important consideration is the prevention of HBV infection, the HBV carrier state, and the wide spectrum of associated acute and chronic sequelae. Indeed, implementable measures are now available that could eventually lead to the prevention of HBV infection. The commercially available vaccines against HBV infection have been shown to be safe and effective (Szmuness et al., 1980; Stevens et al., 1984). Their use in newborn infants of HBsAg carrier mothers holds the promise of greatly reducing and potentially eliminating the incidence of HBV infection and HBV-induced chronic liver disease, including HCC (Stevens et al., 1984; Vyas et al., 1984; Zuckerman, 1982). HBV vaccines produced by recombinant DNA technologies are expected to be equally effective as the presently available vaccines derived from the plasma of HBsAg carriers, and substantially less expensive, a prerequisite for its administration on a worldwide scale, particularly in less developed countries where they are needed most. Further, synthetic peptide analogs of HBsAg might eventually prove to be safe and effective vaccines against HBV infection and conceivably provide a tool for immunointervention, resulting in resolution of the HBsAg carrier state (Vyas and Blum, 1984).

Apart from prevention of HBV infection through vaccination strategies, it appears reasonable to recommend measures to eliminate known heptocarcinogens, e.g., aflatoxin B1, and other factors known to favor the development of HCC, e.g., alcohol, cigaret smoking, and others.

Given our knowledge of the etiologic factors involved in hepatocarcinogenesis in humans and the measures available to influence them, one can hope to substantially reduce and eventually eliminate the incidence of HCC, today still the leading cause of death from cancer.

10. Summary and Conclusions

The HBV genome consists of a small circular, partly double-stranded DNA molecule of about 3200 nucleotides in length. The physical structure and localization of the major genes of HBV (gene S encoding HBsAg, gene C encoding HBcAg/HBeAg, gene P encoding DNA polymerase, and gene X encoding HBxAg) have been identified and the complete nucleotide sequence of the HBV genome has been established. The viral genome replicates asymmetrically with separate pathways for the plus and minus strand synthesis, and involves the reverse transcription of an RNA intermediate as a central feature of the replication cycle similar to the RNA-containing retroviruses.

HBV infection in humans is associated with a wide spectrum of clinical presentations, ranging from the inapparent carrier state, acute, fulminant, and various forms of chronic hepatitis, and liver cirrhosis to hepatocellular carcinoma. Currently the specific laboratory diagnosis of HBV infection is based on the serological detection of HBsAg, HBeAg/anti-HBe, anti-HBc, and anti-HBs. Three newly developed molecular hybridization techniques have permitted (i) the direct identification of viral DNA in serum and liver by dot blot analysis, (ii) the characterization of viral nucleic acid sequences with respect to their interaction with the host cells (free, extrachromosomal vs integrated viral DNA) by Southern blots, and (iii) the localization and quantitation of viral nucleic acid sequences at the single cell level by *in situ* hybridization. In addition, immunohistochemical techniques allow the visualization of viral antigens at the tissue level complementing the *in situ* hybridization analyses, so that the biology of HBV can be comprehensively assessed at the genetic (DNA), transcription (RNA), and translation (viral antigens) levels.

With increasing knowledge of the structural and biological characteristics of HBV, we should gain more insight into the pathogenetic mechanisms leading to acute and fulminant liver cell injury, viral persistence, and chronic liver disease, including hepatocellular carcinoma.

The pathogenesis of HCC in man in most areas of the world is closely associated with HBV infection, which is recognized as the major risk factor for developing this malignancy. Viral DNA has been found integrated into the cellular genome of HCC tissues and cell lines derived from them. However, the molecular mechanisms by which HBV in humans and WHV in woodchucks induce the malignant transformation of hepatocytes are not defined as yet. It is even conceivable that the viruses have no direct transforming effect, but rather induce HCC formation indirectly, such as through chronic liver injury and regeneration, possibly in conjunction with other agents, e.g., aflatoxin B1, alcohol, cigaret smoking, and others. The covalent modification of guanine residues by activated form of aflatoxin B1 may permit more precise delineation of the mutagenic and oncogenic role of aflatoxin in HBV-infected individuals.

In view of the poor prognosis of HCC in humans, once clinically detectable, most efforts are directed toward the development of prophylactic measures and preventive strategies. Here, the HBV vaccines presently available and those being developed by recombinant DNA technologies and synthesis of peptide analogs of HBsAg offer a virological approach to the worldwide problem of HBV infection and hold the promise of being the first vaccine to prevent a human malignancy.

Acknowledgments

We would like to thank Dr. A. T. Haase for advice, support, and helpful discussions. The experimental work was supported in part by Liver Center grant AM 26743 and Alpha Therapeutics Corporation, Los Angeles, CA. HEB is a recipient of a Heisenberg Award from the Deutsche Forschungsgemeinschaft.

References

Albin, C. and W. S. Robinson (1980), Protein kinase activity in hepatitis B virus. *J. Virol.* **34**, 297–302.

Alexander, J., E. Beyu, E. W. Geddes, and G. Lecatsas (1976), Establishment of a continuously growing cell line from primary carcinoma of the liver. *S. Afr. Med. J.* **50**, 2124–2128.

Almeida, J. D., D. Rubenstein, and E. J. Stott (1971), New antigen antibody system in Australia antigen positive hepatitis. *Lancet* ii, 1225–1227.

Beasley, R. P. (1982), Hepatitis B virus as the etiologic agent in hepatocellular carcinoma—epidemiologic considerations. Hepatology **2**, 21S–26S.

Beasley, R. P. and L. -Y Hwang (1984), Epidemiology of Hepatocellular Carcinoma, in *Viral Hepatitis and Liver Disease* (Vyas, G. N., J. L. Dienstag, and J. H. Hoofnagle, eds.) Grune and Stratton, New York, pp. 209–224.

Beasley, R. P., L. Y. Hwang, C. C. Lin, and C. S. Chien (1981), Hepatocellular carcinoma and hepatitis B virus. A prospective study of 22,707 men in Taiwan. *Lancet* ii, 1129–1132.

Beasley, R. P., L. -Y. Hwang, C. C. Lin, M. -L. Len, C. E. Stevens, W. Szmuness, and K. -P. Chen (1982), Incidence of hepatitis B virus infection in preschool children in Taiwan. *J. Infect. Dis.* **146**, 198–204.

Berninger, M., M. Hammer, B. Hoyer, and J. L. Gerin (1982), An assay for the detection of the DNA genome of hepatitis B virus in serum. *J. Med. Virol.* **9**, 57–68.

Bishop, J. M. (1982), Oncogenes. *Sci. Am.* **236**, 80–92.

Bishop, J. M. (1983), Cellular oncogenes and retroviruses. *Ann. Rev. Biochem.* **52**, 301–354.

Blum, H. E. (1984), Viral Agents in Liver Disease, in *Viral Hepatitis and Liver Disease*. (Vyas, G. N., J. L. Dienstag, and J. H. Hoofnagle, eds.) Grune and Stratton, New York, pp. 385–394.

Blum, H. E., A. P. Geballe, L. Stowring, A. Figus, A. T. Haase, and G. N. Vyas (1984a), Hepatitis B Virus DNA in Nonhepatocytes: Demonstration of Viral DNA in Spleen, Bile Duct Epithelium, and Vascular Elements by *In Situ* Hybridization, in *Viral Hepatitis and Liver Disease*, (Vyas, G. N., J. L. Dienstag, and J. H. Hoofnagle, eds.) Grune and Stratton, New York, p. 634.

Blum, H. E., A. T. Haase, J. D. Harris, D. Walker, and G. N. Vyas (1983a), Asymmetric replication of hepatitis B virus DNA in human liver: Demonstration of cytoplasmic minus-strand DNA by Southern blot analyses and *in situ* hybridization. *Hepatology* 3, 840.

Blum, H. E., A. T. Haase, and G. N. Vyas (1984b), Molecular pathogenesis of hepatitis B virus infection: Simultaneous detection of viral DNA and antigens in paraffin embedded liver sections. *Lancet* ii, 771–775.

Blum, H. E., L. Stowring, A. Figus, C. K. Montgomery, A. T. Haase, and G. N. Vyas (1983b), Detection of hepatitis B virus DNA in hepatocytes, bile duct epithelium, and vascular elements by *in situ* hybridization. *Proc. Natl. Acad. Sci. USA* 80, 6685–6688.

Blumberg, B. S., B. Larouze, and W. T. London (1975), The relation of infection with the hepatitis B agent to primary hepatic carcinoma. *Am. J. Pathol.* 81, 669–682.

Bonino, F., B. Hoyer, J. Nelson, R. Engle, G. Verme, and J. L. Gerin (1981), Hepatitis B virus DNA in the sera of HBsAg carriers: A marker of active hepatitis B virus replication in the liver. *Hepatology* 1, 386–391.

Brechot, C., M. Hadchouel, J. Scotto, F. Degos, P. Charnay, C. Trepo, and P. Tiollais (1981a), Detection of hepatitis B virus DNA in liver and serum: A direct appraisal of the chronic carrier state. *Lancet* ii, 765–768.

Brechot, C., M. Hadchouel, J. Scotto, M. Fonck, F. Potet, G. N. Vyas, and P. Tiollais (1981b), State of hepatitis B virus DNA in hepatocytes of patients with hepatitis B surface antigen-positive and -negative liver diseases. *Proc. Natl. Acad. Sci. USA* 78, 3906–3910.

Brechot, C., C. Lugassy, A. Dejean, P. Pontisso, V. Thiers, P. Berthelot, and P. Tiollais (1984), Hepatitis B Virus DNA in Infected Human Tissues, in *Viral Hepatitis and Liver Disease*, (Vyas, G. N., J. L. Dienstag, and J. H. Hoofnagle, eds.) Grune and Stratton, New York, pp. 395–409.

Brechot, C., B. Nalpas, A. -M. Courouce, G. Duhamel, P. Callard, F. Carnot, P. Tiollais, and P. Berthelot (1982a), Evidence that hepatitis B virus has a role in liver-cell carcinoma in alcoholic liver disease. *N. Engl. J. Med.* 306, 1384–1387.

Brechot, C., C. Pourcel, M. Hadchouel, A. Dejean, A. Louise, J. Scotto, and P. Tiollais (1982b), State of hepatitis B virus DNA in liver diseases. *Hepatology* 2, 27S–34S.

Brechot, C., C. Pourcel, A. Louise, B. Rain, and P. Tiollais (1980), Presence of integrated hepatitis B virus DNA sequences in cellular DNA of human hepatocellular carcinoma. *Nature* 286, 533–535.

Chakraborty, P. R., N. Ruiz-Opazo, D. Shouval, and D. A. Shafritz (1980), Identification of integrated hepatitis B virus DNA and expression of viral RNA in an HBsAg-producing human hepatocellular carcinoma cell line. *Nature* 286, 531–533.

Charnay, P., E. Mandart, A. Hampe, F. Fitoussi, P. Tiollais, and F. Galibert (1979), Localization of the viral genome and nucleotide sequence of the gene coding for the major polypeptide of the hepatitis B surface antigen (HBsAg). *Nucl. Acids Res.* 7, 335–346.

Chen, D. -S., B. H. Hoyer, J. Nelson, R. H. Purcell, and J. L. Gerin (1982a), Detection and properties of hepatitis B viral DNA in liver tissues from patients with hepatocellular carcinoma. *Hepatology* **2**, 42S–46S.

Chen, D. S., J. C. Sheu, J. L. Sung, M. Y. Lai, C. S. Lee, C. T. Su, Y. M. Tsang, S. W. How, T. H. Wang, J. Y. Yu, T. H. Yang, C. Y. Wang, and C. Y. Hsu (1982b), Small hepatocellular carcinoma—A clinicopathological study in thirteen patients. *Gastroenterology* **83**, 1109–1119.

Chen, D. -S., J. -L. Sung, J. -C. Shen, M. -Y. Lai, S. -W. How, H. -C. Hsu, C. -S. Lee, and T. -C. Wei (1984), Serum alpha-fetoprotein in the early stage of human hepatocellular carcinoma. *Gastroenterology* **86**, 1404–1409.

Chien, M. -C., M. Y. Tong, J. -K. Lo, J. -K. Lee, D. R. Milich, G. N. Vyas, and B. L. Murphy (1981), Hepatitis B viral markers in patients with primary hepatocellular carcinoma in Taiwan. *J. Natl. Cancer Inst.* **66**, 475–479.

Chlebowski, R. T., M. J. Tong, J. Weissman, J. B. Block, K. P. Ramming, J. M. Weiner, J. R. Bateman, and J. S. Chlebowski (1984), Hepatocellular carcinoma: Diagnostic and prognostic features in North American patients. *Cancer* **53**, 2701–2706.

Cooper, G. M. (1982), Cellular transforming genes. *Science* **218**, 801–806.

Dane, D. S., C. H. Cameron, and M. Briggs (1970), Virus-like particles in serum of patients with Australia antigen associated hepatitis. *Lancet* **ii**, 695–698.

Dejean, A., C. Brechot, P. Tiollais, and S. Wain-Hobson (1983), Characterization of integrated hepatitis B viral DNA cloned from a human hepatoma and the hepatoma cell line PLC/PRF/5. *Proc. Natl. Acad. Sci. USA* **80**, 2505–2509.

Dejean, A., G. Carloni, C. Brechot, P. Tiollais, and S. Wain-Hobson (1982), Organization and expression of hepatitis B sequences cloned from hepatocellular carcinoma tissue DNA. *J. Cell. Biochem.* **20**, 293–301.

Dejean, A., C. Lugassy, S. Zafrani, P. Tiollais, and C. Brechot (1984), Detection of hepatitis B virus DNA in pancreas, kidney, and skin of two human carriers of the virus. *J. Gen. Virol.* **65**, 651–655.

Delius, H., N. M. Gough, C. H. Cameron, and K. Murray (1983), Structure of the hepatitis B virus genome. *J. Virol.* **47**, 337–343.

Denison, E. K., R. L. Peters, and T. B. Reynolds (1971), Familial hepatoma with hepatitis-associated antigen. *Ann. Intern. Med.* **74**, 391–394.

Edman, J. C., P. Gray, P. Valenzuela, L. B. Rall, and W. J. Rutter (1980), Integration of hepatitis B virus sequences and their expression in a human hepatoma cell. *Nature* **286**, 535–538.

Elfassi, E., J. -L. Romet-Lemonne, M. Essex, M. Frances-McLane, and W. A. Haseltine (1984), Evidence of extrachromosomal forms of hepatitis B viral DNA in a bone marrow culture obtained from a patient recently infected with hepatitis B virus. *Proc. Natl. Acad. Sci. USA* **81**, 3526–3528.

Figus, A., H. E. Blum, G. N. Vyas, S. De Vergilis, A. Cao, M. Lippi, E. Lai, and A. Balestrieri (1984), Hepatitis B viral nucleotide sequences in non-A, non-B or hepatitis B virus-related chronic liver disease. *Hepatology*, pp. 364–368.

Fowler, M. J. F., J. Monjardino, K. N. Tsiquaye, A. J. Zuckerman, and H. C. Thomas (1984), The mechanism of replication of hepatitis B virus: Evidence of asymmetric replication of the two DNA strands. *J. Med. Virol.* **13**, 83–91.

Fung, Y. -KT. C. C. Lai, S. Todd, D. Ganem, and H. E. Varmus (1984), An Amplified Domain of Cellular DNA Containing a Subgenomic Insert of Hepatitis B Virus DNA in a Human Hepatoma, in *Viral Hepatitis and Liver Disease* (Vyas, G. N., J. L. Dienstag, and J. H. Hoofnagle, eds.) Grune and Stratton, New York, pp. 633.

Galibert, F., T. N. Chen, and E. Mandart (1982), Nucleotide sequence of a cloned woodchuck hepatitis virus genome: Comparison with the hepatitis B virus sequence. *J. Virol.* **41,** 51–65.

Galibert, F., E. Mandart, F. Fitoussi, P. Tiollais, and P. Charnay (1979), Nucleotide sequence of the hepatitis B virus genome (subtype ayw) cloned in E. coli. *Nature* **281,** 646–650.

Galloway, D. A. and J. K. McDougall (1983), The oncogenic potential of herpes simplex viruses: Evidence for a "hit-and-run" mechanism. *Nature* **302,** 21–24.

Gerin, J. L. (1984), The Woodchuck (Marmota Monax): An Animal Model of Hepatitis B-Like Infection and Disease, in *Advances in Hepatitis Research* (Chisari, F. V., ed.) Masson Publishing USA, New York.

Gerlich, W. and W. S. Robinson (1980), Hepatitis B virus contains protein attached to the 5' terminus of its complete strand. *Cell* **21,** 801–809.

Goudeau, A., P. Maupas, P. Coursaget, J. Crucker, J. -P. Chiron, F. Denis, and I. Diop Mar (1979) Hepatitis B virus antigens in human primary hepatocellular carcinoma tissues. *Int. J. Cancer* **24,** 421–429.

Goudeau, A., P. Maupas, P. Coursaget, J. Crucker, J. -P. Chiron, F. Denis, I. Diop Mar, and P. Demba N'Diaye (1981), Detection of hepatitis B virus antigens in hepatocellular carcinoma tissues. *Prog. Med. Virol.* **27,** 77–87.

Goyette, M., C. J. Petropoulos, P. R. Shank, and N. Fausto (1983), Expression of a cellular oncogene during liver regeneration. *Science* **219,** 510House of Equations12.

Heyward, W. L., T. R. Bender, A. P. Lanier, D. P. Francis, B. J. McMahon, and J. E. Maynard (1982), Serological markers of hepatitis B virus and alpha-fetoprotein levels proceding primary hepatocellular carcinoma in Alaskan Eskimos. *Lancet* ii, 889–891.

Hruska, J. F., D. A. Clayton, J. L. R. Rubenstein, and W. S. Robinson (1977), Structure of hepatitis B Dane particle DNA before and after the Dane particle polymerase reaction. *J. Virol.* **21,** 666–672.

Irvin, T. R. and G. N. Wogan (1984), Quantitation of aflatoxin B 1 adduction within the ribosomal RNA gene sequences of rat liver DNA. *Proc. Natl. Acad. Sci. USA* **81,** 664–668.

Kaplan, P. M., R. L. Greenman, J. L. Gerin, R. H. Purcell, and W. S. Robinson (1973), DNA polymerase associated with human hepatitis B antigen. *J. Virol.* B12, 995–1005.

Kew, M. C. (1982), Tumors of the Liver, in *Hepatology* (Zakim, D. and T. D. Boyer, eds.) Saunders, Philadelphia.

Kew, M. C. (1984), The Possible Etiologic Role of Hepatitis B Virus in Hepatocellular Carcinoma: Evidence from Southern Africa, in *Advances in Hepatitis Research* (Chisari, F. V., ed.) Masson Publishing USA, New York.

Koike, K., M. Kobayashi, H. Mizusawa, E. Yoshida, K. Yaginuma, and M. Taira (1983), Rearrangement of the surface antigen gene of hepatitis B virus integrated in the human hepatoma cell lines. *Nucleic Acids Res.* **11,** 5391–5402.

Koshy, R., A. B. L. Freytag von Loringhoven, S. Koch, O. Marquardt, and P. H. Hofschneider (1984), Structure and Function of Integrated HBV Genes in the Human Hepatoma Cell Line PLC/PRF/5, in *Viral Hepatitis and Liver Disease* (Vys, G. N., J. L. Dienstag, and J. H. Hoofnagle, eds.) Grune and Stratton, New York, pp. 265–273.

Koshy, R., S. Koch, A. B. L. Freytag von Loringhoven, R. Kahmann, K. Murray, and P. H. Hofschneider (1983), Integration of hepatitis B virus DNA: Evidence for integration in the single-stranded gap. *Cell* **34,** 215–223.

Koshy, R., P. Maupas, R. Mueller, and P. H. Hofschneider (1981), Detection of hepatitis B virus-specific DNA in the genomes of human hepatocellular carcinoma and liver cirrhosis tissues. *J. Gen. Virol.* **57**, 95–109.

Lai, C. L., K. C. Lam, K. P. Wong, P. C. Wu, and D. Todd (1981), Clinical features of hepatocellular carcinoma: Review of 211 patients in Hong Kong. *Cancer* **47**, 2746–2755.

Landers, T. A., H. B. Greenberg, and W. S. Robinson (1977), Structure of hepatitis B Dane particle DNA and nature of the endogenous DNA polymerase reaction. *J. Virol.* **23**, 368–376.

Larouze, B., W. T. London, G. Saimot, B. G. Werner, E. D. Lustbader, M. Payet, and B. S. Blumberg (1976), Host response to hepatitis B infection in patients with primary hepatic carcinoma and their families. A case/control study in Senegal, West Africa. *Lancet* ii, 534–538.

Lieberman, H. M., D. R. LaBreque, M. C. Kew, S. J. Hadziyannis, and D. A. Shafritz (1983), Detection of hepatitis B virus DNA directly in human serum by a simplified molecular hybridization test; comparison to HBeAg/anti-HBe status in HBsAg carriers. *Hepatology* **3**, 285–291.

Liebman, H. A., B. C. Furie, M. J. Tong, R. A. Blanchard, K. -J. Ko, S. -D. Lee, M. S. Coleman, and B. Furie (1984), Des-y-Carboxy (abnormal) prothrombin as a serum marker of primary hepatocellular carcinoma. *New Engl. J. Med.* **310**, 1427–1431.

Lie-Injo, L. E., M. Balasegaram, C. G. Lopez, and A. R. Herrera (1983), Hepatitis B virus DNA in liver and white blood cells of patients with hepatoma. *DNA* **2**, 299–301.

Lutwick, L. I. and W. S. Robinson (1977), DNA synthesis in the hepatitis B Dane particle DNA polymerase reaction. *J. Virol.* **21**, 96–104.

MacKay, P., J. Lees, and K. Murray (1981), The conversion of hepatitis B core antigen synthesized in E. coli into e antigen. *J. Med. Virol.* **8**, 237–243.

Mandart, E., A. Kay, and E. Galibert (1984), Nucleotide sequence of a cloned duck hepatitis B virus genome: Comparison with woodchuck and human hepatitis B virus sequences. *J. Virol.* **49**, 782–792.

Marion, P. L., L. S. Oshiro, D. C. Regnery, G. A. Scullard, and W. S. Robinson (1980a), A virus in Beechey ground squirrel that is related to hepatitis B virus of humans. *Proc. Natl. Acad. Sci. USA* **77**, 2941–2945.

Marion, P. L., F. H. Salazar, J. J. Alexander, and W. S. Robinson (1980b), State of hepatitis B viral DNA in a human hepatoma cell line. *J. Virol.* **33**, 795–806.

Marquardt, O., A. B. L. Freytag von Loringhoven, and G. Froesner (1984), Expression of hepatitis B virus core antigen gene is induced in human hepatoma cells by their growth in nude mice. *J. Gen. Virol.* **65**, 1443–1448.

Marquardt, O., V. Zaslavsky, and P. H. Hofschneider (1982), Evidence for non-chromosomal hepatitis B virus surface (HBsAg)- and core antigen (HBcAg)-specific DNA sequences in a hepatoma cell line. *J. Gen. Virol.* **61**, 105–109.

Mason, W. S., C. Aldrich, J. Summers, and J. M. Taylor (1982), Asymmetric replication of duck hepatitis B virus DNA; Free minus-strand DNA. *Proc. Natl. Acad. Sci. USA* **79**, 3997–4001.

Mason, W. S., G. Seal, and J. Summers (1980), Virus of Pekin ducks with structural and biological relatedness to human hepatitis B virus. *J. Virol.* **36**, 829–836.

McCollum, R. W. and A. J. Zuckerman (1981), Viral hepatitis: Report on a WHO informal consultation. *J. Med. Virol.* **8**, 1–29.

Miller, R. H. and W. S. Robinson (1983), Integrated hepatitis B virus DNA sequences specifying the major viral core polypeptide are methylated in

PLC/PRF/5 cells. *Proc. Natl. Acad. Sci. USA* **80**, 2534–2538.

Mitamura, K., B. H. Hoyer, A. Ponzetto, J. Nelson, R. H. Purcell, and J. L. Gerin (1982), Woodchuck hepatitis virus DNA in woodchuck liver tissues. *Hepatology* **2**, 47S–50S.

Monjardino, J., M. J. F. Fowler, L. Montano, I. Weller, K. N. Tsiquaye, A. J. Zuckerman, D. M. Jones, and H. C. Thomas (1982), Analysis of hepatitis virus DNA in the liver and serum of HBe antigen positive chimpanzee carriers. *J. Med. Virol.* **9**, 189–199.

Monjardino, P. J., M. J. F. Fowler, and H. C. Thomas (1983), Defective hepatitis B virus DNA molecules detected in a stable integration pattern in a hepatoma cell line, and in induced tumours and derived cell lines. *J. Gen. Virol.* **64**, 2299–2303.

Muench, K. F., R. P. Misra, and M. Z. Humayun (1983), Sequence specificity in aflatoxin B1–DNA interactions. *Proc. Natl. Acad. Sci. USA* **80**, 6–10.

Nayak, N. C., A. Dhar, R. Sachdeva, A. Mittal, H. N. Beth, D. Sudarsanam, B. Reddy, U. L. Wagholikar, and C. R. R. M. Reddy (1977), Association of human hepatocellular carcinoma and cirrhosis with hepatitis B surface and core antigen in the liver. *Int. J. Cancer* **20**, 643–654.

Novi, A. M. (1981), Regression of aflatoxin B1 induced hepatocellular carcinomas by reduced glutathione. *Science* **212**, 541–542.

Ogston, C. W., G. J. Jonak, C. E. Rogler, S. M. Astrin, and J. Summers (1982), Cloning and structural analysis of integrated woodchuck hepatitis virus sequences from hepatocellular carcinomas of woodchucks. *Cell* **29**, 385–394.

Ohbayashi, A., M. Okochi, and M. Mayumi (1972), Familial clustering of asymptomatic carriers of Australia antigen and patients with chronic liver disease or primary liver cancer. *Gastroenterology* **62**, 618–625.

Okuda, K. and I. Mackay, eds. (1982), *Hepatocellular Carcinoma.* International Union against Cancer, Technical Report Series, Volume 74, Geneva.

Ono, Y., H. Onda, R. Sasada, K. Igarashi, Y. Sugino, and K. Nishioka (1983), The complete nucleotide sequence of the cloned hepatitis B virus DNA; subtypes adr and adw. *Nucleic Acids Res.* **11**, 1747–1757.

Pasek, M., T. Goto, W. Gilbert, B. Zink, H. Schaller, P. MacKay, G. Leadbetter, and K. Murray (1979), Hepatitis B virus genes and their expression in E coli. *Nature* (Lond.) **282**, 575–579.

Payet, M., R. Camain, and P. Pene (1956), Le cancer primitif du foie; etude critique a propos de 240 cas. *Rev. Intern. d'Hepatol.* **6**, 1–86.

Peters, R. L., A. P. Afroudakis, and D. Tatter (1977), The changing incidence of association of hepatitis B with hepatocellular carcinoma in California. *Amer. J. Clin. Pathol.* **68**, 1–7.

Pontisso, P., M. C. Poon, P. Tiollais, and C. Brechot (1984), Detection of hepatitis B virus DNA in human blood mononuclear cells. *Brit. Med. J.* **288**, 1563–1566.

Popper, H., M. A. Gerger, and S. N. Thung (1982), The relation of hepatocellular carcinoma to infection with hepatitis B and related viruses in man and animals. *Hepatology* **2**, 1S–9S.

Prince, A. M. (1975), The Hepatitis B Antigen, in *The Liver: Normal and Abnormal Functions* (Becker, F. F., ed.) Marcel Dekker, New York.

Prince, A. M., W. Szmuness, J. Michon, J. Demaille, G. Diebolt, J. Linhard, C. Quenum, and M. Sankale (1975), A case control study of the association between primary liver cancer and hepatitis B infection in Senegal. *Int. J. Cancer* **16**, 376–383.

Reddy, P. J., R. D. Reynolds, E. Santos, and M. Barbacid (1982), A point mutation is responsible for the acquisition of transforming properties by the T 24 human bladder carcinoma oncogene. *Nature* (Lond.) **300**, 149–152.

Robinson, W. S. (1977), The genome of hepatitis B virus. *Ann. Rev. Microbiol.* **31**, 357–377.

Robinson, W. S., D. A. Clayton, and R. I. Greenman (1974), DNA of a human hepatitis B virus candidate. *J. Virol.* **14**, 384–391.

Robinson, W. S. and R. L. Greenman (1974), DNA polymerase in the core of the human hepatitis B virus candidate. *J. Virol.* **13**, 1231–1236.

Robinson, W. S., R. H. Miller, L. Klote, P. L. Marion, and S. -C. Lee (1984), Hepatitis B Virus and Hepatocellular Carcinoma, in *Viral Hepatitis and Liver Disease* (Vyas, G. N., J. L. Dienstag, and J. H. Hoofnagle, eds.) Grune and Stratton, New York, pp. 245–263.

Rogler, C. E. and J. Summers (1984), Cloning and structural analysis of integrated woodchuck hepatitis virus sequences from a chronically infected liver. *J. Virol.* **50**, 832–837.

Romet-Lemonne, J. -L., M. F. McLane, E. Elfassi, W. A. Haseltine, J. Azocar, and M. Essex (1983), Hepatitis B virus infection incultured human lymphoblastoid cells. *Science* **221**, 667–669.

Rowley, J. D. (1983), Human oncogene locations and chromosome aberrations. *Nature* **301**, 290–291.

Sattler, F. and W. S. Robinson (1979), Hepatitis B viral DNA molecules have cohesive ends. *J. Virol.* **32**, 226–233.

Scotto, J., M. Hadchouel, C. Hery, J. Yvart, P. Tiollais, and C. Brechot (1983), Detection of hepatitis B virus DNA in serum by a simple spot hybridization technique: Comparison with results for other viral markers. *Hepatology* **3**, 279–294.

Shafritz, D. A. (1982), Hepatitis B virus DNA molecules in the liver of HBsAg carriers: Mechanistic considerations in the pathogenesis of hepatocellular carcinoma. *Hepatology* **2**, 35S–41S.

Shafritz, D. A. and M. C. Kew (1981), Identification of integrated hepatitis B virus DNA in human hepatocellular carcinomas. *Hepatology* **1**, 1–8.

Shafritz, D. A. and H. M. Lieberman (1984), The molecular biology of hepatitis B virus. *Ann. Rev. Med.* **35**, 219–232.

Shafritz, D. A., H. M. Lieberman, K. J. Isselbacher, and J. R. Wands (1982), Monoclonal radioimmunoassays for hepatitis B surface antigen: Demonstration of hepatitis B virus DNA or related sequences in serum and viral epitopes in immune complexes. *Proc. Natl. Acad. Sci. USA* **79**, 675–5679.

Shafritz, D. A. and C. E. Rogler (1984), Molecular Characterization of Viral Forms Observed in Persistent Hepatitis Infections, Chronic Liver Disease and Hepatocellular Carcinoma in Woodchucks and Humans, in *Viral Hepatitis and Liver Disease*. (Vyas, G. N., J. L. Dienstag, and J. H. Hoofnagle, eds.) Grune and Stratton, New York, pp. 225–243.

Shafritz, D. A., D. Shouval, H. I. Sherman, S. I. Hadzyannis, and M. C. Kew (1981), Integration of hepatitis B virus DNA into the genome of liver cells in chronic liver disease and hepatocellular carcinoma. *N. Engl. J. Med.* **306**, 1067–1073.

Siddiqui, A. (1983), Hepatitis B virus DNA in Kaposi sarcoma. *Proc. Natl. Acad. Sci. USA* **80**, 4861–4864.

Siddiqui, A., F. Sattler, and W. S. Robinson (1979), Restriction endonuclease cleavage map and location of unique features of the DNA of hepatitis B virus, subtype adw2. *Proc. Natl. Acad. Sci. USA* **76**, 4664–4668.

Slamon, D. J., J. B. Kernion, I. D. Verma, and M. J. Cline (1984), Expression of cellular oncogenes in human malignancies. *Science* **224**, 256–262.

Southern, E. M. (1975), Detection of specific sequences among DNA fragments separated by gel electrophoresis. *J. Mol. Biol.* **98**, 503–517.

Steiner, P. E., and J. N. P. Davis (1957), Cirrhosis and primary liver cancer in Uganda, Africa. *Brit. J. Cancer* **11**, 523–534.

Stevens, C. E., P. E. Taylor, M. J. Tong, P. T. Toy, and G. N. Vyas (1984), Hepatitis B Vaccine: An Overview, in*Viral Hepatitis and Liver Disease* (Vyas, G. N., J. L. Dienstag, and J. H. Hoofnagle, eds.) Grune and Stratton, New York, pp. 275–291.

Summers, J., A. O'Connell, P. Maupas, A. Goudeau, P. Coursaget, and J. Drucker (1978), Hepatitis B virus DNA in primary hepatocellular carcinoma tissue. *J. Med. Virol.* **2**, 207–214.

Summers, J., A. O'Connell, and I. Millman (1975), Genome of hepatitis B virus: Restriction enzyme cleavage and structure of DNA extracted from Dane particles. *Proc. Natl. Acad. Sci. USA* **72**, 4597–4601.

Summers, J. and W. S. Mason (1982), Replication of the genome of a hepatitis B-like virus by reverse transcription of an RNA intermediate. *Cell* **29**, 403–415.

Summers, J., J. Smolec, and R. Snyder (1978), A virus similar to human hepatitis B virus associated with hepatitis and hepatoma in woodchucks. *Proc. Natl. Acad. Sci. USA* **75**, 4533–4537.

Szmuness, W. (1978), Hepatocellular carcinoma and hepatitis B virus: Evidence for a causal relationship. *Prog. Med. Virol.* **24**, 40–69.

Szmuness, W., H. J. Alter, and H. E. Maynard (1982), Viral Hepatitis. Franklin Institute Press, Philadelphia.

Szmuness, W., C. E. Stevens, E. J. Harley, E. A. Zang, W. R. Oleszko, D. C. William, R. Sadovsky, J. M. Morrison, and A. Kellner (1980), Hepatitis B vaccine: Demonstration of efficacy in a controlled clinical trial in a high-risk population in the United States. *N. Engl. J. Med.* **303**, 833–841.

Szmuness, W., C. E. Stevens, H. Ikram, M. I. Much, E. J. Harley, and B. Hollinger (1978), Prevalence of Hepatitis B virus infection and hepatocellular carcinoma in Chinese-Americans. *J. Infec. Dis.* **137**, 822–829.

Tabor, E., R. J. Gerety, C. L. Vogel, A. C. Bayley, P. P. Anthony, C. H. Chan, and L. J. Barker (1977), Hepatitis B virus infection and primary hepatocellular carcinoma. *J. Natl. Cancer Inst.* **58**, 1197–1200.

Takahashi, K., Y. Akahana, T. Gotanda, T. Mishiro, M. Imai, Y. Miyakawa, and M. Mayumi (1979), Demonstration of hepatitis B e antigenin the core of Dane particles. *J. Immunol.* **122**, 275–279.

Tang, Z. -Y. Y. -Y. Ying, and T. -J. Gu (1982), Hepatocellular carcinoma: Changing concepts in recent years. *Prog. Liver Dis.* **VII**, 637–647.

Tepfer, B. D. C. (1972), Hepatoma and HAA. *Ann. Intern. Med.* **76**, 145–146.

Thung, S. N., M. A. Gerber, E. Sarno, and H. Popper (1979), Distribution of five antigens in hepatocellular carcinoma. *Lab. Invest.* **41**, 101–105.

Tiollais, P., P. Charnay, and G. N. Vyas (1981), Biology of hepatitis B virus. *Science* **213**, 406–411.

Tiollais, P., A. Dejean, C. Brechot, M. -L. Michel, P. Sonigo, and S. Wain-Hobson (1984), Structure of Hepatitis B Virus DNA, in*Viral Hepatitis and Liver Disease* (Vyas, G. N., J. L. Dienstag, and J. H. Hoofnagle, eds.) Grune and Stratton, New York, pp. 49–65.

Tiollais, P. and S. Wain-Hobson (1984), Molecular Genetics of the Hepatitis B Virus, in *Advances in Hepatitis Research* (Chisari, F. V., ed.) Masson Publishing USA, New York.

Tong, M. J., R. T. Chlebowski, J. Y. Weissman, and J. R. Bateman (1981), Frequency and treatment of primary hepatocellular carcinoma in Los Angeles. *Prog. Med. Virol.* **27**, 6–13.

Tong, M. J., J. M. Weiner, M. W. Ashcavai, and G. N. Vyas (1979), Evidence for clustering of hepatitis B virus infection in families of patients with primary hepatocellular carcinoma. *Cancer* **44**, 2338–2342.

Twist, M. E., H. F. Clark, D. P. Aden, B. B. Knowles, and S. A. Plotkin (1981), Integration pattern of hepatitis B virus DNA squences in human hepatoma cell lines. *J. Virol.* **37**, 239–243.

Valenzuela, P., M. Quiroga, J. Zaldivar, P. Gray, and W. J. Rutter (1980), The Nucleotide Sequence of the Hepatitis B Viral Genome and the Identification of the Major Polypeptides, in *Animal Virus Genetics* (Fields, B., R. Jaenisch, C. F. Fox, eds.) Academic Press, New York.

Varmus, H. E. (1982), Form and function of retriviral proviruses. *Science* **216**, 812–820.

Varmus, H. E. (1984), Do hepatitis B viruses make a genetic contribution to primary hepatocellular carcinoma? in *Viral Hepatitis and Liver Disease* (Vyas, G. N., J. L. Dienstag, and J. H. Hoofnagle, eds.) Grune and Stratton, New York, pp. 411–414.

Velasco, M., R. Sorenson, A. Daiber, A. Carmona, and R. Katz (1971), Primary carcinoma of the liver associated with Australia antigen. *Lancet* i, 1183–1184.

Vyas, G. N. (1974), Evidence against recessive inheritance of susceptibility to the chronic carrier state for hepatitis B antigen. *Nature* **248**, 159–160.

Vyas, G. N. and H. E. Blum (1984), Hepatitis B virus infection: Current concepts of chronicity and immunity. *Western J. Med.* **140**, 754–762.

Vyas, G. N., J. L. Dienstag, and J. H. Hoofnagle, eds. (1984), *Viral Hepatitis and Liver Diseases*, Grune and Stratton, New York, pp. 1–728.

Wain-Hobson, S. (1984), Molecular Biology of the Hepadna Viruses, in *Advances in Hepatitis Research* (Chisari, F. V., ed.) Masson Publishing USA, New York.

Wands, J. R., H. M. Lieberman, E. Muchmore, K. J. Isselbacher, and D. A. Shafritz (1982), Detection and transmission in chimpanzees of hepatitis B virus-related agents formerly designated "non-A, non-B" hepatitis. *Proc. Natl. Acad. Sci. USA* **79**, 7552–7556.

Weiser, B., D. Ganem, C. Seeger, and H. E. Varmus (1983), Closed circular viral DNA and asymmetrical heterogeneous forms in liver from animals infected with ground squirrel hepatitis virus. *J. Virol.* **48**, 1–9.

Yoakum, G. H. (1984), Protoplast-fusion: A method to transfect human cells for gene isolation, oncogene testing and construction of specialized cell lines. *BioTechniques* **2**, 24–30.

Yoakum, G. H., B. E. Korba, J. F. Lechner, T. Tokiwa, A. F. Gazdar, T. Seeley, M. Siegel, L. Leeman, H. Autrup, and C. C. Harris (1983), High-frequency transfection and cytopathology of the hepatitis B virus core antigen gene in human cells. *Science* **222**, 385–389.

Yu, M. C., T. Mack, R. Hanisch, R. L. Peters, B. E. Henderson, and M. C. Pike (1983), Hepatitis, cigarette smoking, alcohol consumption and hepatocellular carcinoma in Los Angeles. *Cancer Res.* **43**, 6077–6078.

Zaslavsky, V., O. Marquardt, T. -K. Wong, and P. H. Hofschneider (1980), Hepatitis B virus (HBV)-specific structures found in cytoplasmic extracts of cells producing HBV surface antigen (HBsAg) in vitro. *J. Gen. Virol.* **51**, 341–349.

Zuckerman, A. J. (1982), Virological approach to the prevention of primary liver cancer. *Hepatology* **2**, 67S–71S.

Kaposi's Sarcoma

Acquired Immunodeficiency Syndrome (AIDS) and Associated Viruses

Thomas J. Spira

1. Introduction

Since the initial description of the "multiple idiopathic pigmented hemangiosarcoma" by Moricz Kaposi in 1872 (Kaposi, 1872), this tumor now known as Kaposi's sarcoma (KS) has been relatively uncommon in Europe and North America, and relatively common in parts of central Africa. In recent years, however, there has been a resurgence of interest in KS in North America and Europe since its epidemic occurrence associated with the acquired immunodeficiency syndrome (AIDS) (CDC, 1981a,b). In this chapter we will attempt to review the association of viruses with both "classical" or preepidemic KS, and "epidemic" or AIDS-associated KS.

2. Kaposi's Sarcoma

2.1. Description

Classical KS usually presents as reddish-purple to brown macules, plaques, or nodules, most commonly on the lower or upper extremities. These lesions often become symmetric in distribution and can be accompanied by edema. They are usually painless and may often go unnoticed by the individual. The disease rarely has systemic symptoms and usually progresses slowly with coalescence of lesions that may ulcerate. Visceral involvement is uncommon.

2.2. Epidemiology

2.2.1. Europe and North America

In Europe and North America, the incidence of KS gradually increases from childhood with a majority of cases occurring in the fifth through the seventh decades of life. With increasing age there is also a striking increase in the proportion of males to females, with approximately a 10:1 ratio in the peak ages. The majority of cases are in those with an Eastern or Southern European background, most commonly Italians and Eastern European or Ashkenazic Jews. This is true both in Europe and North America.

2.2.2. Africa

African KS differs from that seen in Europe and North America in a number of ways. The incidence curve in Africa is bimodal, with an initial peak in the first decade of life followed by a drop in incidence during the second decade, then with a gradual increase in incidence in the following decades (Davies and Lothe, 1962). In Africa there is a geographic area centering in the black populations of Uganda and surrounding areas—western Kenya and Tanzania and eastern Zaire and Rwanda-Burundi, where KS constitutes up to 10% of all tumors diagnosed. It also differs in its clinical course, with an increased frequency of lymphadenopathic involvement in childhood, and an aggressive, more rapidly progressive disease in adults with fungating, ulcerating lesions and deep tissue invasion.

2.3. Relation to Immunosuppression

Kaposi's sarcoma also occurs with an increased frequency in situations of primary or secondary immunosuppression (Penn, 1983). This is seen most commonly in the period following renal transplantation, in which it comprises over 3% of all *de novo* neoplasms. In addition, it has been found to develop secondary to other malignancies—especially lymphoproliferative disease. Iatrogenic immunosuppression using such agents as corticosteroids and/or azathioprine has also been associated with an increased incidence of KS. Because of the association of KS with immunosuppression, it has been called by some an opportunistic neoplasm analogous to the opportunistic infections associated with immunosuppression. In addition, there have been instances of regression of KS following cessation of immunosuppressive therapy. This has raised the speculation that KS is not a true malignancy.

3.   Kaposi's Sarcoma and AIDS

3.1.   Introduction

In the summer of 1981, a recent upsurge in the numbers of individuals diagnosed with KS was first appreciated in New York City (CDC, 1981b). These individuals did not fall into the usual age group for KS in the US, nor did they have any obvious cause of immunosuppression to account for the development of KS. Upon further investigation it was found that almost all of these cases of KS were occurring in homosexual or bisexual males between the ages of 20 and 50. Almost simultaneously, in both Los Angeles and New York City additional individuals were being diagnosed with a variety of opportunistic infections, most commonly *Pneumocystis carinii* pneumonia, again without any obvious cause of immunosuppression to account for these infections. These individuals, like those developing KS, were also found to be homosexual or bisexual males or intravenous drug users. As this epidemic was investigated, it was found that these individuals were all profoundly immunodeficient, and that those with the opportunistic infections presented more severely than those presenting initially with only KS.

This disease is now known as the acquired immunodeficiency syndrome (AIDS). Over the following 4 yr of investigations, it was determined that this epidemic began in 1978 or 1979 in the US, and currently, in addition to the homosexual or bisexual males and intravenous drug abusers, involves recent Haitian immigrants to the US, hemophiliacs, recipients of blood transfusions, and sexual partners and infants of the above. AIDS in these risk groups has also been identified in other parts of the world. Of special interest has been the relatively high incidence of this disease in Haiti and more recently the reports of AIDS occurring in Central Africa, especially in Zaire and surrounding areas.

3.2.   Epidemiology

Although KS appears to be an opportunistic neoplasm associated with the immunodeficiency of AIDS, there are striking differences in incidence among the groups at high risk for AIDS. The majority of AIDS-associated KS is seen among homosexual or bisexual males (74%) and is seen more so in those without, rather than with, a history of IV drug use (46% vs 28%), whereas only 16% occurs in heterosexuals with IV drug use—more frequently in females (13%) than males (4%). The higher proportion of female IV drug users compared to heterosexual male IV drug users is in contrast to the overall male preponderance in both classical and AIDS-related KS. These differences are currently unexplained (Des Jarlais et al., 1984).

4. KS and HLA

4.1. DR5 Associations

The presence of a genetic susceptibility to the development of both classical and AIDS-associated KS has been suggested by studies of their association with certain histocompatibility locus antigens (HLA) phenotypes. Initially AIDS-associated KS in New York City was found to have a strong association with HLA-DR5 and HLA-Bw35 (Friedman-Kien et al., 1982; Pollack et al., 1983b). Further study of the association with DR5 found that this also occurred in classical KS. Since most classical KS and many of the AIDS-associated KS occurred in individuals of Italian or Ashkenazic Jewish background, the DR5 association with AIDS-associated and classical KS was found to be most significant in these ethnic subpopulations. In those of British or Northern European background, DR2 was associated with AIDS-associated KS (Pollack et al., 1983a). The relative significance of the DR5 association has dropped in New York City as additional cohorts of AIDS-associated KS patients have been studied (Rubinstein et al., 1984). This has been a result of the heterogeneity in the ethnic composition of these cohorts, with more individuals of Italian and Ashkenazic Jewish background being in the earliest cohort. Studies in Los Angeles have confirmed the DR5 association of AIDS-associated KS, which was also present after the exclusion of patients of Black, Ashkenazic Jewish, or Hispanic background, although at a lower level of significance ($0.05 < p < 0.10$) (Prince et al., 1984). In contrast, HLA-DR3 has been found to be decreased in frequency in several studies, but did not always reach statistical significance (Pollack et al., 1983b; Prince et al., 1984).

The HLA-DR5 association with classical KS has recently been confirmed in a more homogeneous population in Sardinia (Contu et al., 1984). Although the population has a high frequency of DR5, 66.6% of the classical KS patients had DR5 compared to 23.1% of controls ($p < 0.001$). An association with DR1 was also found, although this was not as significant as that for DR5 ($p < 0.05$), and a negative association with DR3 was also found ($p = 0.0055$).

4.2. Other Associations

Other HLA associations with KS have been described. The original association found with Bw35 has lost its significance after correction for the number of antigens tested (Rubinstein et al., 1984). Aw23 and Bw49 have been found to be significantly increased in KS patients in one study. A29 and Bw44, which are in linkage disequilibrium, have also been found to be increased (Prince et al., 1984). A trend toward decreased frequency of B8 has also been noted (Pollack et al., 1983b; Prince et al., 1984).

4.3. HLA-DR Associated Diseases

The association of KS with HLA-DR5 in some populations and possibly DR2 in others suggests that genetic susceptibility to the disease-causing agent is carried by a HLA gene in linkage disequilibrium with these loci. DR5 and DR2 have already been associated with resistance to insulin-dependent diabetes in similar populations (Bach et al., 1982). A protective effect of B8 and DR3, if confirmed, may be similar to that postulated for testicular carcinoma (Pollack et al., 1982). It is of interest that a DR5 association has also been reported in individuals with the lymphadenopathy stage of AIDS (Enlow et al., 1983). Further studies are necessary to determine whether these or other HLA associations are also found in other populations developing KS, such as in Africa, where both endemic and AIDS-associated KS is now occurring.

5. KS and CMV

5.1. Viral Particles and Antigen

Human cytomegalovirus (CMV) has been associated with KS on serologic grounds and by the detection of CMV-like particles, CMV antigen, and the CMV genome in tumor material. In 1972, Giraldo et al. (1972b) reported on a detailed study of eight of 51 cell lines derived from KS tumor, lymph node, or skin biopsies. five of the eight lines were found to contain herpes-type viral particles detected by electron microscopy. A common antigen precipitated by sera with high anti-CMV activity but low Epstein-Barr virus (EBV) activity was found in these lines. In four lines, an antigen precipitated by sera from Burkitt's lymphoma patients with high anti-EBV activity but low anti-CMV activity was also found (Giraldo et al., 1972a).

5.2. Seroepidemiology

Seroepidemiologic studies of European, American, and African KS have shown that all patients studied had CMV-neutralizing antibody present (Giraldo et al., 1975, 1978). Seventy-five percent of European KS patients (mainly with regressive disease) had higher titers of anti-CMV antibody by indirect hemagglutination (IHA) than melanoma patients or matched controls. This relationship was also found, although it was less marked, when antibody was measured by complement fixation. There was no similar finding for EBV or Herpes simplex virus (HSV) type 1 or 2. Among African KS patients (mainly with progressive disease), no such association was found with either CMV, EBV, or HSV 1 or 2. This lack of association in African patients may be a result of the high prevalence of seropositivity to these agents in these populations, such as that found in the African controls studied. African KS patients did have significantly lower geometric mean titers of anti-CMV antibody when compared to European KS patients. American KS patients were similar to the European patients in having significantly higher geometric mean titers of anti-CMV antibody by IHA compared to melanoma patients and normal controls. This therefore confirms the specific serologic association of CMV with at least nonAfrican KS.

5.3. CMV Genomic Material

The application of techniques of molecular biology to the association of CMV to KS has led to some intriguing findings. Zur Hausen et al. (1974) attempted to hybridize DNA from KS tissue with radioactive complementary RNA (cRNA) synthesized in vitro with E. coli RNA polymerase from Herpesvirus group DNA. CMV cRNA did not hybridize with DNA from KS tissue. In contrast, EBV cRNA hybridized with DNA from nasopharyngeal carcinoma tissue and lymphoid cells from patients with infectious mononucleosis. These negative results do not eliminate the role of CMV in KS, but may be a result of limitations in the methodology, both in regard to sensitivity in detecting genomic material in cells, as well as in not being able to detect fragments of viral DNA not transcribed in the in vitro generation of the cRNA probe.

Giraldo and Beth (1980), using different methods, have detected CMV DNA in three of eight KS tumor biopsies by DNA–DNA hybridization, two at a level of 0.35 genome/cell and one at one copy of 2.5% genome/cell. By anti-complement immunofluorescence, CMV antigen was found mainly in the nucleus of seven of 31 KS tumor biopsies and four of 12 early passage KS cell lines (Boldogh et al., 1981). Hybridization studies using a more sensitive [^{32}P]-labeled CMV DNA probe have found three of 10 KS DNA's homologous to the probe at a level of 0.7 to 1.0 genome/cell. *In situ* RNA–DNA cytohybridization studies found virus-specific RNA in five of 10 biopsies. Similar studies with EBV and HSV 1 or 2 probes were negative.

5.4. AIDS-Associated KS and CMV

Although all of the above studies were done on material from classical KS, some recent studies have examined material from AIDS-associated KS. Drew et al. (1982), although finding both IgG (nine of nine) and IgM (seven of nine antibodies to CMV in homosexual men with KS, failed to obtain a positive culture in eight of eight tested. In contrast, DNA–RNA *in situ* hybridization detected CMV RNA in two of three and immunofluorescence detected CMV antigen in six of nine. Three biopsies of normal tissue from KS patients were negative. Spector et al. (1984), using a set of cloned and well-characterized subgenomic fragments of CMV as hybridization probes by the Southern blot technique, found CMV sequences in AIDS-associated KS material at a level of one copy/five cells to less than one copy/50 cells. In one patient, CMV sequences were also detected in uninvolved skin and lung, but not in liver, spleen, heart, testes, lymph node, or bone marrow (Fenoglio et al., 1982). Although finding CMV sequences, these results showed no evidence for selective retention, amplification, or integration of specific CMV fragments in this material.

More recently, Ruger et al. (1984), using cloned probes of DNA from CMV that were selected to exclude clones with virus-host cell homology, failed to detect CMV DNA in KS tissue of two African patients. This technique, which would identify 70.4% of the CMV genome, has a sensitivity of 0.1 copy/cell if the sequence complexity would be equivalent to the length of one cloned virion DNA probe. The result suggests that KS does not require high complexity CMV-DNA, although this does not eliminate possible involvement of the virus in KS because short sequences have been implicated in oncogenic transformation.

In summary, although there is evidence of an association of CMV with KS on seroepidemiologic grounds and based on findings of CMV sequences in KS tissue, the precise role of CMV in this neoplasm remains to be elucidated.

6.   AIDS-Etiologic Agent

6.1.   Background

Although the specific nature of the association of CMV and KS is still unclear, there has been significant progress during the past 2 yr in our understanding of the etiology of AIDS and consequently AIDS-associated KS. One of the prime hypotheses underlying AIDS investigations was that it was caused by an infectious agent.

6.2.   CMV

An early candidate for the AIDS agent was CMV, since CMV infection was highly prevalent among some of the groups at risk for AIDS, especially among homosexual men. Additional implicating factors included knowledge that CMV infection could be immunosuppressive and can cause an abnormal T-cell subset ratio; CMV could be transmitted through sexual contact and blood transfusion, presumed routes of AIDS transmission; and CMV was associated with the development of KS. Strains of CMV from epidemic KS patients have been examined to determine whether a specific strain was associated with this disease. Huang (1984) has studied five strains from epidemic KS patients and four from AIDS-related opportunistic infection patients and has found that although sharing some common DNA restriction patterns, none have identical DNA fragment fingerprints. He concluded that the degree of heterogeneity probably precluded a relation to the epidemic. This did not however exclude the possibility of a set of "transforming gene(s)" occurring at the subgenomic level, or that CMV may carry gene functions that can assist the replication and expression of another defective virus that in turn causes KS and/or AIDS.

6.3.   Retroviruses

6.3.1.   HTLV-I

As other candidate agents were proposed, retroviruses, similar to feline leukemia virus, causing both immunosuppression and lymphoproliferative disease in animals, were suggested as a possible cause of AIDS. The prototype for this type of virus in man is the human T-cell leukemia virus I (HTLV-I), which is thought to cause adult T-cell leukemia/lymphoma endemic in parts of southwestern Japan.

Initial studies looking for antibodies to this virus revealed that a subset of AIDS patients in fact did have antibodies against HTLV-I. As with any putative AIDS agent, it was necessary to ensure that this association was not because HTLV-I was an opportunistic agent in these immunodeficient patients. In addition, it was necessary to study other groups of individuals in high-risk groups for AIDS for evidence of infection. Using an assay detecting antibodies to an antigen on the membrane of HTLV-I infected cells, Essex et al. (1983a) found that 25% of AIDS patients and 26% of patients with the lymphadenopathy syndrome (LAS) associated with AIDS had such antibodies. In contrast, less than 1% of healthy controls or those at risk for opportunistic infections for other reasons had detectable antibody. Similarly, Gallo et al. (1983) cultured HTLV-I from peripheral blood lymphocytes of a US patient with AIDS and obtained two other HTLV-I isolates from peripheral blood lymphocytes of two cases of AIDS in France. Strengthening this association were the findings of Gelmann et al. (1983) who discovered integrated proviral HTLV-I DNA sequences in the fresh (uncultured) lymphocytes and in T cells cultured with T-cell growth factor of two of 33 patients with AIDS analyzed by Southern blot hybridization with a radiolabeled cloned HTLV-I DNA probe.

Further support for the association of an HTLV-like virus with AIDS came from a series of seroepidemiologic studies. Essex et al. (1983b) found that between 5 and 19% of hemophiliacs in four different areas of the US had antibodies to HTLV-I-infected cells compared to less than 1% of control populations. Similarly, in a study of sera from New York hemophiliacs collected between 1976 and 1981 and from Georgia hemophiliacs collected in 1983, Evatt et al. (1983) found that 11% of the former and 16% of the latter had antibodies to HTLV-I-associated membrane antigens. Those with antibody also had significantly fewer T-helper lymphocytes, compared to those lacking antibody. Studies of transfusion-associated AIDS also found that 7.7% of donors to individuals who developed AIDS following blood transfusions had antibodies to HTLV-I-associated membrane antigens compared to 0.3% of random donors. In addition, nine of 12 sets of donors to these individuals included a donor who was antibody positive. Six of these nine donors were also suspected of being the source of the AIDS on epidemiologic and immunologic grounds (Jaffe et al., 1984).

6.3.2. LAV

Simultaneous to the initial reports of the association of HTLV and AIDS, investigators from the Institute Pasteur in Paris reported the isolation of a retrovirus that they initially thought belonged to the family of HTLV, but later found to be distinct from HTLV subgroups I and II (Barré-Sinoussi et al., 1983). This isolate came from lymph node lymphocytes cultured from a homosexual male with the lymphadenopathy syndrome now associated with AIDS. This virus, originally described as a typical type-C RNA tumor virus and called lymphadenopathy-associated virus (LAV), was subsequently also isolated from peripheral blood lymphocytes of several AIDS patients in a number of high-risk groups both in Europe and the US (Barré-Sinoussi et al., 1983). It was similar to the other HTLV strains in that it budded from the cell membrane of infected cells, contained a magnesium preferring reverse transcriptase, and contained a major core protein (p25) of similar size to that of HTLV-I. It differed from HTLV-I and -II in that the core protein was immunologically distinct and type-specific antibodies to the p19 and p24 core proteins of HTLV-I did not react with virus-producing cells, whereas serum from the patient from whom the LAV was isolated did react. Further characterization of LAV found it to be morphologically distinct from HTLV-I with a core diameter about half that of HTLV-I (41 vs 91 nm), and to resemble in some aspects type-D retroviruses such as the Mason-Pfizer virus. It also resembled a horse retrovirus, equine infectious anemia virus (EIAV), and horse sera having antibodies to EIAV precipitated the p25 core protein of LAV. On the other hand, it was clearly not the same as EIAV since it did not grow on equine dermis cells, and human sera with activity against LAV did not react with EIAV core antigen (Montagnier et al., 1984).

6.3.3. HTLV-III

Following the reports of the isolation of LAV, investigators at the National Institutes of Health reported the isolation of HTLV variants from patients with AIDS and pre-AIDS (Popovic et al., 1984). These variants were cytopathic and could be cultivated more readily in a susceptible T-cell line (HT) derived from an adult with lymphoid leukemia. They were lymphotrophic for T helper (T4) cells, had a reverse transcriptase similar to HTLV-I and -II, reacted with serum from AIDS patients, and induced syncytia. They were named collectively HTLV-III, HTLV now indicating a human T-cell lymphotropic virus.

Once identified, attempts were made to culture HTLV-III from larger numbers of AIDS patients and those in high-risk groups. Forty-eight isolates were obtained of which 26 were from 72 AIDS patients, 18 from 21 pre-AIDS patients, three from four mothers of children with AIDS, and one from 22 healthy homosexuals. No isolates were obtained from 115 healthy heterosexuals. This frequency of isolation of HTLV-III is probably an underestimate of its incidence, since some specimens had been received in unsatisfactory condition (Gallo et al., 1984).

6.3.4. ARV

In addition to the isolations of LAV and HTLV-III from lymphocytes of individuals with AIDS, lymphadenopathy syndrome, and those asymptomatic but in high-risk groups for AIDS, investigators at the University of California, San Francisco have isolated a similar retrovirus from individuals with AIDS that they call AIDS-related virus (ARV). Antibody to ARV was detected in 100% of 86 AIDS patients and the virus was grown from the blood of 54% of 41 patients with KS and 50% of 10 with the lymphadenopathy syndrome (Levy et al., 1984).

For the purpose of discussion we will consider LAV, HTLV-III, and ARV to be strains of the same AIDS-associated virus and refer to them collectively as LAV/HTLV-IIII/ARV.

6.3.5. Seroepidemiology

Antibodies to HTLV-III have been detected frequently in AIDS and pre-AIDS patients (Sarngadharan et al., 1984). By an enzyme-liked immunosorbant assay (ELISA) using a sucrose density gradient purified HTLV-III, 87.8% of AIDS patients, 78.6% of pre-AIDS patients, and 0.6% of healthy controls had antibody detected. The previously detected antibody to HTLV-I in sera of AIDS patients recognized the p65 antigen encoded by the *env* gene of HTLV-I and also recognized the p65 antigen of HTLV-III (Schüpbach et al., 1984). Sera not recognizing the p65 antigen recognized the p55, p48, p41, p39, and p24 antigens. Heteroantisera against the different HTLV subgroups, when reacted with the different strains, gave a pattern of reactivity that would indicate that HTLV-III is antigenically more closely related to HTLV-II than to HTLV-I.

Further seroepidemiologic studies of LAV/HTLV-III/ARV have been conducted in many of the risk groups for AIDS. Utilizing the Western blot assay, in addition to the already-described ELISA, Safai et al. (1984) have found that 100% of 34 AIDS sera were positive. Eighty-four percent of 19 patients with the lymphadenopathy syndrome and 21% of 14 healthy homosexual men were also positive. Kalyanaraman et al. (1984) using a radioimmunoprecipitation assay (RIPA) for antibody to the p25 core protein of LAV found that in a study cohort of homosexual males recruited from sexually transmitted diseases clinics in San Francisco, only 1% of 100 had antibody in 1978, although this had increased to 25% of 48 in 1980, and to 65% of 215 in 1984. Of the 126 who had no symptoms or clinical signs of AIDS or related conditions in 1984, 55% had antibody. A more recent study of a random sample of single men, aged 25–54, in parts of San Francisco where AIDS is most prevalent (Anderson and Levy, 1985) found that 37% of single men with homosexual contacts had antibodies to ARV. This difference in prevalence, which is lower than that of the previous study, is likely to be a result of differences in the recruitment of study participants. Groopman et al. (1985) have recently reported a 21% incidence of antibodies to HTLV-III in asymptomatic homosexual males in Boston, a city with a lower incidence of AIDS than New York City, San Francisco, or Los Angeles. In Europe, antibody prevalence in homosexuals varies from one area to another, with 10% in Zurich, 17% in London, 25% in Paris, and 39% in West Germany (Schüpbach et al., 1985; Cheingsong-Popov et al., 1984; Mathez et al., 1984; Hehlmann et al., 1985).

Studies of intravenous (IV) drug abusers have been limited compared to those of homosexuals. Spira et al. (1984) have reported that 58% of 86 recent heavy IV drug abusers in New York City had antibody to LAV by RIPA. Similarly, Weiss et al. (1985) reported that 46% of 56 sea from IV drug abusers in New York City had antibody to HTLV-III by ELISA. Intravenous drug abusers in cities such as San Francisco and Chicago with a lower incidence of AIDS in IV drug abusers compared to New York City have about a 10% incidence of antibodies to LAV (Spira et al., 1985). There is also a great difference in prevalence in IV drug users in different parts of Europe. London reports a 1.5% prevalence, whereas West Germany and Zurich report 34 and 36%, respectively (Cheingsong-Popov et al., 1984; Schüpbach et al., 1985; Hunsmann et al., 1985).

Individuals with hemophilia A in the US appear to have a high prevalence rate of antibodies to LAV/HTLV-III. Ramsey et al. (1984) found that 72% of 25 asymptomatic hemophiliacs (all factor VIII concentrate users) had antibody to LAV as detected by the Western blot technique. In Montreal, Tsoukas et al. (1984) have found that 56% were positive for antibodies to HTLV-III, and Melbye et al. (1984) has reported a 64% prevalence in Denmark. That the rise in the prevalence of antibodies to this virus has paralleled the epidemic of AIDS in this population has been documented both in the US and Europe (Evatt et al., 1985; Gurtler et al., 1984; Machin et al., 1985), and the virus has also been isolated from hemophiliacs (Vilmer et al., 1984; Palmer et al., 1984).

Whereas Haitians have been classified as having an increased incidence of AIDS, seroepidemiologic studies of antibody prevalence in this population is scarce. Gazzolo et al. (1984) studied Haitian immigrants in French Guiana in 1983 and found a 7.1% prevalence of antibodies to HTLV-III by ELISA. Preliminary data from a case-control study of AIDS in Haitians in the US indicates a prevalence of about 6%. These low prevalence figures contrast to the high prevalence in other populations at risk and would appear to indicate that all Haitians are not at equal risk of exposure to the virus.

The prevalence of antibodies of LAV/HTLV-III/ARV in non-risk group populations in both the US and Europe is under 1%. Currently, the long-term prognosis of those who are antibody positive and are asymptomatic or who have only mild symptoms is still unclear. Since AIDS has a long incubation period, it may be several years until this question is answered.

6.3.6. T-Helper Cell Tropism

Although all the human retroviruses appear to be tropic for T-helper lymphocytes, LAV has been shown to be specifically cytopathic for this subpopulation of T-lymphocytes (Klatzmann et al., 1984). Studies of a healthy hemophiliac carrier of LAV showed virus particles and reverse transcriptase activity only in cultures of T-helper lymphocytes. Even in these T-helper cell cultures, only about 10% of the cells appeared to be infected, possibly as a result of a heterogeneity of the T-helper cell subset. Alternatively, only a subpopulation of these cells contain virus at detectable levels. In vitro infection of cells from normal individuals yielded similar results. This demonstration of LAV's tropism for, and cytopathic effect on, T-helper cells is consistent with what is seen in vivo in

AIDS patients. There is progressive elimination of the T-helper cell population in peripheral blood, as well as in lymph nodes, with the development of the immunodeficiency of severe AIDS (i.e., KS or opportunistic infection).

6.3.7. DNA Sequencing

Recent DNA sequencing of the prototype isolates of LAV, HTLV-III, and ARV has shown that LAV and HTLV-III differ in only 1.5% of their nucleotides, whereas ARV differs in about 6% of its nucleotides from LAV and HTLV-III (Wain-Hobson et al., 1985; Ratner et al., 1985; Sanchez-Pescador et al., 1985). This significant nucleotide homology suggests that LAV, HTLV-III, and ARV are strains of the same virus.

7. African KS and AIDS

With the identification of the putative etiologic agent for AIDS, investigators have been able to expand on the initial clinical studies finding a difference between endemic African KS and presumed AIDS-associated KS. Antibodies to HTLV-III were found in 91% of 22 "atypical" or presumed AIDS-associated KS sera, and 87% of 15 with AIDS-related disorders sera compared to 24% of 17 endemic KS sera and 2% of 158 control sera from individuals in Zambia (Bayley et al., 1985). Similar results were obtained in Uganda, with all of four "atypical" KS sera being antibody positive, compared to 8% of 13 endemic KS sera, and 20% of 51 control sera. These data support the contention that "atypical" or AIDS-associated KS, although histologically identical to endemic African KS, is both clinically, by its more aggressive course and poor response to therapy, and seroepidemiologically, by the high prevalence of antibodies to HTLV-III, distinct from the latter.

8. Summary

In summary, the study of Kaposi's sarcoma as a possible virus-associated tumor has received new impetus with the increased incidence of KS associated with AIDS. AIDS-associated KS has confirmed the association of KS with immunodeficiency, either drug-induced or induced in this case by the AIDS virus.

However, the differences in the incidence of KS among the various AIDS risk groups must still be explained. It is likely that individuals developing KS in either situation have a common cofactor that is associated with susceptibility to the development of KS, whether genetic (HLA-DR5), viral (CMV), or some other still unrecognized factor. The precise mechanisms of these interactions still remain to e elucidated.

References

Anderson, R. E., and J. A. Levy (1985), Prevalence of antibodies to AIDS-associated retrovirus in single men in San Francisco. *Lancet* 1, 217.

Bach, F. H., M. Segall, S. Rich, and J. Barbosa (1982), HLA and susceptibility to type I diabetes. *Tissue Antigens* 20, 28–32.

Barré-Sinoussi, F., J. C. Chermann, F. Rey, M. T. Nugeyre, S. Chamaret, J. Gruest, C. Dauguet, C. Axler-Bliin, F. Vézinet-Brun, C. Rouzioux, W. Rozenbaum, and L. Montagnier (1983), Isolation of a T-lymphotropic retrovirus from a patient at risk for acquired immune deficiency syndrome (AIDS). *Science* 220, 868–871.

Bayley, A. C., R. Cheingsong-Popov, A. G., Dalgleish, R. G. Downing, R. S. Tedder, and R. A. Weiss (1985), HTLV-III serology distinguishes atypical and endemic Kaposi's sarcoma in Africa. *Lancet* 1, 359–361.

Boldogh, I., E. Beth, E. S. Huang, S. K. Kyalwazi, and G. Giraldo (1981), Kaposi's sarcoma. IV Detection of CMV DNA, CMV RNA and CMNA in tumor biopsies. *Int. J. Cancer* 28, 469–474.

CDC (1981a), Pneumocystis pneumonia—Los Angeles. *MMWR* 30, 250–252.

CDC (1981b), Kaposi's sarcoma and pneumocystis pneumonia among homosexual men—New York City and California. *MMWR* 30, 305–308.

Cheingsong-Popov, R., R. A. Weiss, A. Dalgleish, R. S. Tedder, D. J. Jeffries, D. C. Schanson, R. B. Ferns, F. M. Briggs, I. V. D. Weller, S. Mitton, M. W. Adler, C.Farthing, A. B. Lawrence, B. G. Gazzard, J. Webber, J. R. W. Harris, A. J. Pinching, J. Craske, and J. A. J. Barbara (1984), Prevalence of antibody to human T-lymphotropic virus type III in AIDS and AIDS-risk patients in Britain. *Lancet* 2, 477–480.

Contu, L., D. Cerimele, A. Pintus, F. Cottoni, and G. La Nasa (1984), HLA and Kaposi's sarcoma in Sardinia. *Tissue Antigens* 23, 240–245.

Davies, J. N. P., and F. Lothe (1962), Kaposi's Sarcoma in African Children in *Symposium on Kaposi's Sarcoma* (Ackerman, L. V. and J. F. Murray, eds.) Karger, New York.

Des Jarlais, D. C., M. Marmor, P. Thomas, M. Chamberland, S. Zolla-Pazner, and D. J. Sencer (1984), Kaposi's sarcoma among four different AIDS risk groups. *N. Engl. J. Med.* 310, 1119.

Drew, W. L., R. C. Miner, J. L. Ziegler, J. H. Gullett, D. I. Abrams, M. A. Conant, E. S. Huang, J. R. Groundwater, P. Volberding, and L. Mintz (1982), Cytomegalovirus and Kaposi's sarcoma in young homosexual men. *Lancet* 1, 125–127.

Enlow, R. W., A. Nunez Roldan, P. Lo Galbo, D. Mildvan, V. Mathur, and R. J. Winchester (1983), Increased frequency of HLA-DR5 in lymphadenopathy stage of AIDS. *Lancet* 2, 51–52.

Essex, M., M. F. McLane, T. H. Lee, L. Falk, C. W. S. Howe, J. I. Mullins, C. Cabradilla, and D. P. Francis (1983a), Antibodies to cell membrane antigens associated with human T-cell leukemia virus in patients with AIDS. *Science* 220m, 859–862.

Essex, M., M. F. McLane, T. H. Lee, N. Tachigana, J. I. Mullins, J. Kreiss, C. K. Kasper, M. C. Poon, A. Landay, S. F. Stein, D. P. Francis, C. Cabradilla, D. N. Lawrence, and B. L. Evatt (1983b), Antibodies to human T-cell leukemia virus membrane antigens (HTLV-MA) in hemophiliacs. *Science* 221, 1061–1064.

Evatt, B. L., D. P. Francis, M. F. McLane, T. H. Lee, C.Cabradilla, S. F. Stein, D. N. Lawrence, J. S. McDougal, T. J. Spira, J. I. Mullens, and M. Essex (1983), Antibodies to human T cell luekemia virus-associated membrane antigens in hemophiliacs: Evidence for infection before 1980. *Lancet* 2, 698–701.

Evatt, B. L., E. D. Gomperts, J. S. McDougal, and R. B. Ramsay (1985), Coincidental appearance of LAV/HTLV-III antibodies in hemophiliacs and the onset of the AIDS epidemic. *N. Engl. J. Med.* 312, 483–486.

Fenoglio, C. M., M. W. Oster, P. Lo Gerfo, T. Reynolds, R. Edelson, J. A. K. Patterson, E. Madeiros, and J. K. McDougall (1982), Kaposi's sarcoma following chemotherapy for testicular cancer in a homosexual man: Demonstration of cytomegalovirus RNA in sarcoma cells. *Hum. Pathol.* 13, 955–959.

Friedman-Kien, A. E., L. J. Laubenstein, P. Rubinstein, E. Buimovici-Klein, M. Marmor, R. Stahl, I. Spigland, K. Soo Kim, and S. Zolla-Pazner (1982), Disseminated Kaposi's sarcoma in homosexual men. *Ann. Intern. Med.* 96, 693–700.

Gallo, R. C., S. Z. Salahuddin, M. Popovic, G. M. Shearer, M. Kaplan, B. F. Haynes, T. J. Palker, R. Redfield, J. Oleske, B. Safai, G. White, P. Foster, and P. D. Markham (1984), Frequent detection and isolation of cytopathic retroviruses (HTLV-III) from patients with AIDS and at risk for AIDS. *Science* 224, 500–503.

Gallo, R. C., P. S. Sarin, E. P. Gelmann, M. Robert-Guroff, E. Richardson, V. S. Kalyanaraman, D. Mann, G. D. Sidhu, R. E. Stahl, S. Zolla-Pazner, J. Leibowitch, and M. Popovic (1983), Isolation of human T-cell leukemia virus in acquired immune deficiency syndrome (AIDS). *Science* 220, 865–867.

Gazzolo, L., A. Gessain, Y. Robin, M. Robert-Guroff, and G. de-The, (1984), Antibodies to HTLV-III in Haitian immigrants in French Guiana. *N. Engl. J. Med.* 311, 1252–1253.

Gelmann, E. P., M. Popovic, D. Blayney, H. Masur, G. D. Sidhu, R. E. Stahl, and R. C. Gallo (1983), Proviral DNA of a retrovirus, human T-cell leukemia virus, in two patients with AIDS. *Science* 220, 862–865.

Giraldo, G., and E. Beth (1980), The Relationship of Cytomegalovirus to Certain Human Cancers, Particularly to Kaposi's Sarcoma, in *The Role of Viruses in Human Cancer*, Vol. 1 (Giraldo, G., and E. Beth, eds.) Elsevier North Holland, Amsterdam.

Giraldo, G., E. Beth, P. Coeur, C. L. Vogel, and D. S. Dhru (1972a), Kaposi's sarcoma: A new model in the search for viruses associated with human malignancies. *J. Nat. Cancer Inst.* 49, 1495–1507.

Giraldo, G., E. Beth, and F. Haguenau (1972b), Herpes-type virus particles in tissue culture of Kaposi's sarcoma from different geographic regions. *J. Nat. Cancer Inst.* 49, 1509–1526.

Giraldo, G., E. Beth, W. Henle, G. Henle, V. Mike, B. Safai, J. M. Huraux, J. McHardy, and G. de-The (1978), Antibody patterns to herpesvirus in Kaposi's sarcoma. II. Serological association of American Kaposi's sarcoma with cytomegalovirus. *Int. J. Cancer* **22**, 126–131.

Giraldo, G., E. Beth, and E. S. Huang (1980), Kaposi's sarcoma and its relationship to cytomegalovirus (CMV). III. CMV DNA and DMV early antigens in Kaposi's sarcoma. *Int. J. Cancer* **26**, 23–29.

Giraldo, G., E. Beth, F. M. Kourilsky, G. Henle, V. Mike, J. M. Huraux, H. K. Anderson, M. R. Gharbi, S. K. Kyalwazi, and A. Puissant (1975), Antibody patterns to herpesviruses in Kaposi's sarcoma: Serological association of European Kaposi's sarcoma with cytomegalovirus. *Int. J. Cancer* **15**, 839–848.

Groopman, J. E., K. H. Mayer, M. G. Sarngadharan, D. Ayotte, A. L. DeVico, R. Finberg, A. H. Sliski, J. Davis Allan, and R. C. Gallo (1985), Seroepidemiology of human T-lymphotropic virus type III among homosexual men with the acquired immunodeficiency syndrome or generalized lymphadenopathy and among asymptomatic controls in Boston. *Ann. Intern. Med.* **102**, 334–337.

Gurtler, L. G., D. Wernicke, J. Eberle, G. Zoulek, F. Deinhardt, and W. Schramn (1984), Increase in prevalence of anti-HTLV-III in haemophiliacs. *Lancet* **2**, 1275–1276.

Hehlmann, R., G. Krech, V. Erfle, H. Piechowiak, G. Kruger, and F. D. Goebel (1985), IgG-antibodies to HTLV-III in patients with AIDS, LAS, and persons at risk of AIDS in West Germany. *Blut* **50**, 13–18.

Huang, E. S. (1984), Cytomegalovirus: Its oncogenes and Kaposi's sarcoma. *Antibiot. Chemother.* **32**, 27–42.

Hunsmann, G., J. Schneider, H. Bayer, R. Kurth, A. Werner, H. D. Brede, V. Erfle, W. Mellert, H. R. Brodt, L. Bergmann, I. Helm, I. Scharrer, W. Kreuz, H. Berthold, P. Wernet, E. M. Schneider, K. Schimpf, U. Egli, U. Bienzle, H. Schmitz, P. Kern, G. Kruger, H. Rosakat, E. Lechler, E. Seifried, P. Hellstern, W. Schneider, E. Holzer, F. D. Goebel, and R. Hehlmann (1985), Seroepidemiology of HTLV-III (LAV) in the Federal Republic of Germany. *Klin. Wochenschr.* **63**, 233–235.

Jaffe, H. W., D. P. Francis, M. F. McLane, C. Cabradilla, J. W. Curran, B. W. Kilbourne, D. N. Lawrence, H. Haverkos, T. J. Spira, R. Y. Dodd, J. Gold, D. Armstrong, A. Ley, J. Groopman, T. H. Lee, and M. Essex (1984), Transfusion-associated AIDS: Serologic evidence of human T-cell leukemia virus infection of donors. *Science* **223**, 1309–1312.

Kaposi, M. (1872), Idiopathisches multiples pigmentsarkom der haut. *Arch. Dermatol. Syph.* **4**, 265–273.

Kalyanaraman, V. S., C. D. Cabradilla, J. P. Getchell, R. Narayanan, E. H. Braff, J. C. Cherman, F. Barré-Sinoussi, L. Montagnier, T. J. Spira, J. Kaplan, D. Fishbein, H. W. Jaffe, J. W. Curran, and D. P. Francis (1984), Antibodies to the core protein of lymphadenopathy-associated virus (LAV) in patients with AIDS. *Science* **225**, 321–323.

Klatzmann, D., F. Barré-Sinoussi, M. T. Nugeyre, C. Dauguet, E. Vilmer, C. Griscelli, F. Brun-Vézinet, C. Rouzioux, J. C. Gluckman, J. C. Chermann, and L. Montagnier (1984), Selective tropism of lymphadenopathy associated virus (LAV) for helper-inducer T lymphocytes. *Science* **225**, 59–63.

Levy, J. A., A. D. Hoffman, S. M. Kramer, J. A. Lanois, J. M. Shimabukuro, and L. S. Oskiro (1984), Isolation of lymphocytopathic retroviruses from San Francisco patients with AIDS. *Science* **225**, 840–842.

Machin, S. J., B. A. McVerry, R. Cheingsong-Popov, and R. S. Tedder (1985), Seroconversion for HTLV-III since 1980 in British haemophiliacs. *Lancet* **1**, 336.

Mathez, D., J. Leibowitch, S. Matheron, A. G. Saimot, P. Catalan, and D. Zaguri (1984), Antibodies to HTLV-III associated antigens in populations exposed to AIDS virus in France. *Lancet* 2, 460.

Melbye, M., R. J. Biggar, J. C. Chermann, L. Montagnier, S. Stenbjer, and P. Ebbesen (1984), High prevalence of lymphadenopathy virus (LAV) in European haemophiliacs. *Lancet* 2, 40–41.

Montagnier, L., C. Dauguet, C. Axler, S. Chamaret, J. Gruest, M. T. Nugeyre, F. Rey, F. Barré-Sinoussi, and J. C. Chermann (1984), A new type of retrovirus isolated from patients presenting with lymphadenopathy and acquired immune deficiency syndrome: Structural and antigenic relatedness with equine infectious anemia virus. *Ann. Virol.* 135, 119–134.

Palmer, E. L., R. B. Ramsey, P. F. Feorino, A. K. Harrison, C. Cabradilla, D. F. Francis, M. C. Poon, and B. L. Evatt (1984), Human T-cell leukemia virus in lymphocytes of two hemophiliacs with the acquired immunodeficiency syndrome. *Ann. Intern. Med.* 101, 293–297.

Penn, I. (1983), Kaposi''s sarcoma in immunosuppressed patients. *J. Clin. Lab. Immunol.* 12, 1–10.

Pollack, M. S., B. Safai, and B. Dupont (1983a), HLA-DR5 and DR2 are susceptibility factors for acquired immunodeficiency syndrome with Kaposi's sarcoma in different ethnic subpopulations. *Dis. Markers* 1, 135–139.

Pollack, M. S., B. Safai, P. L. Myskowsky, J. W. M. Gold, J. Pandey, and B. Dupont (1983b), Frequencies of HLA and GM immunogenetic markers in Kaposi's sarcoma. *Tissue Antigens* 21, 1–8.

Pollack, M. S., D. Vugrin, W. Hennessy, H. W. Herr, B. Dupont, and W. F. Whitmore, Jr. (1982), HLA antigens in patients with germ cell cancers of the testis. *Cancer Res.* 42, 2470–2473.

Popovic, M., M. G. Sarngadharan, E. Read, and R. C. Gallo (1984), Detection, isolation, and continuous production of cytopathic retroviruses (HTLV--III) from patients with AIDS and pre-AIDS. *Science* 224, 497–500.

Prince, H. E., R. W. Schroff, G. Ayoub, S. Han, M. S. Gottlieb, and J. L. Fahey (1984), HLA studies in acquired immune deficiency syndrome patients with Kaposi's sarcoma. *J. Clin. Lab. Immunol.* 4, 242–245.

Ramsay, R. B., E. L. Palmer, J. S. McDougal, V. S. Kalyanaraman, D. W. Jackson, T. L. Chorba, R. C. Holman, and B. L. Evatt (1984), Antibody to lymphadenopathy-associated virus in haemophiliacs with and without AIDS. *Lancet* 2, 397–398.

Ratner, L., W. Hasetine, R. Patarca, K. J. Livak, B. Starich, S. F. Josephs, E. R. Doran, J. A. Rafalski, E. A. Whitehorn, K. Baumeister, L. Ivanoff, S. R. Petteway, Jr., M. L. Pearson, J. A. Lautenberger, T. S. Papas, J. Ghrayeb, N. T. Chang, R. C. Gallo, and R. Wong-Staal (1985), Complete nucleotide sequence of the AIDS virus, HTLV-III. *Nature* 313, 277–284.

Rubinstein, P., W. M. Rothman, and A. Friedman-Kien (1984), Immunologic and immunogenetic findings in patients with epidemic Kaposi's sarcoma. *Antibiot. Chemother.* 32, 87–98.

Ruger, R., R. Colimon, and B. Fleckenstein (1984), Search for DNA sequences of human cytomegalovirus in Kaposi's sarcoma tissues with cloned probes. *Antibiot. Chemother.* 32, 43–47.

Safai, B., J. E. Groopman, M. Popovic, J. Schupbach, M. G. Sarngadharan, K. Arnett, A. Sliski, and R. C. Gallo (1984), Seroepidemiological studies of human T-lymphotropic retrovirus type III in acquired immunodeficiency syndrome. *Lancet* 1, 1438–1440.

Sanchez-Pescador, R., M. D. Power, P. J. Barr, K. S. Steimer, M. M. Stempien, S. L. Brown-Shimer, W. W. Gee,A. Renard, A. Randolph, J. A. Levy, D. Dina, and P. A. Luciw (1985), Nucleotide sequence and expression of an AIDS-associated retrovirus (ARV-2). *Science* **227**, 484–492.

Sarngadharan, M. G., M. Popovic, L. Bruch, J. Schupbach, and R. C. Gallo (1984), Antibodies reactive with human T-lymphotropic retroviruses (HTLV-III) in the serum of patients with AIDS. *Science* **224**, 506–508.

Schupbach, J., O. Haller, M. Vogt, R. Luthy, H. Joller, O. Oelz, M. Popovic, M. G. Sarngadharan, and R. C. Gallo (1985), Antibodies to HTLV-III in Swiss patients with AIDS and pre-AIDS and in groups at risk for AIDS. *N. Engl. J. Med.* **312**, 265–270.

Schupbach, J., M. Popovic, R. V. Gilden, M. A. Gonda, M. G. Sarngadharan, and R. C. Gallo (1984), Serological analysis of a subgroup of human T-lymphotropic retroviruses (HTLV-III) associated with AIDS. *Science* **224**, 503–505.

Spector, D. H., S. B. Shaw, L. J. Hock, D. Abrams, and M. S. Gottlieb (1984), Association of Human Cytomegalovirus With Kaposi's Sarcoma, *J. Cell. Biochem. Suppl. 8A*, 10.

Spira, T. J., D. C. Des Jarlais, D. Bokos, R. Onichi, D. Kiprov, and V. S. Kalyanaraman (1985) HTLV-III/LAV antibodies in intravenous drug (IV) abusers—Comparison of high and low risk areas for AIDS. *Program, International Conference on Acquired Immunodeficiency Syndrome*, Dept. of Health and Human Services, Atlanta, GA.

Spira, T. J., D. C. Des Jarlais, M. Marmor, S. Yancovitz, S.Friedman, J. Garber, H. Cohen, C. Cabradilla, and V. S. Kalyanaraman (1984), Prevalence of antibody to lymphadenopathy-associated virus among drug-detoxification patients in New York. *J. Engl. J. Med.* **311**, 467–468.

Tsoukas, C., F. Gervais, J. Shuster, P. Gold, M. O'Shaughnessy, and M. Robert-Guroff (1984), Association of HTLV-III antibodies and cellular immune status of hemophiliacs. *N. Engl. J. Med.* **311**, 1514–1515.

Vilmer, E., C. Rouzioux, F. Vézinet-Brun, A. Fischer, J. C. Chermann, F. Barré-Sinoussi, C. Gazengel, C.Dauguet, P. Mani gne, C. Griscelli, and L. Montagnier (1984), Isolation of new lymphotrophic retovirus from two siblings with haemophilia B, one with AIDS. *Lancet* **1**, 753–757.

Wain-Hobson, S., P. Sonigo, O. Danos, S. Cole, and M. Alizon (1985), Nucleotide sequence of the AIDS virus, LAV. *Cell* **40**, 9–17.

Weiss, S. H., J. J. Goedert, M. G. Sarngadharan, A. J. Bodner, the AIDS Seroepidemiology Collaborative Working Group, R. C. Gallo, and W. A. Blattner (1985), Screening test for HTLV-III (AIDS agent) antibodies. *J. Am. Med. Assoc.* **253**, 221–225.

zur Hausen, H., H. Schulte-Holthausen, H. Wolfe, K. Dorries, and H. Egger (1974), Attempts to detect virus specific DNA in human tumors. II. Nucleic acid hybridizations with complementary RNA of human herpes group viruses. *Int. J. Cancer* **13**, 657–664.

INDEX